Progress in Inflammation Research

Series Editor

Prof. Dr. Michael J. Parnham
PLIVA
Research Institute
Prilaz baruna Filipovica 25
10000 Zagreb
Croatia

Inflammation and Stroke

Giora Z. Feuerstein

Editor

Springer Basel AG

Editor

Giora Z. Feuerstein
DuPont Pharmaceuticals Company
Cardiovascular Diseases Research
Experimental Station
Route 141 & Henry Clay Road
Wilmington, DE 19880
USA

A CIP catalogue record for this book is available from the Library of Congress, Washington D.C., USA

Deutsche Bibliothek Cataloging-in-Publication Data
Inflammation and stroke / Giora Z. Feuerstein, ed. - Basel ; Boston ; Berlin :
Birkhäuser, 2001
(Progress in inflammation research)
ISBN 978-3-0348-9508-8   ISBN 978-3-0348-8297-2 (eBook)
DOI 10.1007/978-3-0348-8297-2

ISBN 978-3-0348-9508-8

Cover illustration: Inflammation in brain following stroke. The figure depicts a brain capillary in the ischemic zone of rat cortex subjected to 12 h of ischemia. The capillary contains neutrophils at various stages of adhesion and migration into the brain parenchyma, as follows: 0. Neutrophil aggregates inside the capillary, possibly activated by endovascular stimuli associated with ischemia; 1. Neutrophil in loose contact with the endothelium, probably non-commited to migration; 2. Neutrophil permanently attached and possibly committing for irreversible adhesion to the endothelium; 3. Neutrophil firmly attached and spread over an endothelial cell preparing for migration across the endothelium; 4. Neutrophil migrating through the endothelial layer; 5. Neutrophil that have exited from capillary into the brain parenchyma. Taken together, all stages of inflammatory cell adhesion and migration from the systemic circulation into the ischemic brain tissue can be observed in rat model of stroke. (Wang X, Feuerstein GZ (2000) The role of immune and inflammatory mediators in CNS injury. *Drug News & Perspectives* 13: 133–140, with permission)

© 2001 Springer Basel AG
Originally published by Birkhäuser Verlag in 2001

Printed on acid-free paper produced from chlorine-free pulp. TCF ∞
Cover design: Markus Etterich, Basel

ISBN 978-3-0348-9508-8

9 8 7 6 5 4 3 2 1

Contents

Inflammatory cells in stroke

Inflammatory cytokines, interleukins and chemokines in stroke and CNS trauma

Inflammation in cerebral thrombosis, angiogenesis and matrix regulation: a new perspective in stroke research and therapeutics

List of contributors

Raymond T. Bartus, Alkermes, Inc., 64 Sidney Street, Cambridge, MA 02139, USA; e-mail: raymond.bartus@alkermes.com

Yaara Ben-Yosef, Neuroimmunology Research Unit, Carmel Medical Center, Haifa 34362, Israel; e-mail: millera@tx.technion.ac.il

John R. Bethea, The Miami Project to Cure Paralysis, Departments of Neurological Surgery, University of Miami School of Medicine, P.O. Box 016960 (R-48), Miami, FL 33101, USA; e-mail: jbethea@miami.edu

Clara Braker, Neuroimmunology Research Unit, Carmel Medical Center, Haifa 34362, Israel; e-mail: millera@tx.technion.ac.il

Pak H. Chan, Neurosurgical Laboratories, Departments of Neurosurgery, Neurology and Neurological Sciences, and Program in Neurosciences, Stanford University, 1201 Welch Road, Room 314, Stanford, CA 94305, USA; e-mail: phchan@leland.stanford.edu

Michael Chopp, Department of Neurology, Henry Ford Health System, MI 48202, and Oakland University, Physics Department, Rochester, MI 48307, USA; e-mail: chopp@neuro.hfh.edu

E. Sander Connolly, Columbia University Department of Medicine, Department of Neurological Surgery, 630 W 168th St., New York, NY 10032, USA; e-mail: esc5@columbia.edu

Jean-Christophe Copin, Neurosurgical Laboratories, Departments of Neurosurgery, Neurology and Neurological Sciences, and Program in Neurosciences, Stanford University, 1201 Welch Road, Room 314, Stanford, CA 94305, USA, and Divisions of Surgical and Medical Critical Care, Departments of Medicine, Anesthesiology, Pharmacology and Surgical Critical Care Medicine, Geneva University Hospital, 1211 Geneva 14, Switzerland; e-mail: jean-christophe.copin@medecine.unige.ch

Reginald L. Dean III, Alkermes, Inc., 64 Sidney Street, Cambridge, MA 02139, USA; e-mail: reggie.dean@alkermes.com

Gregory del Zoppo, Department of Molecular and Experimental Medicine, The Scripps Research Institute,10550 North Torrey Pines Rd., MEM 132, La Jolla, CA 92037, USA; e-mail: grgdlzop@hermes.scripps.edu

W. Dalton Dietrich, The Miami Project to Cure Paralysis, Departments of Neurological Surgery and Neurology, University of Miami School of Medicine, P.O. Box 016960 (R-48), Miami, FL 33101, USA; e-mail: ddietrich@miami.edu

Dwaine F. Emerich, Alkermes, Inc., 64 Sidney Street, Cambridge, MA 02139, USA; e-mail: dwaine.emerich@alkermes.com

Yvan Gasche, Neurosurgical Laboratories, Departments of Neurosurgery, Neurology and Neurological Sciences, and Program in Neurosciences, Stanford University, 1201 Welch Road, Room 314, Stanford, CA 94305, USA, and Divisions of Surgical and Medical Critical Care, Departments of Medicine, Anesthesiology, Pharmacology and Surgical Critical Care Medicine, Geneva University Hospital, 1211 Geneva 14, Switzerland; e-mail: yvan-gasche@medecine.unige.ch

John M. Hallenbeck, Stroke Branch, National Institute of Neurological Disorders and Stroke, National Institutes of Health, 36 Convent Drive MSC 4128, Building 36, Room 4A03, Bethesda, Maryland 20892-4128, USA; e-mail: hallenbj@ninds.nih.gov

Costantino Iadecola, Department of Neurology, University of Minnesota, Box 295 UMHC, 420 Delaware St SE, Minneapolis, MN 55455, USA; e-mail: iadec001@tc.umn.edu

Bernhard H.J. Juurlink, Department of Anatomy and Cell Biology, College of Medicine, University of Saskatchewan, 107 Wiggins Road, Saskatoon, SK S7N 5E5, Canada; e-mail: juurlink@duke.usask.ca

Hiroyuki Kato, Departments of Neurology and Neuroendovascular Therapy, Field of Neuroscience, Tohoku University School of Medicine, 1-1 Seiryo-machi, Aoba-ku, Sendai 980-8574, Japan; e-mail: katoh@mail.cc.tohoku.ac.jp

John A. Kessler, Davee Department of Neurology and Clinical Neurological Sciences, Northwestern University School of Medicine, Abbott Hall, Room 1120, 710 North Lake Shore Drive, Chicago, Illinois 60611, USA; e-mail: jakessler@northwestern.edu

Thomas Kossmann, Research Division and Trauma Division, Department of Surgery, University Hospital, Rämistrasse 100, 8091 Zürich, Switzerland; e-mail: thomas.kossmann@chi.usz.ch

Philipp M. Lenzlinger, University of Pennsylvania, Department of Neurosurgery, 3320 Smith Walk, 105 Hayden Hall, Philadelphia, PA 19104-6316, USA; e-mail: lenzling@mail.med.upenn.edu, and
Research Division and Trauma Division, Department of Surgery, University Hospital, Rämistrasse 100, 8091 Zürich, Switzerland

Perttu J. Lindsberg, Neuroscience Program, Rm B409b, Biomedicum Helsinki, P.O. Box 700, 00290 Helsinki, Finland; e-mail: perttu.lindsberg@hus.fi

Sarah A. Loddick, Biological Sciences, 1.124, Stopford Building,University of Manchester, Manchester M13 9PT, UK; e-mail: sarah.loddick@man.ac.uk

Tracy McIntosh, Department of Neurosurgery, University of Pennsylvania, and Veterans Administration Medical Center, 105 Hayden Hall, 3320 Smith Walk, Philadelphia, PA 19104-6316, USA; e-mail: mcintosh@seas.upenn.edu

Mark F. Mehler, Departments of Neurology, Neuroscience and Psychiatry, Albert Einstein College of Medicine, Rose F. Kennedy Center for Research in Mental Retardation and Developmental Disabilities, Room 401, 1410 Pelham Parkway South, Bronx, New York 10461, USA; e-mail: mehler@aecom.yu.edu

Ariel Miller, Neuroimmunology Research Unit, Lady Davis Carmel Medical Center, 7 Michal St., Haifa, 34362, Israel, and Rappaport Institute for Research in the Medical Sciences, Haifa, and Faculty of Medicine, Technion-Israel Institute of Technology, Haifa, Israel; e-mail: millera@tx.technion.ac.il

Maria Cristina Morganti-Kossmann, Research Division and Trauma Division, Department of Surgery, University Hospital, Rämistrasse 100, 8091 Zürich, Switzerland; e-mail: cristina.kossmann@chi.usz.ch

Daniel C. Morris, Department of Emergency Medicine, Henry Ford Health System, Detroit, MI 48202, USA; e-mail: morris@neuro.hfh.edu

Elaine E. Peters, Cardiovascular Sciences, DuPont Pharmaceuticals Company, Experimental Station E400/6220E, Route 141 & Henry Clay Road, Wilmington, DE 19880, USA; e-mail: elaine.e.peters@dupontpharma.com

David J. Pinsky, Columbia University Department of Medicine, Divisions of Cardiology & Circulatory Physiology, 630 W 168th St., New York, NY 10032, USA; e-mail: djp5@columbia.edu

Nikolaus Plesnila, Massachusetts General Hospital, Harvard Medical School, Charlestown 02129, USA, and Institut für Chirurgische Forschung, Marchioninistrasse 15, 81366 München, Germany; e-mail: plesnila@icf.med.uni-muenchen.de

Ricardo Prado, Department of Neurology, University of Miami School of Medicine, P.O. Box 016960 (R-4-5), Miami, FL 33101, USA

Richard M. Ransohoff, The Lerner Research Institute, Cleveland Clinic Foundation, 9500 Euclid Avenue, Cleveland, OH 44195-5244, USA; e-mail: ransohr@cesmtp.ccf.org

Jane Relton, Biogen, Inc., 14 Cambridge Center, Cambridge, MA 02142, USA

Gary A. Rosenberg, Department of Neurology, University of New Mexico Health Sciences Center, 915 Camino de Salud, Albuquerque, NM 87131, USA; e-mail: grosenberg@salud.unm.edu

Nancy J. Rothwell, Biological Sciences, 1.124, Stopford Building, University of Manchester, Manchester M13 9PT, UK; e-mail: nancy.rothwell@man.ac.uk

Christl A. Ruetzler, Stroke Branch, National Institute of Neurological Disorders and Stroke, National Institutes of Health, 36 Convent Drive MSC 4128, Building 36, Room 4A03, Bethesda, MD 20892-4128, USA; e-mail: ruetzlec@ninds.nih.gov

Ann Marie Schmidt, Departments of Pathology, Surgery, Medicine and Physiology and Cellular Biophysics of Columbia University College of Physicians & Surgeons, 630 West 168th Street, New York, NY 10032, USA

Sarah Shapiro, Immunology Research Unit, Carmel Medical Center, Haifa 34362, Israel

Anna-Leena Sirén, Max-Planck-Institute for Experimental Medicine, Hermann-Rein Str. 3, 37075 Goettingen, Germany; e-mail: siren@em.mpg.de

Michal Schwartz, Deptartment of Neurobiology, The Weizmann Institute of Science, 76100 Rehovot, Israel; e-mail: michal.schwartz@weizmann.ac.il

Esther Shohami, Department of Pharmacology, School of Pharmacy, The Hebrew University of Jerusalem, Jerusalem 91120, Israel; e-mail: esty@cc.huji.ac.il

Danica B. Stanimirovic, Institute for Biological Sciences, National Research Council of Canada, Montreal Road Campus, Bldg. M-54, Ottawa, ON K1A 0R6, Canada; e-mail: Danica.Stanimirovic@nrc.ca

David M. Stern, College of Physicians & Surgeons, Columbia University, 630 W 168th St., New York, NY 10032, USA; e-mail: dms9@columbia.edu

Xinkang Wang, Cardiovascular Diseases Research, DuPont Pharmaceuticals Company, Experimental Station 400/3420B, (Rt. 141 & Henry Clay Road,) Wilmington, DE 19880-0400, USA; e-mail: xinkang.wang@dupontpharma.com

Shi Du Yan, Department of Pathology, P & S 17-410, College of P & S of Columbia, 630 West 168th Street, New York, New York 10032, USA; e-mail: sdy1@columbia. edu

V. Wee Yong, Departments of Oncology & Clinical Neurosciences, University of Calgary, 330 Hospital Drive NW, Calgary, Alberta T2N 4N1, Canada; e-mail; vyong@ucalgary.ca

Introduction

New opportunities for stroke prevention and therapeutics: a hope from anti-inflammatory drugs?

Giora Z. Feuerstein and Xinkang Wang

Cardiovascular Disease Research, DuPont Pharmaceuticals, Experimental Station, Route 141 & Henry Clay Road, Wilmington, DE 19880, USA

Stroke is the third leading cause of death in most developed countries and the leading cause of cardiovascular death in Japan and China [1]. Stroke management is a leading health burden in all developed countries considering loss of productive years and rehabilitation costs. Epidemiological studies conducted over the past 10 years consistently demonstrated a steady reduction in the incidence of stroke in developed countries until the very recent years, when the incidence seemed to plateau [1, 2]. This remarkable reduction in the incidence of strokes is attributed to many factors, including (i) effective management of risk factors such as hypertension and diabetes [3], (ii) prevention of thromboembolic events with anticoagulant treatment, (coumadin for chronic atrial fibrillation) [4] and antiplatelet agents (aspirin, clopidogrel) for secondary prevention [5, 6], (iii) reduction of atherosclerosis burden by lipid lowering agents and physical activity and [7], and (iv) better understanding of environmental, psychological (stress) and behavioral (smoking and dietary habits) factors. In fact, effective treatment of hypertension, smoking cessation and anticoagulation alone have been estimated to prevent ~75% of stroke events in the USA [8].

While the incidence of stroke has declined steadily over the past decades, progress in treatment of acute stroke has been disappointing. At the turn of the 21st century, management of patients with acute stroke is still largely conservative, featuring clinical assessment, preservation of vital function and elimination of obvious causes such as emboli and hemodynamic factors. Only a minority of patients with acute ischemic stroke benefit from specific therapy with thrombolytics (~ 2–5%) since the therapeutic window is narrow (limited to 3 h post onset of stroke) and major adverse events (in particular, intracerebral hemorrhage). In only one area of stroke management, diagnosis, has substantial progress been made in light of the remarkable progress in imaging techniques that better assess the nature and location of the ischemic event [9–11].

The failure of the medical and pharmaceutical community to provide improved management for acute stroke patients is in particular striking in view of the enormous resources that have been applied to invent, develop and apply new therapeutics for stroke. Table 1 summarizes the scope of clinical trials that have been con-

Inflammation and Stroke, edited by Giora Z. Feuerstein
© 2001 Birkhäuser Verlag Basel/Switzerland

Table 1 - Recent stroke trials

Drug	Mechanism	Time/ Route	Status phase	Ref.
Lubeluzole	Blocks glutamate and NO release	6–8 h/iv	III negative	[12]
Enlimomab	Anti-ICAM antibody	6 h/iv	III negative	[13]
Citicoline	Radical scavenger	24 h/po	III negative	[14]
Fosphenytoin	Membrane stabilizer/Na⁺ channel inhibitor	6 h/iv	III negative	[15]
Cerestat	Glutamate antagonist	6 h/iv	III terminated	22th Stroke Meeting,1997
Cervene	Opioid κ receptor antagonist	6 h/iv	III terminated	[16]
Trilizad	Free radical scavenger	6 h/iv	III negative	[17]
Nimodipine	L calcium channel antagonist	24–48 h/iv	III negative	[18]
Eliprodil	NMDA antagonist	6 h/iv	III stopped	[15]
GM1 ganglioside	Ganglioside	48 h/iv	III negative	[19]
Selfotel	NMDA antagonist	6 h/iv	III terminated	[20]
Gavestynel	Glycine antagonist	6 h/iv	III negative	[21]

NMDA, N-methyl-D-aspartate; NO, nitric oxide; ICAM, intercellular adhesion molecule; GM1, ganglioside

ducted over the past decade by various pharmaceuticals firms. These trials have explored the efficacy of various agents that have been intensely researched in many experimental paradigms that feature components of the human stroke condition. Yet, none of the clinical trials conducted with neuroprotective agents resulted in benefits to the patients. This disappointing reality has raised many questions regarding the schemes and strategies that underwrote the pharmaceutical development of drugs for stroke. In this regard, one of the most pressing issues is whether the molecular targets that have been chosen for manipulation by the agents that failed in the trails were indeed the proper ones. Inspection of the compounds that have been used in phase III studies, as summarized in Table 1, suggest that so far, inhibitors and antagonists of excitotoxic neurotransmitters such as glutamate and its co-activators, glycine, have not produced the expected benefits. Other targets such as adhesion molecule (ICAM-1), ion channels (Ca^{2+}, Na^+) and oxygen radicals have not as yet demonstrated efficacy either. The reasons for the choices of these targets, largely based on research in the 1970–1980s, is depicted in Figure 1 where pathways of neuronal damage are shown. Figure 1, a highly simplified representation of the enormously complex perturbations of brain neurochemistry by ischemia, focuses on

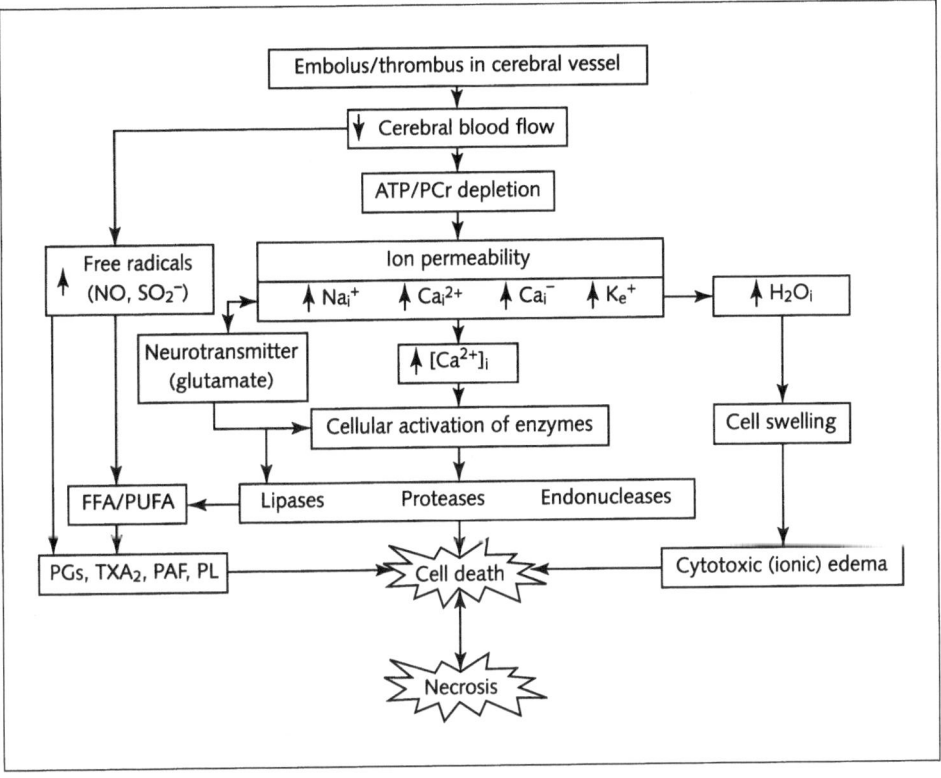

Figure 1

Schematic diagram illustrating changes occurring in thromboembolic cerebral ischemia that contribute to loss of cellular integrity and tissue destruction/infarction.

three major molecular pathways: (i) The accumulation of Na^+/Ca^{2+} ions consequent to loss of membrane potential and unregulated ion fluxes; (ii) massive release of neurotransmitters that are excitotoxic – of which glutamate was held as the "primary suspect", and (iii) oxidative stress that leads to radical formations, lipid peroxidation and indiscriminate membrane and organelle damage. These events have been well documented and provided basis for clinical development of specific compounds largely represented in Table 1. However, as shown in Figure 2, the timeframe for activation and action of the molecular targets used in table 1 is likely to be a major reason that these pharmacological agents failed in clinical development. Figure 2 provides a temporal perspective to this issue; clearly, at the time of patients' availability for treatment in a medical facility (usually beyond 3 h after the onset of the ischemic event) the early biochemical events that result from loss of membrane

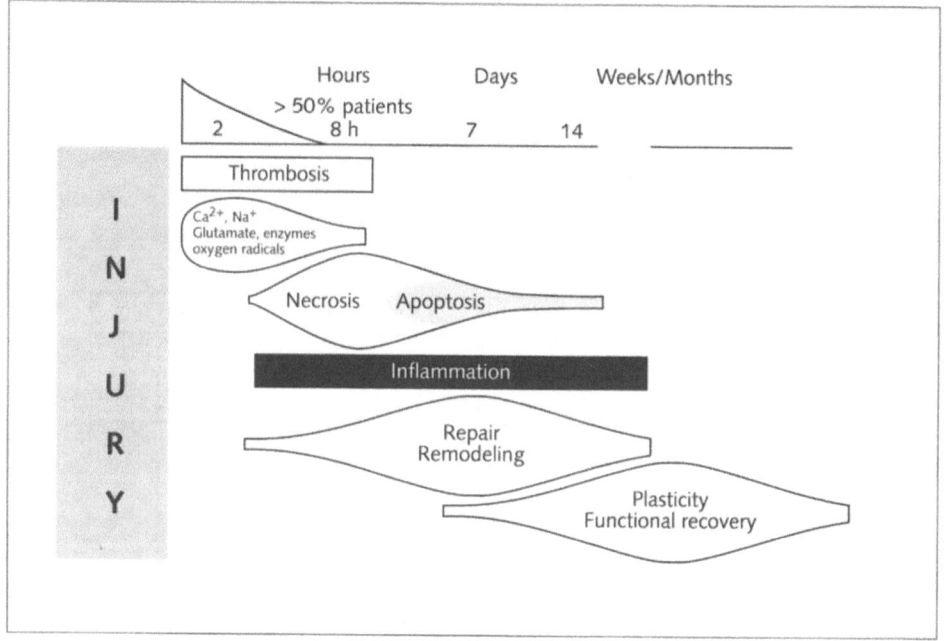

Figure 2
Schematic diagram depicting the dynamic changes following ischemic stroke

potential- ion fluxes, excitotoxic mediators release and radicals formation have long exercised their effect. Several hours after the ischemic attack, new molecular and biochemical events are emerging which include *de novo* gene expression, protein synthesis and cellular events not seen in the normal healthy brain tissue. These cellular components include activation of microglia and infiltration of blood borne leukocytes across the blood brain barrier into the brain. In brief, an acute inflammatory reaction that is initiated a few hours after brain ischemia that lasts for several days is in effect. At that time brain cells commence an extensive transcription and translation of genes that express inflammatory mediators such as cytokines and chemokines, which together induce an inflammatory milieu in the ischemic region (Fig. 3).

The inflammatory reaction induced by an ischemic challenge to brain tissue has been well documented in experimental as well as clinical studies which are extensively reviewed in respective chapters in this book. It is important though to keep in mind that the inflammatory reaction at large is designed as a defense mechanism against invading toxic organisms and noxious agents as well as providing for "tissue cleansing" and repair. This fundamental role of the inflammatory reaction in preserving tissue health poses the issue of whether or not inflammatory cells and

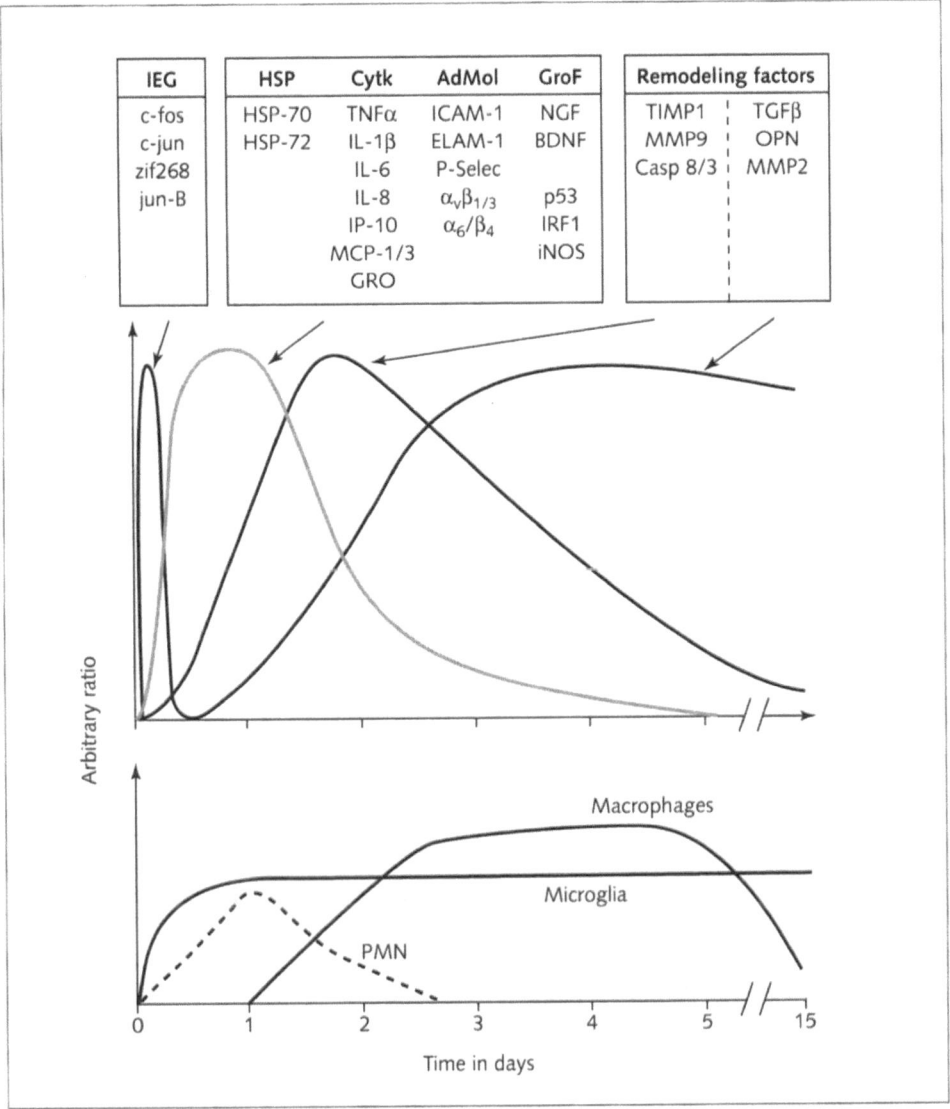

Figure 3

Gene expression in rat ischemic cortex after middle cerebral artery occlusion. Four waves of ischemic gene expression include early response genes/transcription factors (wave 1), heat shock proteins, pro-inflammatory mediators and growth factors (wave 2), proteinases and proteinase inhibitors (wave 3) and delayed remodeling proteins (wave 4). The leukocyte wave, including early polymorphonuclear (PMN) neutrophils and later monocytes/macrophages infiltration, as well as activated microglia, is illustrated in the lower panel. Astrocyte activation (gliosis) occurs following leukocyte infiltration in the ischemic brain tissue.

mediators that are present in the injured brain are "friend or foe". Several chapters in this book will address the multifaceted role of the inflammatory reaction in this perspective, at time, with opposing positions. Thus, the overall objective of this book on the role of inflammation in stroke is not to take a one-sided position on the matter, but to provide the readers with data and opinions regarding the significance of inflammation in an ischemic brain lesion.

Inflammatory cells are known to produce and release factors that have diverse effects on cells and tissue viability and death. Cytokines are pleiotrophic factors that can induce cell death as well as cell survival and growth. TNFα is an example of such cytokines which may have opposing effects on brain functions and cell integrity. For example, TNFα may disrupt the blood brain barrier (BBB) and increase edema formation and inflammatory cell influx into the lesion site, thereby increase damage and cell death. On the other hand, TNFα, via its growth-promoting effect, may induce a state of "tolerance" (or pre-conditioning) that provides brain cells better capacity to sustain injury. Furthermore, TNFα may be involved in brain damage in acute situations, yet provide salutary effects for long-term recovery. Finally, some mediators (e.g., thrombin) [22] have been shown to act "positively" (i.e., provide protection) at low doses while exerting "negative" effects at high doses. Thus, the emerging concepts on inflammatory cells and mediators in ischemic brain injury, as will be unfolding in this book, point to the possibility that the role inflammation plays in brain injury is rather complex; the nature of the mediator, their concentration, the context of their production (what other mediators are present that act in concert to synergize or modulate each other action) as well the temporal relationships to the ischemic injury, are likely to be very important.

In summary, the book on "inflammation and stroke" provides the opportunity for readers interested in stroke research to review the most current information that supports (or refutes) a possible role of inflammatory cells and mediators in brain ischemia (stroke). Special emphasis was placed on the diverse biological and pathological aspects of inflammation and the potential for salutary as well as detrimental components of this reaction. It is hoped that further research on the role of inflammatory mediators in stroke will lead to new strategies and formulas for novel preventive and therapeutics for stroke.

References

1   Heart and Stroke Statistical Update, American Heart Association (1999).
2   Wolf PA, Kannel WB, D'Agostino RB (1998) Epidemiology of stroke. In: MD Ginsberg, J Bogousslavsky (eds): *Cerebrovascular disease: Pathophysiology, diagnosis and management*. Blackwell Science, USA, 834–849
3   Yusuf S, Sleight P, Pogue J, Bosch J, Davies R, Dagenais G (2000) Effects of an angiotensin-converting-enzyme inhibitor, ramipril, on cardiovascular events in high-risk

patients. The Heart Outcomes Prevention Evaluation Study Investigators. *New Engl J Med* 342: 145–153

4   Atrial Fibrillation Investigators (1994) Risk factors for stroke and efficacy of antithrombotic therapy in atrial fibrillation: analysis of poled data from five randomized controlled trials. *Arch Intern Med* 154: 1449–1457

5   Barnett HT (1990) Aspirin in stroke prevention: an overeview. *Stroke* 21 (suppl IV): IV40–IV43

6   Hass WK, Easton JD, Adams HP Jr, Pryse-Phillips W, Molony BA, Anderson S, Kamm B (1989) A randomized trial comparing ticlopidine hydrochloride with aspirin for the prevention of stroke in high-risk patients. Ticlopidine Aspirin Stroke Study Group. *New Engl J Med* 321: 501–507

7   Plehn JF, Davis BR, Sacks FM, Rouleau JL, Pfeffer MA, Bernstein V, Cuddy TE, Moye LA, Piller LB, Rutherford J et al (1999) Reduction of stroke incidence after myocardial infarction with pravastatin: the Cholesterol and Recurrent Events (CARE) study. The Care Investigators. *Circulation* 99: 216–223

8   Wolf PA, Grotta JC (2000) Cerebrovascular diseases. *Circulation* 102: IV75–IV80

9   Neumann-Haefelin T, Moseley ME, Albers GW (2000) New magnetic resonance imaging methods for cerebrovascular disease: emerging clinical applications. *Ann Neurol* 47: 559–570

10 Wityk RJ, Beauchamp NJ Jr (2000) Diagnostic evaluation of stroke. *Neurol Clin* 18: 357–378

11 Tong DC, Albers GW (2000) Diffusion and perfusion magnetic resonance imaging for the evaluation of acute stroke: potential use in guiding thrombolytic therapy. *Curr Opin Neurol* 13: 45–50

12 Diener HC, Cortens M, Ford G, Grotta J, Hacke W, Kaste M, Koudstaal PJ, Wessel T (2000) Lubeluzole in acute ischemic stroke treatment: A double-blind study with an 8-hour inclusion window comparing a 10-mg daily dose of lubeluzole with placebo. *Stroke* 31: 2543–2351

13 DeGraba TJ (1998) The role of inflammation after acute stroke: utility of pursuing anti-adhesion molecule therapy. *Neurology* 51: S62–S68

14 Clark WM, Williams BJ, Selzer KA, Zweifler RM, Sabounjian LA, Gammans RE (1999) A randomized efficacy trial of citicoline in patients with acute ischemic stroke. *Stroke* 30: 2592–2597

15 Morgenstern LB, Pettigrew LC (1997) Brain protection – human data and potential new therapies. *New Horiz* 5: 397–405

16 Clark WM, Raps EC, Tong DC, Kelly RE (2000) Cervene (Nalmefene) in acute ischemic stroke: final results of a phase III efficacy study. The Cervene Stroke Study Investigators. *Stroke* 31: 1234–1239

17 Haley EC Jr, Kassell NF, Apperson-Hansen C, Maile MH, Alves WM (1997) A randomized, double-blind, vehicle-controlled trial of tirilazad mesylate in patients with aneurysmal subarachnoid hemorrhage: a cooperative study in North America. *J Neurosurg* 86: 467–474

18   Ahmed N, Nasman P, Wahlgren NG (2000) Effect of intravenous nimodipine on blood pressure and outcome after acute stroke. *Stroke* 31 (6): 1250–1255

19   Candelise L, Ciccone A (2000) Gangliosides for acute ischaemic stroke. Cochrane Database Syst Rev 2: CD000094

20   Davis SM, Lees KR, Albers GW, Diener HC, Markabi S, Karlsson G, Norris J (2000) Selfotel in acute ischemic stroke: possible neurotoxic effects of an NMDA antagonist. *Stroke* 31: 347–354

21   Lees KR, Asplund K, Carolei A, Davis SM, Diener HC, Kaste M, Orgogozo JM, Whitehead J (2000) Glycine antagonist (gavestinel) in neuroprotection (GAIN International) in patients with acute stroke: a randomised controlled trial. GAIN International Investigators. *Lancet* 355: 1949–1954

22   Striggow F, Riek M, Breder J, Henrich-Noack P, Reymann KG, Reiser G (2000) The protease thrombin is an endogenous mediator of hipocampal neuroprotection against ischemia at low concentrations but causes degeneration at high concentrations. *Proc Natl Acad Sci USA* 97 (5): 2264–2269

Inflammation in stroke and CNS trauma – experimental and clinical evidence

Clinical evidence of inflammation as a risk factor in ischemic stroke

Perttu J. Lindsberg

Department of Neurology, Helsinki University Central Hospital, Haartmaninkatu 4, P.O. Box 340, 00290 Helsinki, Finland, and Neuroscience Program, Rm B409b, Biomedicum Helsinki, Haartmaninkatu 4, P.O. Box 700, 00290 Helsinki, Finland

Inflammatory transformation of cerebral vasculature

Stationing of inflammatory cells in healthy cerebral vessels

Before the development of early atherosclerotic lesions, inflammatory cells (macrophages, T lymphocytes) can be found in the subendothelial layer of human cerebrovasculature in major arteries such as the carotid artery bifurcation as well as in perivascular spaces of small cerebral vessels [1, 2]. It is believed that mechanisms of immune function are stimulated and launch the development of inflammatory cell infiltrates within vascular walls of human blood vessels [3]. Which mechanisms of cell-cell adhesion or diapedesis are crucial for this process in healthy, noninflamed cerebral vasculature, remain unclear at this point. However, the view of intact blood-brain barrier (BBB) as a major obstacle for the entry of leukocytes has changed dramatically [2]. Presence of monocyte/macrophage lineage cells and T lymphocytes in cerebral perivascular and parenchymal locations has been observed to continue from development through maturity. This is actively regulated by endothelium, both in health and disease, and serves homeostatic functions such as immune surveillance and removal of apoptotically expired cells. It was recently demonstrated that besides being expressed on the luminal endothelial surface, chemotactic factors such as monocyte chemotactic protein MCP-1 and macrophage inflammatory protein-1α (MIP-1α) have specific and separate binding sites along the parenchymal surface of human cerebral microvessels [4]. These factors can be released by resident glial cells and transported to receptors on the vascular endothelium. Chemotactic factors and molecules mediating leukocyte adhesion exert chemotaxis and transmigration across the BBB and orchestrate cell entry to perivascular/subendothelial locales.

Although the significance of this early "subendothelial" or "perivascular" stationing of inflammatory cells for clinical CNS diseases is unclear, they are equipped for signaling toward endothelial cells and smooth muscle cells, and for releasing proliferative or lytic substances in the face of systemic challenges. Presumably these

Inflammation and Stroke, edited by Giora Z. Feuerstein
© 2001 Birkhäuser Verlag Basel/Switzerland

cells (macrophage/ monocyte lineage cells, T lymphocytes) can receive receptor stimulation and become activated upon humoral changes, and can then release proinflammatory mediators or growth factors, such as interleukins, TNFα, interferons, and TGFβ. Some of these mediators drive the inflammatory process further, and can make the endothelial cell surface proadhesive and procoagulant. At this important point, novel gene expression has occurred, and the endothelial cell has become activated. This early inflammatory step occurs also in small vessels. Interestingly, markers of inflammatory endothelial activation, plasma levels of soluble adhesion molecules (sICAM-1, sE-selectin) were elevated both in large intracranial artery disease and small artery disease (subcortical vascular encephalopathy) [5].

Stroke risk factors and inflammation

It is likely that vessel-based inflammatory cells participate and respond to known long-term risk factors for human stroke such as hypertension, hypercholesterolemia, diabetes mellitus, obesity and smoking. These risk factors have been linked to increased markers of endothelial inflammatory changes in otherwise healthy patient populations [6–8] and in patients with additional cardiovascular risk factors or a history of cerebral infarction [7, 9]. To this end, common cardiovascular risk factors have been demonstrated to increase systemic levels of TNFα [10, 11], an example of a cytokine that strongly augments adhesion molecule-dependent transendothelial migration of lymphocytes in monolayer models of human cerebral endothelium [12]. This response is most likely related to activation of circulating monocytes, which regulate the level of systemic TNFα. Clearly, cholesterol is one of the factors activating monocytes, where it steadily becomes accumulated as the cells transform into macrophages and eventually foam cells. Hypercholesterolemia has been shown to increase several markers of activation both in inflammatory cells and in endothelium [13]. This may stem from increased transcription of nuclear factor κB (NF-κB), a gene that regulates many of the inflammatory vascular effects also in hypercholesterolemia [14].

Arterial hypertension is one of the the most robust risk factors for stroke, and antihypertensives have a prominent effect in secondary prevention of stroke. Although hypertension causes a host of non-inflammatory physiological perturbations, convincing evidence exists of the association of chronically and acutely elevated blood pressure with markers of inflammation. Serum levels of circulating sICAM-1 and sVCAM-1 and sE-selectin have been reported to be increased in patients with essential hypertension [15, 16]. Acute hypertension induced by cold pressor test in normotensive and hypertensive patients increased serum levels of sICAM-1, sVCAM-1 and sE-selectin, but did not influence the expression of adhesion molecules in circulating monocytes and lymphocytes [17]. However, chronic hypertension with structural organ remodeling is associated with signs of activation in monocytes obtained from peripheral blood [18]. Another interesting study suggested that circulating monocytes from patients with hypertension are preactivated if compared to non-hypertensive controls. Upon stimulation with lipopolysaccharide (LPS) or angiotensin II, these monocytes released significantly more TNFα than those in normotensives [19].

Cigarrette smoking is generally held to be immunosuppressive, but in association with a pro-hemostatic risk factor, it may also be pro-inflammatory. Monocyte expression of tissue factor (TF) was found to be increased in women who smoke, and increased even more in those using oral contraceptives, which was based on induction of NF-κB in monocytes [20]. Even moderate smoking was observed to increase circulating levels of sICAM-1 and decrease the amount of activated monocytes in circulation, supposedly to indicate pro-adhesive effects [21]. In a population with ischemic cerebrovascular disease, smokers had increased levels of sICAM-1 and sE-selectin [5]. To summarize, stroke risk factors may thrust the early interaction between inflammatory cells and the surrounding resident cerebrovascular cells to a long run track leading to atherogenesis in large arteries and intimal thickening and local thrombosis in small arteries.

Atherosclerosis as an inflammatory process

As observed already by Virchow, development of atherosclerotic vascular lesions includes an immune-mediated inflammatory response [22]. Migration of inflammatory cells, mononuclear cells, mast cells, and lymphocytes into the vascular wall is today considered a hallmark of a human atherosclerotic plaque in the cerebrovasculature, as elsewhere ([23–26, reviewed in [27]). This process associates with the progressive deposition of modified lipids in the subendothelial layers [27]. When low-density lipoproteins (LDL) are caught in an artery, they become oxidized and phagocytosed by macrophages, which leads to formation of lipid peroxides, accumulation of cholesterol esters and formation of foam cells [27, 28] Autopsy evidence of young children and even fetuses indicates that appearance of early fatty streaks in blood vessels associates with infiltration of foam cells and T cells [29, 30], but this phenomenon is not necessarily associated with the eventual development of atherosclerosis. However, migration of inflammatory cells to the vascular wall must intimately be associated with the cause of vascular transformation leading to atherosclerosis. Oxidized LDL stimulates chemotactic effects and can increase the expression of macrophage colony-stimulating factor and MCP-1 synthesized by endothelial cells [31, 32]. Oxidized LDL can also upregulate the expression of adhesion molecules on human endothelial cells [33] and promote the transmigration of monocytes [34]. LDL may therefore augment the inflammatory response by stimulating chemokines and recruit new monocytes into the atherosclerotic lesion. Once the circulating monocyte has become a tissue macrophage, oxidized LDL inhibits its chemotaxis, presumably to prevent its exit from the vascular wall [35].

Is cerebrovascular atherosclerosis also an infectious disease?

Infectious agents were first implicated in atherosclerosis by Saikku et al. [36], when they associated serological evidence of *Chlamydia pneumoniae* infection with myocardial ischemia and infarction. Subsequent serological data have indicated that *C. pneumoniae* infection may predispose also to atherosclerotic carotid artery disease and cerebrovascular insults [37–39]. Other microbial pathogens such as herpes and cytomegaloviruses and *Helicobacter pylori* bacteria have also been suggested to be associated with atherosclerosis, but evidence of their potential relation to stroke is scanty. Recent studies based on immunohistochemistry and RT-PCR have verified the presence of *C. pneumoniae* micro-organisms in carotid artery plaques [40–42]. Furthermore, the intima-media thickness of carotid arteries measured by ultrasound in men with cardiovascular risk factors was associated with seropositivity for *C. pneumoniae* [43], although the same phenomenon was not confirmed in a normal population between 30 and 70 years of age [44].

Although the reviewed clinical evidence supports a role for *C. pneumoniae* in atherosclerotic cerebrovascular disease, little information exists on the timing of infection of the vascular sites through the evolution of atherosclerosis. Interestingly, it was shown that human macrophage/monocyte lineage cells infected with *C. pneumoniae* degenerated into foam cells [45], an early indication of atherosclerotic plaque formation in young subjects [29, 30]. Possibly, infection of macrophages with *C. pneumoniae* enhances the smooth muscle cell proliferation and local inflammmatory response in atherosclerotic plaques through cytokines or low density lipoproteins. To this end, it was recently shown that human endothelial and smooth muscle cells infected with *C. pneumoniae* had increased the expression of TF, PAI-1 and IL-6. Concomitantly, NF-κB was activated in the same cells [46]. Since antibiotics have been shown to reduce the prevalence of *C. pneumoniae* positivity in carotid endarterectomy specimens studied by PCR [47], we may soon discover whether antimicrobial therapy will influence the rates of cerebrovascular incidents in the long term. Before specific antimicrobial interventions have been shown effective in preventing cerebrovascular morbidity, the causative role of microbes in atherosclerotic cerebrovascular lesions remains putative.

Inflammatory cells in plaque growth and destabilation

Based on analysis of 5393 carotid bifurcation angiograms from 3007 patients with carotid artery stenosis, it was recently reported that some individuals have a systemic predisposition to irregularity and rupture of atherosclerotic plaques that is independent of traditional vascular risk factors [48]. Could inflammatory processes explain this? Continued dysfunction of the vascular endothelium in the presence of macrophages and T cells leads to compensatory vascular changes, smooth muscle cell proliferation and recruitment of more macrophages and lymphocytes from the blood to multiply within the atherosclerotic lesion. This further enhances the inflammatory changes of the endothelium and plaque maturation by locally released factors such as cytokines, chemokines, and growth factors [27]. As the atherosclerotic lesion grows this leads to formation of the so-called fibrous cap overlying the lipid-laden plaque core. Evidence from carotid artery plaques, a common source of artery-to-artery cerebral emboli, indicates that asymptomatic carotid plaques are more commonly morphologically so-called fibrous "hard" plaques, whereas symptomatic plaques are more commonly lipid-laden "soft" plaques [49, 50], although this view has been disputed [51]. However, it is believed that the fibrous "cap" protects the plaque from rupturing and causing *in situ* thrombosis. In human carotid arteries, mast cells capable of releasing matrix-degrading proteases, such as matrix metalloproteinases and elastases, are present in the "shoulder" region of the fibrous cap and may thus cause plaque rupture and intraplaque hemorrhages [26]. Preliminary evidence from our hospital suggests that mast cell infiltration may associate with symptomatic carotid artery plaques (Lehtonen-Smeds et al. submitted). Clearly, much more abundant macrophages may also play an important role in plaque destabilation.

Systemic inflammation and stroke

Clinical inflammatory states and stroke risk

It is well-known that systemic infectious diseases, such as respiratory and dental infections and streptococcal, staphylococcal and enterobacterial infections, are linked to stroke risk [52–54]. Similar association has thereafter been shown by various groups, indicating that infection during the preceding week is a risk factor for stroke [55–58]. It is likely that the systemic inflammatory response in the host rather than the microbial invasion *per se* is responsible for this elevated stroke risk. Clinical evidence for systemic inflammation as a risk factor for stroke is supported by data from the Physicians Health Study, where baseline blood concentration of C reactive protein (CRP) predicted the risk of myocardial infarction and stroke [59]. It was also found that the risk reduction afforded by aspirin was largest in the group with highest concentration of CRP, which suggests that inflammation promotes platelet aggregation.

Several other mechanisms have been indicated to link inflammation with prothrombotic state. In a study of victims of stroke preceded by an infectious/inflammatory condition, Macko et al. found several immunohematologic variables to indicate a prothrombotic state. The level of circulating antithrombotic activated protein C (APC) was decreased in stroke subjects and those with an antecendent infection/inflammation and the lowest concentrations of APC. Furthermore, the same cohort had elevated levels of plasma C4b-binding protein and distinctively lower ratio of active tissue plasminogen activator to plasminogen activator inhibitor levels [60]. Although Grau et al. did not confirm differences in a large number of factors of hemostasis and fibrinolysis in stroke patients with and without infection [61], Ameriso et al. found increased D-dimer levels in stroke patients with infections [62]. To summarize, since systemic changes in hemostatic parameters have not been consistently found in these studies, mild infections may increase the level of procoagulant factors among which local vascular procoagulant effects dominate over robust systemic changes.

Septic states and stroke risk

Septic states permit the entry of bacteria and LPS into the blood stream, which has profound effects favoring thrombosis *in vivo*. For example, TNFα is released during septic states, resulting in procoagulant changes in vascular endothelium [63]. It stimulates the endothelial surface to produce TF, which activates the extrinsic pathway of blood coagulation [64]. Furthermore, it reduces the secretion of thrombomodulin, which diminishes the anticoagulant effect of protein C [65]. Finally, TNFα blocks the fibrinolytic system by liberating PAI-1 [65]. In septic patients, systemically increased levels of TNFα have been correlated to antithrombin III and PAI-1 [63]. Changes in hemostasis and fibrinolysis explain the tremendously increased risk for ischemic stroke in patients with endocarditis and high risk of recurrences [67].

Tempering the inflammation – is there a lesson in statins?

Statins are a group of antihyperlipidemic compounds that inhibit the HMG CoA reductase (3-hydroxy-3-methylglutaryl coenzyme A) (e.g., simvastatin, pravastatin, fluvastatin, cerivastatin) that effectively decrease the blood level of LDL and triglycerides, and raise HDL. They have been found in several large-scale studies to substantially reduce cardiovascular morbidity (roughly by 30%) and mortality in with mildly hyperlipidemic or even normolipemic patient cohorts [66]. Importantly, the risk of stroke has also been found to be decreased by 32% in patients treated with pravastatin after myocardial infarction [69]. It is now commonly believed that the beneficial effects of statins are not solely mediated by lipid-lowering, but also effects on systemic signs of inflammatory parameters have been observed in clinical studies [70]. It is through recent investigations of the effects of statins on both systemic parameters and local plaque composition, that we have really started to understand the clinical significance of the multifaceted inflammatory processes contributing to atherosclerosis and associated thrombotic events. Pravastatin was recently reported to decrease the plasma concentration of C-reactive protein [71], which is a sensitive systemic marker of inflammation found to independently associate with myocardial infarction and stroke [59, 72]. Statin therapy also reduced the expression of soluble adhesion molecules P-selectin and ICAM-1 in hyperlipemic patients [73] and is reported to reduce cytokine production [74].

There is recent evidence that statins (lovastatin, simvastatin) inhibit the expression of monocyte chemoattractant protein 1 (MCP-1) in human endothelial cells and monocytes upon stimulation by lipopolysaccharide (LPS) or whole bacteria [75], which suggests that statins might inhibit the early stationing of inflammatory cells in vascular sites. In accordance, atorvastatin inhibited the expression of the proinflammatory regulator NF-κB and the chemokines interferon-inducible protein 10 (IP-10) and MCP-1 in isolated smooth muscle cells and mononuclear leukocytes [76]. Lovastatin was reported to bind to the domain I of human LFA-1 thereby inhibiting leukocyte adhesion through interaction of LFA-1 and ICAM-1 [77]. Furthermore, statins were shown to inhibit the production and gene expression of cyclooxygenase-2, IL-1β and IL-6 in human endothelial cells [78]. Additional effects of statins on platelet-thrombus interaction, hemostasis and on improvement of nitric oxide dependent endothelial function also need to be taken into consideration [79, 80]. Lastly, cerivastatin was recently shown to inhibit production of MCP-1, IL-8 during co-incubation with *C. pneumoniae* to infect monocytes obtained from volunteers [81], an observation which fits well with the infectious hypothesis of atherosclerotic plaque genesis. Taken together, these data suggest that the substantial ameliorating effect which statins have on the risk of cardiovascular insults and stroke is largely mediated through multi-faceted anti-inflammatory systemic and local vascular effects. Future studies may reveal additional aspects of the effects of different statins on the inflammatory pathogenesis of cerebrovascular atherosclerosis that may help us target and tailor their use in a selected patient group, which is chronically predisposed to unstable atherosclerotic plaques [48].

Conclusion

Starting from continuous or transitory presence of inflammatory cells in the cerebral vascular and non-vascular sites, as yet unknown stimuli lead to activation of the endothelium, in small cerebral microvessels and/or intracranial and extracranial arteries. Longstanding risk factors and genetic predispositions may lead to a gradual process of circulating mononuclear inflammatory cells entering the subendothelial/perivascular locales, and to aggravation of the proinflammatory and procoagulant endothelial effects. Responsiveness of the cerebrovasculature to various systemic or local challenges such as acute infections is thus transformed, and may lead to local thrombosis in small intracranial vessels. Infections with microbes like *C. pneumoniae* may enhance or even initiate this process in larger arteries and contribute to cell infiltration and maturation of atherosclerotic plaques. Inflammatory cells are always present in these plaques and respond to further systemic stimuli by releasing proteases of matrix constituents, and may trigger plaque rupture and large arterial thromboemboli/thrombosis. Future studies need to address whether inhibition of inflammatory cells and changes, or long-standing antimicrobial therapies will reduce the risk of ischemic stroke and offer effective adjuncts to platelet deaggregant, anticoagulant and statin therapies already in clinical use.

Acknowledgements

The author is supported by grants from the University of Helsinki, Helsinki University Central Hospital, the Sigrid Jusélius Foundation, Maire Taponen Foundation and the Finnish Academy.

References

1   Endres M, Laufs U, Merz H, Kaps M (1997) Focal expression of intercellular adhesion molecule-1 in the human carotid bifurcation. *Stroke* 28: 77–82

2   Perry VH, Anthony DC, Bolton SJ, Brown HC (1997) The blood-brain barrier and the inflammatory response. *Mol Med Today* 3: 337341

3   van der Wal AC, Das PK, Bentz van de Berg D, van der Loos CM, Becker AE (1989) Atherosclerotic lesions in humans: *in situ* immunophenotypic analysis suggesting an immune mediated response. *Lab Invest* 61: 166–170

4   Andjelkovic AV, Spencer DD, Pachter JS (1999) Visualization of chemokine binding sites on human brain microvessels. *J Cell Biol* 145: 403–412

5   Fassbender K, Bertsch T, Mielke O, Mühlhauser F, Hennerici M (1999) Adhesion molecules in cerebrovascular diseases: Evidence for an inflammatory endothelial activation in cerebral large- and small-vessel disease. *Stroke* 30: 1647–1650

6   Rohde LE, Hennekens CH, Ridker PM (1999) Cross-sectional study of soluble intercellular adhesion molecule-1 and cardiovascular risk factors in apparently healthy men. *Arterioscler Thromb Vasc Biol* 19: 1595–1599

7   Hackman Ayasunori A, Insull W Jr., Pownall H, Smith L, Dunn K, Gotto AM Jr., Ballantyne CM (1996) Levels of soluble adhesion molecules in patients with dyslipidemia. *Circulation* 93: 1334–1338

8   Ferri C, Desideri G, Valenti M, Bellini C, Pasin M, Santucci A, De Mattia G (1999) Early upregulation of endothelial adhesion molecules in obese hypertensive men. *Hypertension* 34: 568–573

9   Kawamura T, Umemura T, Kanai A, Uno T, Matsumae H, Sano T, Sakamoto N, Sakakibara T, Nakamura J, Hotta N (1998) The incidence and characteristics of silent cerebral infarction in elderly diabetic patients: Association with serum-soluble adhesion molecules. *Diabetologia* 41: 911–917

10   Bruunsgaard H, Skinhøj P, Pedersen AN, Schroll M, Pedersen BK (2000) Ageing, tumour necrosis factor-a (TNF-a) and atherosclerosis. *Clin Exp Immunol* 121: 255–260

11   Lechleitner M, Koch T, Herold M, Dzien A, Hoppichler F (2000) Tumour necrosis factor-a plasma level in patients with type I diabetes mellitus and its association with glycaemic control and cardiovascular risk factors. *J Int Med* 248: 67–76

12   Wong D Prameya R, Dorovini-Zis (1999) *In vitro* adhesion and migration of T lymphocytes across monolayers of human brain microvessel endothelial cells: regulation b ICAM-1, VCAM-1, E-selectin and PECAM-1. *J Neuropathol Exp Neurol* 58: 138–152

13   Lefer DJ, Granger DN (1999) Monocyte rolling in early atherogenesis: vital role in lesion development. *Circul Res* 84: 1353–1355

14   Wilson SH, Caplice NM, Simari RD, Holmes DR Jr, Carlson PJ, Lerman A (2000) Activated nuclear factor kB is present in the coronary vasculature of experimental hypercholesterolemia. *Atherosclerosis* 148: 23–30

15   Blann AD, Tse W, Maxwell SJ, Waite MA (1994) Increased levels of the soluble adhesion molecule E-selectin in essential hypertension. *J Hypertension* 12: 925–928

16   deSouza CA, Dengel DR, Macko RF, Cox K, Seals DR (1997) Elevated levels of circulating cell adhesion molecules in uncomplicated essential hypertension. *Am J Hypertension* 10: 1335–1341

17   Buemi M, Allegra A, Aloisi C, Corica F, Alonci A, Ruello A, Montalto G, Frisina N (1997) Cold pressor test raises serum concentrations of ICAM-1, VCAM-1, and E-selectin in normotensive and hypertensive patients. *Hypertension* 30: 845–847

18   Porreca E, Di Febbo C, Mincione G, Reale M, Baccante G, Guglielmi MD, Cuccurullo F, Colletta G (1997) Increased transforming growth factor-beta production and gene expression by peripheral blood monocytes of hypertensive patients. *Hypertension* 30: 134–139

19   Dorffel Y, Latsch C, Stuhlmüller B, Schreiber S, Scholze S, Burmeister GR, Scholze J (1999) Preactivated peripheral blood monocytes in patients with essential hypertension. *Hypertension* 34: 113–117

20   Holschermann H, Terhalle HM, Zakel U, MausU, Parviz B, Tillmans H, Haberbosch W (1999) Monocyte tissue factor expression is enhanced in women who smoke and use oral contraceptives. *Thromb Haemost* 82: 1614–1620

21   Bergmann S, Siekmeier R, Mix CD, Jaross W (1998) Even moderate cigarrette smoking influences the pattern of circulating monocytes and the concentration of sICAM-1. *Resp Physiol* 114: 269–275

22   Virchow R (1856) Der atheromatöse Prozess der Arterien. *Wien Med Wochenschr* 6: 825

23   Jonasson L, Holm J, Skalli O, Bondjers G, Hansson GK (1986) Regional accumulations of T cells, macrophages, and smooth muscle cells in the human atherosclerotic plaque. *Arteriosclerosis* 6: 131–138

24   van der Wal AC, Becker AE, van der Loos CM, Tigger AJ, Das PK (1994) Fibrous and lipid-rich atherosclerotic plaques are part of interchangeable morphologies related to inflammation: a concept. *Coron Art Dis* 5: 463–469

25 Kaartinen M, van der Wal AC, van der Loos CM, Piek JJ, Koch KT, Becker AE, Kovanen PT (1998) Mast cell infiltration in acute coronary syndromes: implications for plaque rupture. *J Am Coll Cardiol* 32: 606–612

26 Johnson JL, Jackson CL, Angelini GD, George SJ (1998) Activation of matrix-degrading metalloproteinases by mast cell proteases in atherosclerotic plaques. *Arterioscler Thromb Vasc Biol* 18: 707–715

27 Ross R (1999) Atherosclerosis – an inflammatory disease. *N Engl J Med* 340: 115–126

28 Ylä-Herttuala S, Palinski W, Rosenfeld ME, Parthasarathy S, Carew TE, Butler S, Witztum JL, Steinberg D (1989) Evidence for the presence of oxidatively modified low density lipoprotein in atherosclerotic lesions of rabbit and man. *J Clin Invest* 84: 1086–1095

29 Stary HC, Chandler AB, Glagov ·S, Fuster V, Glagov S, Insull W Jr., Rosenfeld ME, Schwartz CJ, Wagner WD, Wissler RW (1994) A definition of initial, fatty streak, and intermediate lesions of atherosclerosis: a report from the Committee on Vascular Lesions of the Council on Arteriosclerosis, American Heart Association. *Circulation* 89: 2462–2478

30 Napoli C, D'Armiento FP, Mancini FP, Postiglione A, Witztum JL, Palumbo G, Palinski W (1997) Fatty streak formation occurs in human fetal aortas and is greatly enhanced by maternal hypercholesterolemia: intimal accumulation of low density lipoprotein and its oxidation precede monocyte recruitment into early atherosclerotic lesions. *J Clin Invest* 100: 2680–2690

31 Rajavashisth TB, Andalibi A, Territo MC, Berliner JA, Navab M, Fogelman AM, Lusis AJ (1990) Induction of endothelial cell expression of granulocyte and macrophage colony-stimulating factors by modified low-density lipoproteins. *Nature* 344: 254–257

32 Leonard EJ, Yoshimura T (1990) Human monocyte chemoattractant protein-1 (MCP-1). *Immunol Today* 11: 97–101

33 Berliner JA, Territo MC, Sevanian A, Ramin S. Kim JA, Bamshad B, Esterson M, Fogelman AM (1990) Minimally modified low density lipoprotein stimulates monocyte endothelial interactions. *J Clin Invest* 85: 1260–1266

34 Navab M, Imes SS, Hama SY, Hough GP, Ross LA, Bork RW, Valente AJ, Berliner JA, Drinkwater DC, Laks H et al (1991) Monocyte transmigration induced by modification of low density lipoprotein in cocultures of human aortic wall cells is due to induction of monocyte chemotactic protein 1 and is abolished by high density lipoprtotein. *J Clin Invest* 88: 2039–2046

35 Rajamani K, Fisher M, Fisher M (1998) Atherosclerosis: pathogenesis and pathophysiology. In: MD Ginsberg, J Bogousslavsky (eds): *Cerebrovascular disease: pathophysiology, diagnosis, and management*, Blackwell Science, Malden, Mass, 308–318

36 Saikku P, Leinonen M, Mattila K, Ekman M-R, Nieminen MS, Mäkelä PH, Huttunen JK, Valtonen V (1988) Serological evidence of an association of a novel *Chlamydia*, TWAR, with chronic coronary heart disease and acute myocardial infarction. *Lancet* 2: 983–985

37 Melnick SL, Shahar E, Folsom AR, Grayston JT, Sorlie PD, Wang SP, Szklo M (1993)

Past infection by *Chlamydia pneumoniae* strain TWAR and asymptomatic carotid atherosclerosis. *Am J Med 95*: 499–504

38 Wimmer ML, Sandmann-Strupp R, Saikku P, Haberl RL (1996) Association of chlamydial infection with cerebrovascular disease. *Stroke 27*: 2207–2210

39 Cook PJ, Honeybourne D, Lip GYH, Beevers DG, Wise R, Davies P (1998) Chlamydia pneumoniae antibody titers are significantly associated with acute stroke and transient cerebral ischemia. *Stroke 29*: 404–410

40 Grayston JT, Kuo CC, Coulson AS, Campbell LA, Lawrence RD, Lee MJ, Strandness ED, Wang SP (1995) *Chlamydia pneumoniae* (TWAR) in atherosclerosis of the carotid artery. *Circulation 92*: 3397–3400

41 Yamashita K, Ouchi K, Shirai M, Gondo T, Nakazawa T, Ito H (1998) Distribution of Chlamydia pneumoniae infection in the athersclerotic carotid artery. *Stroke 29*: 773–778

42 Esposito G, Blasi F, Allegra L, Chiesa R, Melissano G, Cosentini R, Tarsia P, Dordoni L, Cantoni C, Arosio C, Fagetti L (1999) Demonstration of viable *Chlamydia pneumoniae* in atherosclerotic plaques of carotid arteries by reverse transcriptase polymerase chain reaction. *Ann Vasc Surg 13*: 421–425

43 Schmidt C, Hulthe J, Wikstrand J, Gnarpe H, Gnarpe J, Agewall S, Fagerberg B (2000) Chlamydia pneumoniae seropositivity is associated with carotid artery intima-media thickness. *Stroke 31*: 1526–1531

44 Markus HS, Sitzer M, Carrington D, Mendall MA, Steinmetz H (1999) Chlamydia pneumoniae infection and early asymptomatic carotid atherosclerosis. *Circulation 100*: 832–837

45 Kalayoglu MV, Byrne GI (1998) Induction of macrophage foam cell formation by *Chlamydia pneumoniae. J Infect Dis 177*: 725–729

46 Dechend R, Maass M, Gieffers J, Dietz R, Scheidereit C, Leutz A, Gulba DC (1999) Chlamydia pneumoniae infection of vascular smooth muscle and endothelial cells activates NF-κB and induces tissue factor and PAI-1 expression: a potential link to accelerated arteriosclerosis. *Circulation 100*: 1369–1373

47 Melissano G, Blasi F, Esposito G, Tarsia P, Dordoni L, Arosio C, Tshomba Y,Fagetti L, Allegra L, Chiesa R (1999) Chlamydia pneumoniae eradication from carotid plaques. Results of an open, randomized study. *Eur J Vasc Endovasc Surg 18*: 355–359

48 Rothwell PM, Villagra R, Gibson R, Donders RC, Warlow CP (2000) Evidence of a chronic systemic cause of instability of atherosclerotic plaques. *Lancet 355*: 19–24

49 O'Holleran LW, Kennelly MM, McClurken M, Johnson JM (1987) Natural history of asymptomatic carotid plaque: a five year follow-up study. *Am J Surg 154*: 659–662

50 Avril G, Batt M, Guidoin R, Marois M, Hassen-Khodja R, Daune B, Galiardi JM, Le-Bas P (1991) Carotid endarterectomy plaques: correlations of clinical and anatomic findings. *Ann Vasc Surg 5*: 50–54

51 Hatsukami TS, Ferguson MS, Beach KW, Gordon D, Detmer P, Burns D, Alpers C, Strandness E Jr (1997) Carotid plaque morphology and clinical events. *Stroke 28*: 95–1000

52 Syrjänen J, Valtonen VV, Iivanainen M, Hovi T, Malkamäki M, Mäkelä PH (1986) Association between cerebral infarction and increased serum bacterial antibody levels in young adults. *Acta Neurol Scand* 73: 273–278

53 Syrjänen J, Valtonen VV, Iivanainen M, Kaste M, Huttunen JK (1988) Preceding infection as an important risk factor for ischaemic brain infarction in young and middle aged subjects. *Br J Med* 296: 1156–1160

54 Syrjänen J, Peltola J, Valtonen V, Iivanainen M, Kaste M, Huttunen JK (1989) Dental infections in association with cerebral infarction in young and middle-aged men. *J Int Med* 225: 179–184

55 Grau AJ, Buggle F, Heindl S, Steichen-Wiehn C, Banerjee T, Maiwald M, Rohlfs M, Suhr H, Fiehn W, Becher H et al (1995) Recent infection as a risk factor for cerebrovascular ischemia. *Stroke* 26: 373–379

56 Grau AJ, Buggle F, Ziegler C, Schwarz W, Meuser J, Tasman AJ, Buhler A, Benesch C, Becher H, Hacke W (1997) Association between acute cerebrovascular ischemia and chronic and recurrent infection. *Stroke* 28: 1724–1729

57 Bova IY, Bornstein NM, Korczyn AD (1996) Acute infection as a risk factor for ischemic stroke. *Stroke* 27: 2204–2206

58 Macko RF, Ameriso SF, Barndt R, Clough W, Weiner JM, Fisher M (1996) Precipitants of brain infarction. Roles of preceding infection/inflammation and recent psychological stress. *Stroke* 27: 1999–2004

59 Ridker PM, Cushman M, Stampfer MJ, Tracy RP, Hennekens CH (1997) Inflammation, aspirin, and risks of cardiovascular disease in apparently healthy men. *N Engl J Med* 336: 973–979

60 Macko R, Ameriso SF, Gruber A, Griffin JH, Fernandez JA, Barndt R, Quismorio FP Jr, Weiner JM, Fisher M (1996) Impairments of the protein C system and fibrinolysis in infection-associated stroke. *Stroke* 27: 2005–2011

61 Grau AJ, Buggle F, Steichen-Wiehn C, Heindl S, Banerjee T, Seitz R, Winter R, Forsting M, Werle E, Bode C et al (1995) Clinical and biochemical analysis in infection-associated stroke. *Stroke* 26: 1520–1526

62 Ameriso SF, Wong VLY, Quismorio FP Jr, Fisher M (1991) Immunohematologic characteristics of infection-associated cerebral infarction. Stroke 22: 1004–1009

63 Martinez MA, Pena JM, Fernandez A, Jimenez M, Juarez S, Madero R, Vazquez JJ (1999) Time course and prognostic significance of hemostatic changes in sepsis: relation to tumor necrosis factor-α. *Crit Care Med* 27: 1303–1308

64 Conway EM, Bach R, Rosenberg RD, Konigsberg WH (1989) Tumor necrosis factor enhances expression of tissue factor mRNA in endothelial cells. *Thromb Res* 53: 231–241

65 Moore KL, Esmon CT, Esmon NL (1989) Tumor necrosis factor leads to the internalization and degradation of thrombomodulin from the surface of bovine aortic endothelial cells in culture. *Blood* 73: 159–165

66 van der Poll T, Buller HR, ten Cate H, Wortel CH, Bauer KA, van Deventer SJ, Hack CE, Sauerwein HP, Rosenberg RD, ten Cate JW (1990) Activation of coagulation after

administration of tumor necrosis factor to normal subjects. *New Engl J Med* 322: 1622–1627

67   Hart RG, Foster JW, Luther MF, Kanter MC (1990) Stroke in infective endocarditis. *Stroke* 21: 695–700

68   Velasco JA (1999) After 4S, CARE and LIPID – is evidence-based medicine being practised? *Atherosclerosis* 147 (Suppl 1): S39–S44

69   Plehn JF, Davis BR, Sacks FM, Rouleau JL, Pfeffer MA, Bernstein V, Cuddy TE, Moyé LA, Piller LB, Rutherford J et al for the CARE Investigators (1999) Reduction of stroke incidence after myocardial infarction with pravastatin. The cholesterol and recurrent events (CARE) study. *Circulation* 99: 216–223

70   Ridker PM, Rifai N, Pfeffer MA, Sacks FM, Moyé LA, Goldman S, Flaker GC, Braunwald E for the CARE Investigators (1998) Inflammation, pravastatin, and the risk of coronary events after myocardial infarction in patients with average cholesterol levels. *Circulation* 98: 839–844

71   Ridker PM, Rifai N, Pfeffer MA, Sacks F, Braunwald E for the CARE Investigators (1999) Long-term effects of pravastatin on plasma concentration of C-reactive protein. *Circulation* 100: 230–235

72   Ridker PM, Buring JE, Shih J, Matias M, Hennekens CH (1998) Prospective study of C-reactive protein and the risk of future cardiovascular events among apparently healthy women. *Circulation* 98: 731–733

73   Romano M, Mezzetti A, Marulli , Ciabattoni G, Febo F, Di Ienno S, Roccaforte S, Vignieri S, Nubile G, Milani M et al (2000) Fluvastatin reduces soluble P-selectin and ICAM-1 levels in hypercholesterolemic patients: role of nitric oxide. *J Invest Med* 48: 183–189

74   Rosenson RS, Tangney CC, Casey LC (1999) Inhibition of proinflammatory cytokine production by pravastatin. *Lancet* 353: 983–984

75   Romano M, Diomede L, Sironi M, Massimiliano L, Sottocorno M, Polentarutti N, Guglielmotti A, Albani D, Bruno A, Fruscella P, Salmona M et al (2000) Inhibition of monocyte chemotactic protein-1 synthesis by statins. *Lab Invest* 80: 1095–1100

76   Ortego M, Bustos C, Hernandez-Presa MA, Tunon J, Diaz C, Hernandez G, Egido J (1999) Atorvastatin reduces NF-κB acivation and chemokine expression in vascular smooth muscle cells and mononuclear cells. *Atherosclerosis* 147: 253–261

77   Kallen J, Welzenbach K, Ramage P, Geyl D, Kriwacki R, Legge G, Cottens S, Weitz-Schmidt G, Hommel U (1999) Structural basis for LFA-1 inhibition upon lovastatin binding to the CD11a I-domain. *J Molec Biol* 292: 1–9

78   Inoue I, Goto S, Mizotani , Awata T, Mastunaga T, Kawai S, Nakajima T, Hokari S, Komoda T, Katayama S (2000) Lipophilic HMG-CoA reductase inhibitor has an anti-inflammatory effect: reduction of m-RNA levels for interleukin-1β, interleukin-6, cyclooxygenase-2, and p22phox by regulation of peroxisome proliferator-activated receptor a (PPARa) in primary endothelial cells. *Life Sciences* 67: 863–876

79   Dupuis J, Tardif J-C, Cernacek P, Théroux P (1999) Cholesterol reduction rapidly improves endothelial function after acute coronary sundromes. The RECIFE (Reduction

of cholesterol in ischemia and function of the endothelium) trial. *Circulation* 99: 3227–3233

80 Weissberg P (1999) Mechanisms modifying atherosclerotic disease – from lipids to vascular biology. *Atherosclerosis* 147 (Suppl 1): S3–S10

81 Kothe H, Dalhoff K, Rupp J, Müller A, Kreutzer J, Maass M, Katus HA (2000) Hydroxylmethylglutaryl coenzyme A reductase inhibitors modify the inflammatory response of human macrophages and endothelial cells infected with *Chlamydia pneumoniae*. *Circulation* 101: 1760–1763

Inflammation as a risk factor for stroke: evidence from experimental models

Anna-Leena Sirén

Max-Planck-Institute for Experimental Medicine and the Departments of Neurology and Psychiatry, Georg-August University, 37075 Göttingen, Germany

Prior infection/inflammation as a risk-factor for stroke

The association of preceding systemic infection and ischemic stroke has long been recognized by clinicians [1–7]. In a retrospective study of ischemic stroke in Sweden, stroke incidence exhibited seasonal variability with higher incidence in the colder winter months [1]. Infection was suggested to underlie the increased stroke incidence during winter since, in young adults without established stroke-risk factors, evidence of infection was seen concomitantly with the onset of stroke [1]. Seasonal variability of plasma fibrinogen and factor VII activity in an elderly population in England with increased levels during winter was also related to respiratory infections [8]. Syrjänen et al. [4] demonstrated in Finland that young to middle-aged patients presenting with acute ischemic stroke had a significantly higher prevalence of febrile infections 1 month preceding the stroke. A similar association of ischemic stroke and dental infection in the preceding month was further established in young Finnish men [9]. Evidence of infection less than 1 month before onset of stroke was also reported in 34% of stroke patients of all age groups in southern California by Ameriso et al. [10]. Several case-control studies that have also included older patients, revealed that infection within 1 week before onset of stroke or examination was significantly more common among stroke patients than in control subjects [5–7]. An inflammatory response may also explain why chronic infection with *Chlamydia pneumoniae* is a predisposing risk factor for carotid atherosclerosis and cerebrovascular disease [11–16]. Furthermore, there is evidence that non-infectious inflammation can increase risk for stroke: Macko et al. [5] found that non-infectious inflammatory syndromes associated with an increased stroke risk. Increased cardiovascular mortality has been reported in Swedish patients with seropositive rheumatoid arthritis [17, 18]. Inflammatory activity, as measured by haptoglobin at disease onset was found as a predictor for heart disease and stroke in these patients [18]. The studies summarized here suggest that in addition to the established stroke-risk factors (hypertension, ischemic heart disease, diabetes mellitus, cigarette smoking), prior infection/inflammation may serve as a predisposing factor for ischemic stroke.

Inflammation and Stroke, edited by Giora Z. Feuerstein

Inflammatory mechanisms and increased stroke-risk – role of cytokines

The authors reporting on the association between preceding infection and stroke have proposed that endothelial dysfunction and immunologic mechanisms involving proinflammatory cytokines could explain the increased stroke-risk after bacterial infections [1–7]. Under the influence of cytokines such as interleukin-1 (IL-1) and tumor necrosis factor-α (TNFα) the endothelium undergoes a reversal from an actively anticoagulant and antithrombotic surface to an actively prothrombotic membrane [16, 19–21]. The specific changes include an increased adhesion and transmigration of monocytes and granulocytes, release of prothrombotic factors (von Willebrand factor, platelet-activating factor, tissue factor) and inhibition of anticoagulant mechanisms (thrombomodulin-protein C protein S system, tissue plasminogen activator, prostacyclin) [19]. This possibility is further supported by the evidence suggesting that inflammation is the initial stimulus and promoter of atherogenesis [16]. Direct support for these mechanisms in infection-associated stroke has been provided by the findings that in stroke patients with nosocomial infections plasma levels of IL-6 and sTNFR-55 were significantly elevated [22]. *Chlamydia pneumoniae* infection of human vascular endothelial and smooth muscle cells has been recently reported to activate nuclear-factor-κB and induce IL-6, tissue factor and plasminogen activator inhibitor 1 [23]. Increased procoagulant properties could be demonstrated in patients presenting with infection-associated cerebral infarction as blood fibrinogen and anti-cardiolipin levels as well as generation of fibrin were significantly elevated in stroke patients with prior infection compared to stroke patients without infections [10, 24]. Interestingly, the difference in plasma fibrinogen levels between patients with and without preceding infection was significant only when studied early after stroke, indicating that acute-phase responses in stroke patients early after stroke may reflect prior infection rather than stroke itself, while later these inflammatory responses are more likely related to the cerebrovascular event [10].

Inflammatory mechanisms may also be instrumental to understanding how established risk factors for stroke such as hypertension, aging, diabetes mellitus, and atherosclerosis increase the likelihood for stroke (Tab. 1). Hallenbeck et al. [25] were the first to propose that stroke-risk factors may promote a cytokine-mediated interaction of endothelium with monocytes that prepares local segments of cerebral vessels for subsequent thrombosis or hemorrhage in a manner similar to the localized Shwartzman reaction. Established risk factors for stroke (hypertension, old age, diabetes, genetic stroke-proneness) increased the incidence of ischemia and hemorrhage in brainstem vasculature of rats in response to a "provocative" dose of lipopolysaccharide (LPS) [25]. It was proposed that the stroke risk factor effects may be due to an increased interaction between cerebrovascular endothelium and circulating monocytes [25–27] and many studies have provided indirect evidence that support this working hypothesis: Activation of endothelium and monocytes

Table 1 - Hypothetical sequence of events how stroke-risk factors operate to increase stroke-likelihood via *an inflammatory cytokine-mediated cascade.*

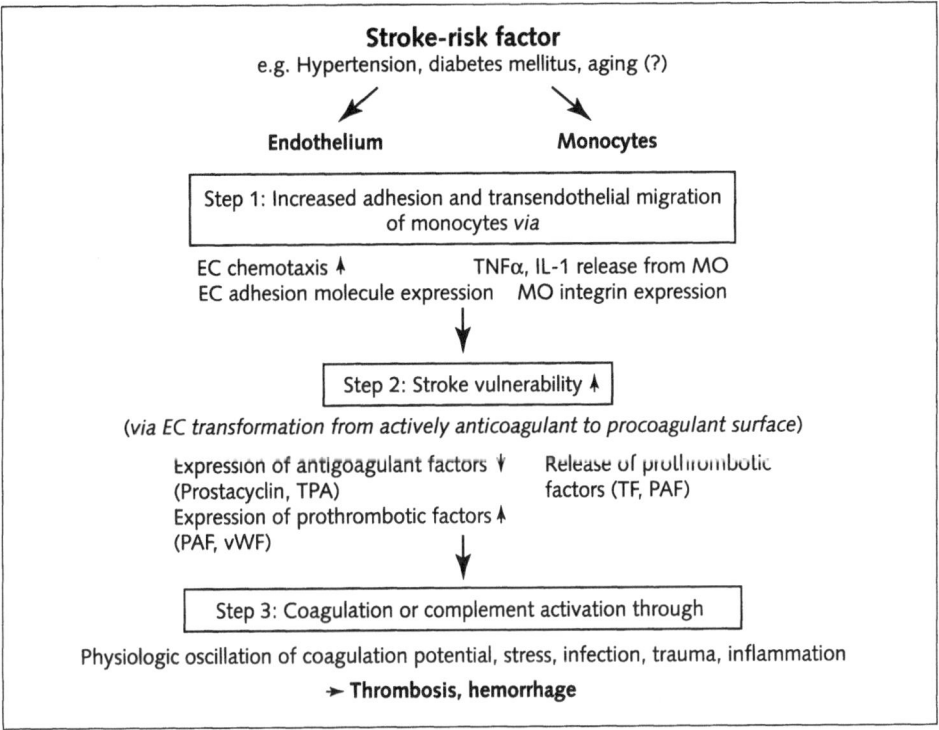

Abbreviations: *EC, endothelium; MO, monocyte; PAF, platelet activating factor; TF, tissue factor; TPA, tissue plasminogen activator; vWF, von Willebrand factor*

and an increased adherence of monocytes to endothelium are induced by hypertension [28–35]. Accordingly, an increased local accumulation of monocyte/macrophages has been found in the brains of aged or stroke prone and hypertensive rats [36], and cells of these rats produced more TNFα in response to stimulation (with LPS) than cells from normotensive control animals [26, 27, 32]. These events may contribute to the increased stroke risk in hypertensive and aged animals, inasmuch as the subendothelial clusters of monocyte/macrophages could transform the overlying endothelial cells from actively anticoagulant to a prothrombotic state *via* increased release of TNFα and IL-1. Direct support for this hypothesis has been provided by the findings that monocyte activation following priming with bacillus Calmette-Guerin (BCG) and the production of TNFα and IL-1 were crucial to the development of neurological deficits and cerebral infarcts after activation of the local Shwartzman reaction [37]. Activation of circulating monocytes was evident after BCG injection in all animals in this study when the spontaneous superoxide production and adhesion receptor expression were used as indices of cell activation. The study [37] further demonstrated that inhibitors of IL-1 and TNF dramatically reduced the development of cerebral infarcts that were provoked by monocyte activating treatments lending further support to the hypothesis that both TNFα and IL-1 may mediate ischemic brain damage and that monocyte activation may predispose brain tissue to ischemia by an exaggerated release of IL-1 and TNFα from monocyte/macrophages located around local blood vessels.

Inflammation plays a pivotal role in the initiation, progression, and activation of atherosclerotic plaques[16,38-40]. It seems also to be involved in the conversion of carotid atherosclerotic plaques from an asymptomatic to a symptomatic state. Thus, expression of the endothelial adhesion molecule ICAM-1 was increased in the high-grade regions of symptomatic *versus* asymptomatic carotid plaques and a differential expression of ICAM-1 was reported in the high-grade *versus* the low-grade region of symptomatic plaques [41]. Plasma sICAM-1 levels were not predictive of symptomatic disease, however, when compared with a risk factor–free, age-matched control group, sICAM-1 was significantly elevated in patients with symptomatic atherosclerosis [41].

References

1   Hindfelt B, Nilsson O (1977) Brain infarction in young adults (with particular reference to pathogenesis). *Acta Neurol Scand* 55: 145–157

2   Ode B, Cronberg S (1976) Infection and intracranial arterial thrombosis [letter]. *Lancet* 2: 863–864

3   Syrjanen J, Valtonen VV, Iivanainen M, Hovi T, Malkamaki M, Makela PH (1986) Association between cerebral infarction and increased serum bacterial antibody levels in young adults. *Acta Neurol Scand* 73: 273–278

4   Syrjanen J, Valtonen VV, Iivanainen M, Kaste M, Huttunen JK (1988) Preceding infection as an important risk factor for ischaemic brain infarction in young and middle aged patients. *Br Med J (Clin Res Ed)* 296: 1156–1160

5   Macko RF, Ameriso SF, Barndt R, Clough W, Weiner JM, Fisher M (1996) Precipitants of brain infarction. Roles of preceding infection/inflammation and recent psychological stress [see comments]. *Stroke*: 27 1999–2004

6   Grau AJ, Buggle F, Heindl S, Steichen-Wiehn C, Banerjee T, Maiwald M, Rohlfs M, Suhr H, Fiehn W, Becher H et al (1995) Recent infection as a risk factor for cerebrovascular ischemia. *Stroke* 26: 373–379

7   Bova IY, Bornstein NM, Korczyn AD (1996) Acute infection as a risk factor for ischemic stroke. *Stroke* 27: 2204–2206

8   Woodhouse PR, Khaw KT, Plummer M, Foley A, Meade TW (1994) Seasonal variations

of plasma fibrinogen and factor VII activity in the elderly: winter infections and death from cardiovascular disease. *Lancet* 343: 435–439

9   Syrjanen J, Peltola J, Valtonen V, Iivanainen M, Kaste M, Huttunen JK (1989) Dental infections in association with cerebral infarction in young and middle-aged men. *J Intern Med* 225: 179–184

10 Ameriso SF, Wong VL, Quismorio FP, Jr., Fisher M (1991) Immunohematologic characteristics of infection-associated cerebral infarction [see comments]. *Stroke* 22: 1004–1009

11 Melnick SL, Shahar E, Folsom AR, Grayston JT, Sorlie PD, Wang SP, Szklo M (1993) Past infection by Chlamydia pneumoniae strain TWAR and asymptomatic carotid atherosclerosis. Atherosclerosis Risk in Communities (ARIC) Study Investigators. *Am J Med* 95: 499–504

12 Wimmer ML, Sandmann-Strupp R, Saikku P, Haberl RL (1996) Association of chlamydial infection with cerebrovascular disease. *Stroke* 27: 2207–2210

13 Cook PJ, Honeybourne D, Lip GY, Beevers DG, Wise R, Davies P (1998) *Chlamydia pneumoniae* antibody titers are significantly associated with acute stroke and transient cerebral ischemia: the West Birmingham Stroke Project. *Stroke* 29: 404–410

14 Fagerberg B, Gnarpe J, Gnarpe H, Agewall S, Wikstrand J (1999) *Chlamydia pneumoniae* but not cytomegalovirus antibodies are associated with future risk of stroke and cardiovascular disease: a prospective study in middle-aged to elderly men with treated hypertension. *Stroke* 30: 299–305

15 Elkind MS, Lin IF, Grayston JT, Sacco RL (2000) *Chlamydia pneumoniae* and the risk of first ischemic stroke : The Northern Manhattan Stroke Study. *Stroke* 31: 1521–1525

16 Ross R (1999) Atherosclerosis is an inflammatory disease. *Am Heart J* 138: S419–S420

17 Wallberg-Jonsson S, Dahlen G, Johnson O, Olivecrona G, Rantapaa-Dahlqvist S (1996) Lipoprotein lipase in relation to inflammatory activity in rheumatoid arthritis. *J Intern Med* 240: 373–380

18 Wallberg-Jonsson S, Johansson H, Ohman ML, Rantapaa-Dahlqvist S (1999) Extent of inflammation predicts cardiovascular disease and overall mortality in seropositive rheumatoid arthritis. A retrospective cohort study from disease onset. *J Rheumatol* 26: 2562–2571

19 Hallenbeck JM (1996) Inflammatory reactions at the blood-endothelial interface in acute stroke. *Adv Neurol* 71: 281–297

20 del Zoppo G, Ginis I, Hallenbeck JM, Iadecola C, Wang X, Feuerstein GZ (2000) Inflammation and stroke: putative role for cytokines, adhesion molecules and iNOS in brain response to ischemia. *Brain Pathol* 10: 95–112

21 Couffinhal T, Duplaa C, Labat L, Lamaziere JM, Moreau C, Printseva O, Bonnet J (1993) Tumor necrosis factor-alpha stimulates ICAM-1 expression in human vascular smooth muscle cells. *Arterioscler Thromb* 13: 407–414

22 Fassbender K, Dempfle CE, Mielke O, Rossol S, Schneider S, Dollman M, Hennerici M (1997) Proinflammatory cytokines: indicators of infection in high-risk patients. *J Lab Clin Med* 130: 535–539

23   Dechend R, Maass M, Gieffers J, Dietz R, Scheidereit C, Leutz A, Gulba DC (1999) *Chlamydia pneumoniae* infection of vascular smooth muscle and endothelial cells activates NF-kappaB and induces tissue factor and PAI-1 expression: a potential link to accelerated arteriosclerosis. *Circulation* 100: 1369–1373

24   Macko RF, Ameriso SF, Gruber A, Griffin JH, Fernandez JA, Barndt R, Quismorio FP, Jr, Weiner JM, Fisher M (1996) Impairments of the protein C system and fibrinolysis in infection-associated stroke. *Stroke* 27: 2005–2011

25   Hallenbeck JM, Dutka AJ, Kochanek PM, Sirén A, Pezeshkpour GH, Feuerstein G (1988) Stroke risk factors prepare rat brainstem tissues for modified local Shwartzman reaction. *Stroke* 19: 863–869

26   Sirén AL, Heldman E, Doron D, Lysko PG, Yue TL, Liu Y, Feuerstein G, Hallenbeck JM (1992) Release of proinflammatory and prothrombotic mediators in the brain and peripheral circulation in spontaneously hypertensive and normotensive Wistar-Kyoto rats. *Stroke* 23: 1643–1650; discussion 1650–1651

27   Sirén AL, Liu Y, Feuerstein G, Hallenbeck JM (1993) Increased release of tumor necrosis factor-alpha into the cerebrospinal fluid and peripheral circulation of aged rats. *Stroke* 24: 880–886; discussion 887–888

28   Schmid-Schonbein GW, Seiffge D, DeLano FA, Shen K, Zweifach BW (1991) Leukocyte counts and activation in spontaneously hypertensive and normotensive rats [see comments]. *Hypertension* 17: 323–330

29   Schroder S, Palinski W, Schmid-Schonbein GW (1991) Activated monocytes and granulocytes, capillary nonperfusion, and neovascularization in diabetic retinopathy. *Am J Pathol* 139: 81–100

30   Veniant M, Clozel JP, Kuhn H, Clozel M (1992) Protective effect of cilazapril on the cerebral circulation. *J Cardiovasc Pharmacol* 19: S94–S99

31   Duplàa C, Couffinhal T, Labat L, Fawaz J, Moreau C, Bietz I, Bonnet J (1993) Monocyte adherence to endothelial cells in patients with atherosclerosis: relationships with risk factors. *Eur J Clin Invest* 23: 474–479

32   Liu Y, Liu T, McCarron RM, Spatz M, Feuerstein G, Hallenbeck JM, Sirén AL (1996) Evidence for activation of endothelium and monocytes in hypertensive rats. *Am J Physiol* 270: H2125–H2131

33   McCarron RM, Wang L, Sirén AL, Spatz M, Hallenbeck JM (1994) Monocyte adhesion to cerebromicrovascular endothelial cells derived from hypertensive and normotensive rats. *Am J Physiol* 267: H2491–H2497

34   McCarron RM, Doron DA, Sirén AL, Feuerstein G, Heldman E, Pollard HB, Spatz M, Hallenbeck JM (1994) Agonist-stimulated release of von Willebrand factor and procoagulant factor VIII in rats with and without risk factors for stroke. *Brain Res* 647: 265–272

35   McCarron RM, Wang L, Sirén AL, Spatz M, Hallenbeck JM (1994) Adhesion molecules on normotensive and hypertensive rat brain endothelial cells. *Proc Soc Exp Biol Med* 205: 257–262

36   Liu Y, Jacobowitz DM, Barone F, McCarron R, Spatz M, Feuerstein G, Hallenbeck JM,

Sirén AL (1994) Quantitation of perivascular monocytes and macrophages around cerebral blood vessels of hypertensive and aged rats. *J Cereb Blood Flow Metab* 14: 348–352

37   Sirén A-L, McCarron RM, Wang L, Garcia-Pinto P, Ruetzler C, Hallenbeck JM (2001) Proinflammatory cytokine expression contributes to brain injury provoked by chronic monocyte activation. *Mol Med* 7: 219–229

38   Alexander RW (1998) Atherosclerosis as disease of redox-sensitive genes. *Trans Am Clin Climatol Assoc* 109: 129–145

39   Chobanian AV, Alexander RW (1996) Exacerbation of atherosclerosis by hypertension. Potential mechanisms and clinical implications [see comments]. *Arch Intern Med* 156: 1952–1956

40   Chappell DC, Varner SE, Nerem RM, Medford RM, Alexander RW (1998) Oscillatory shear stress stimulates adhesion molecule expression in cultured human endothelium. *Circ Res* 82: 532–539

41   DeGraba TJ, Sirén AL, Penix L, McCarron RM, Hargraves R, Sood S, Pettigrew KD, Hallenbeck JM (1998) Increased endothelial expression of intercellular adhesion molecule-1 in symptomatic versus asymptomatic human carotid atherosclerotic plaque. *Stroke* 29: 1405–1410

Inflammatory and immune responses to CNS injury: beneficial and detrimental components

Salutary effect of autoimmune T cells after central nervous system injury

Michal Schwartz

Department of Neurobiology, The Weizmann Institute of Science, 76100 Rehovot, Israel

Cross-talk between the CNS and the immune system

The interaction between the central nervous system (CNS) and the immune system is unique, partly because it is characterized by "immune privilege", involving restriction of local immune responses within the CNS. This phenomenon is probably an evolutionary adaptation developed to protect the intricate neuronal networks of the CNS from potentially disruptive incursion by the immune system [1–3]. An early definition of immune privilege was based on the assumption that the immune system ignores the CNS. This concept of immune ignorance was supported by the poor ability of the CNS to reject allografts, i.e. tissue grafts from the same species but from a different major histocompatibility complex (MHC) haplotype. Immune privilege was thought to be maintained by the harboring of antigens within the CNS and the inability of immune cells to enter the CNS under normal physiological conditions. Any entry of leukocytes was viewed as evidence of pathology [4–8]. Several observations have indicated that the CNS is accessible to immune cells, and that immune privilege is the result of an active barrier, or of several mechanisms collectively endowing the CNS with unique immune characteristics [9–13]. It thus appears that protection of the CNS from pathogen invasion has been achieved at the cost of forfeiting some of the advantages normally bestowed on damaged tissues by the immune system.

Autoimmune T cells have a neuroprotective effect

The healthy CNS is constantly patrolled by T cells, albeit in small numbers [7]. It was suggested that any increase in the numbers of patrolling T cells in the CNS, as in other immune-privileged sites, is kept to a minimum by apoptosis, in which FasL is involved [14, 15]. The active elimination of invading T cells from the immune-privileged CNS is not surprising; what is surprising is that there is any T-cell entry at all. What makes the CNS permissive to patrolling by T cells? Is it the failure to create a mechanism for its prevention [2]? And why are the T cells there at all? Are they present as a safety measure in case they should be needed? If so, this raises other questions: Is entry restricted to T cells of a specific type, and what is their function in the CNS? While these questions still remain unanswered, a recent series of results suggest that – at least after non-pathogenic damage in the CNS – the adaptive immune response serves the function of tissue maintenance and protection. The first unexpected finding was that T cells accumulate at the site of a CNS lesion. Moreover, the accumulation is increased if the insult is accompanied by systemic injection of activated T cells, irrespective of their antigen specificity [14, 16]. The effects of the increased recruitment on the damaged nerve were then studied in an attempt to find out whether the increased accumulation is an outcome of the injurious conditions or is a purposeful (though non-selective) recruitment.

Injury to the CNS is known to lead to neuronal damage as a consequence of degeneration, which results not only from the direct insult but also from destructive processes affecting the extracellular environment of all neurons, including uninjured ones, in the vicinity of the site of injury. The resulting changes include abnormal intracellular shifts of ions such as Na^+ and Ca^{2+}, free radical-associated lipid peroxidation of cell membranes, release of excitotoxic neurotransmitters, depletion of growth factors, and energy loss. The end result is neuronal cell death. The progression of degeneration caused by these abnormal conditions can, in principle, be stopped or at least attenuated by the use of pharmacological agents that neutralize the mediators of toxicity or compete for binding sites on their receptors, or by increasing the resistance of the remaining neurons to the hostile conditions [17, 18].

In an attempt to establish a possible link between the increased post-injury accumulation of T cells (both physiologically and after systemic injection of T cells specific to the relevant antigens) and the ability of the nerve to recover from the injury, we used two models of partial lesion in the rat CNS: partial optic nerve crush and spinal cord contusion. Use of these models made it possible to determine whether recovery would be better or worse in the presence of an increased number of T cells. In rats with partial optic nerve crush, morphological and functional tests yielded another surprising finding, namely that after systemic injection of T cells specific to the CNS self-antigen myelin basic protein (MBP), but not of T cells specific to the non-self antigen ovalbumin, the rate of neuronal survival is significantly higher than in control (PBS-treated) rats [19–21]. The same effect was achieved in the contused spinal cord, where functional recovery (i.e., the outcome of the recovery of the spared neurons minus the ones that degenerate both laterally and longitudinally) was significantly better in rats treated by systemic injection of anti-MBP T cells than in rats treated with anti-ovalbumin T cells or with PBS. Recovery was assessed by behavioral criteria (measurement of locomotor activity), morphological criteria (counting of retrogradely labeled red nuclei), and immunocytochemical staining for neurofilaments [22–25]. These results raised some key questions: is the observed beneficial effect of the autoimmune T cells obtained only at the risk of development of a myelin-related autoimmune disease (e.g. experimental autoimmune encephalitis (EAE) in animals or multiple sclerosis in humans)? Or are autoimmune disease and immune neuroprotection distinct processes mediated by two subpopulations of cells differing in their phenotype and/or antigenic specificity? Alternatively, are the two processes mediated by the same cells, whose activity differs depending on injury-induced changes in the tissue context?

Our results suggest that the T cells which confer neuroprotection are not necessarily only those directed against proteins that destroy myelin. On the contrary, neuroprotection was also exhibited by T cells that are reactive specifically to an epitope, located within the myelin protein, that causes little or no myelin destruction [19]. Using the mouse optic nerve model we recently showed that protection of optic nerve cell bodies and axons from mechanical injury, but not from glutamate toxicity, can be achieved by several myelin-associated proteins in addition to MBP, and in all cases also by non-encephalitogenic epitopes of these proteins [26]. Results of our subsequent experiments further suggest that the immune neuroprotection achieved by passive transfer of T cells can be reproduced by active immunization, provided that both antigen and adjuvant are carefully chosen so as to ensure activation of the relevant T cells at the right time, in the right number, and within the window of opportunity for neuroprotection, i.e., before the neurons are committed to death [21, 22, 26, 27].

Mechanisms underlying the neuroprotective effect of the autoimmune T cells

Analysis of the electrophysiological activity of the rat optic nerve at different times after injury and systemic injection of the anti-MBP T cells showed that neuroprotection was preceded by a transient reduction in nerve conduction. There are several possible explanations for this. The observed neuroprotective effect might be caused, at least in part, by a T-cell-induced transient reduction in the nerve's electrophysiological activity. Induction of a resting state in the damaged nerve was shown to transiently reduce the nerve's metabolic requirements and prevent energy depletion, thus helping to preserve neuronal viability in a manner similar to hypothermia-induced neuroprotection [19]. It is also possible that the neuroprotective activity of the T cells is independent of their effect on the nerve's conductivity.

An alternative or additional mechanism might involve the activity of neurotrophins, shown in a number of studies to participate in the inflammatory response. T cells produce a variety of neurotrophic factors and cytokines [28–31], some or all of which may be supportive and protective after CNS injury [32–34]. We showed that the secretion of neurotrophic factors by T cells, like the secretion of cytokines, is dependent on reactivation of the T cells by their specific antigens in conjunction with antigen-presenting cells. T cells of different antigenic specificities were found by our group to express mRNA and protein specific to nerve growth factor, brain-derived neurotrophic factor, neurotrophin-3, and neurotrophin-4/5. Secretion of these neurotrophins was significantly increased after reactivation of the T cells by their specific antigens [21]. It thus appears that only CNS autoimmune T cells, upon recognizing their antigen, can secrete increased amounts of neurotrophins in injured optic nerves. This would explain why only T cells specific to myelin, or to antigens that cross-react with myelin, have neuroprotective properties in the context of damage to myelinated axons. Support for the feasibility of a neurotrophic mechanism comes from the finding that mRNA for TrkA, TrkB, and p75 receptors is expressed in the injured optic nerve, pointing to an ability of T-cell-derived neurotrophins to mediate their effects *via* these specific receptors [21]. Other studies have pointed to a neuroprotective effect of neurotrophic and other growth factors in spinal cord injuries [35–37].

More recently, we observed that T cells activated by their antigens can bring to the lesion site a battery of proteases capable of reducing the potentially toxic amounts of physiological compounds such as thrombin (Friedmann et al., J. Neuroimmunol., in press). It seems reasonable to suggest that, because of its heterogeneous neuronal subtypes and the complexity of the degenerative process, the injured CNS nerves may respond positively to a variety of factors. Suitably activated T cells might therefore have an advantage over a single-compound therapy by supplying a number of remedial factors, whose production and local secretion are regulated by signals derived locally from the damaged tissue, presumably in accordance with tissue requirements.

Beneficial T cell-dependent immunity is a physiological response evoked by the injury

The results summarized above showed that manipulation of the adaptive response directed against self can be beneficial in the context of CNS trauma. This raised a fundamental question: Does the beneficial effect represent a physiological response, or is it merely the result of an immunological intervention? Experiments in our laboratory showed that splenocytes from rats with a week-old spinal cord contusion exert neuroprotective activity when transferred, after exposure *ex vivo* to MBP, to rats with a newly sustained CNS injury [38]. Moreover, the survival rate of retinal ganglion cells after optic nerve injury was significantly lower in rats devoid of T cells (as a result of having undergone thymectomy at birth) than in normal rats. Additional support came from the use of transgenic mice overexpressing a T-cell receptor for MBP or for ovalbumin. The rate of neuronal survival after crush injury was significantly higher in the former, and significantly lower in the latter, than in matched wild-type controls [38].

One of the compounds responsible for neuronal losses after CNS injury is glutamate, an amino acid which normally serves as a ubiquitous neurotransmitter in brain functions such as learning and memory. When its physiological levels are exceeded, however, it becomes cytotoxic [18, 40–42]. Extracellular glutamate is normally buffered *via* uptake by astrocytes, and is recycled after being converted to glutamine [43–45]. Under abnormal conditions, caused for example by acute or chronic CNS insults, the local buffering capacity is apparently insufficient to control the inevitable increase in glutamate above a certain threshold and thus death of neurons occurs. Studies in our laboratory have shown that glutamate, when injected intravitreally into rats at different concentrations, exerts an effect in a dose-dependent manner, on the ability of the immune system to counteract the cytotoxicity. This was demonstrated by comparing retinal ganglion cell death in normal mice and nude mice [47]. Thus, for any given amount of glutamate injected intravitreally, more retinal ganglion cells died in the mice deprived of mature T cells than in the matched wild-type controls [48]. The lower survival rate in the nude mice could be counteracted, at least in part, by the transfer of splenocytes from the wild-type mice [49].

We suggest that immune neuroprotection may be viewed as a mechanism for recruitment of a second line of defense when the local control mechanism is inadequate. It seems reasonable to assume that this additional adaptive mechanism, unlike the constitutive local mechanisms, is evoked not as a specific response to challenge by a single potentially toxic compound, but as a general feature of any endogenous compound that has an essential physiological function but is cytotoxic when present in excessive amounts. The specificity of the T cells associated with grey matter lesion, as in the case of glutamate toxicity, has yet to be determined (Schori et al, *J Neuroimmunol; in press*).

Taken together, our findings in connection with neuroprotective autoimmunity thus appear to ascribe an additional function, hitherto unrecognized, to the immune system. Up to now the adaptive immune response has been viewed as a defensive mechanism that evolved to provide a versatile backup when the innate immune response (involving macrophages) to foreign invasion is unequal to the task. Our studies provide evidence that stressful conditions, caused by a pathological increase in potentially toxic compounds (e.g. glutamate), might exceed the constitutive capacity of the adaptive immune system (expressed here by the response to self-antigens) to provide neuroprotective immunity. An inadequate autoimmune response will lead, on the one hand, to a lack of beneficial autoimmunity and hence accelerated degeneration, and on the other hand to a possible predisposition to autoimmune disease. This pattern of immune inadequacy can be compared to the breakdown of the normally protective immune response in the face of an overwhelming infective process, resulting in recurrence of the infection. Our preliminary results suggest that the same T cells can mediate both autoimmune neuroprotection and autoimmune disease [46]. For the former, however, additional T cells, presumably of regulatory nature are needed (Kipnis et al., unpublished observations). The presence of regulatory T cells might explain the inverse relationship observed between protective autoimmunity and susceptibility to autoimmune disease [47]. According-ly, an inverse relationship was found between the ability of rats with optic nerve crush injury to sustain a beneficial endogenous protective response and their sus-ceptibility to development of an autoimmune disease [47].

The prospect of T-cell-mediated autoimmunity as therapy for degenerative diseases

The observed autoimmune neuroprotection of undamaged fibers and of cell bodies of damaged fibers in the hostile post-traumatic extracellular environments of the rat spinal cord and optic nerve leads us to believe that such neuroprotection will prove to be a feature of other degenerative events as well [19, 22, 23, 26].

Since the neuroprotective immune response operating under conditions of non-pathogenic damage is directed against self-antigens, it must be well controlled in order to avoid exceeding the risk threshold and thus inducing an autoimmune dis-ease. Our studies have shown that wherever this risk exists it can be outweighed by the benefit, provided that the immune response is well controlled. In a recent study aimed at achieving an autoimmune neuroprotective response without the accompa-nying risk, we found that the synthetic copolymer known as Copolymer 1 (Cop 1), consisting of the amino acids Glu, Ala, Lys and Tyr, and widely used as a bystander immunosuppressive drug, can evoke passive or active T-cell-mediated autoimmuni-ty that is neuroprotective. T cells specific to Cop-1 were found to accumulate in the uninjured CNS, a feature typical of autoimmune T cells. It therefore seems likely that the anti-Cop-1 T cells are cross-activated by CNS-associated antigens (e.g. MBP) in the damaged area, an event that seems to be necessary for displaying neu-roprotection [48]. Our experiments have shown that the use of this polypeptide for active immunization results in significant protection of the optic nerve from mechanical or biochemical insult [48, 49]. The marked neuroprotection obtained when the insult is directly caused by glutamate [49], a common mediator of toxici-ty in numerous nerve disorders, led us to consider immunization with Cop-1 as a potential approach to the treatment of degeneration caused by various risk factors. Our most recent data show that Cop-1 immunization attenuates the loss of retinal ganglion cells in the rat model of a neurodegenerative disease such as glaucoma [49], as well as the neuronal degeneration in a rat model of closed head injury [47].

Discussion

The adaptive immune response has generally been considered as an immune activi-ty that enables the organism to cope with stressful conditions caused by pathogens. Thus, immunologists have viewed the functions of the adaptive immune response as neutralizing pathogens, preventing pathogen invasion of the tissue, or counteracting the damage caused by pathogens that manage to invade. The damage caused by trauma, however, does not involve pathogens, and was therefore not viewed by immunologists as posing the type of danger to the tissue that necessitates an adaptive immune response.

Opinions differ as to the mechanisms by which self becomes invisible to the immune system (for example by clonal deletion, anergy, or tolerance) [50–55]. Some authors have proposed that autoimmunity, once established, might be harmless or even useful. In the "danger signal" theory, which basically argues against discrimination between self and non-self in characterizing the signals triggering a beneficial immune response, the response to self is viewed as a by-product of a response to a pathogen, a side-effect that soon decays in the absence of a second signal to maintain it [56]. On the basis of our results, we suggest that the anti-self immune activity evoked in response to trauma in the CNS is a purposeful physiological event. If trauma can indeed act as a stress signal that activates a helpful immune response, a number of questions arise: Does this occur in all tissues? If not, why not? Does the trauma-related stress signal vary from tissue to tissue? Since the role of the immune system is tissue protection, defense and maintenance, does the signal always operate for the organism's benefit? How is it related to autoimmune disease?

It is possible that what determines whether or not a purposeful autoimmune response will be activated depends on what poses the greater threat to the organism: the trauma-induced damage that leads to degeneration and tissue loss, or the risk of the negative side-effect of the autoimmune response. Our finding that autoimmunity has a neuroprotective function after CNS trauma [14, 19–22] is particularly interesting in view of the well-known catastrophic consequences of trauma to the CNS as compared with other tissues, and hence the importance of arresting the progression of CNS damage. Because terminally damaged neurons are irreplaceable, loss of cells is more devastating in the CNS than in any other tissue. Accordingly, trauma in the CNS potentially poses more of a threat to the individual than trauma in any other tissue, and the distress signal elicited by trauma in the CNS can therefore be expected to be more profound. For example, the traumatized CNS might transmit – in addition to the signal sent by the damage itself – a second, as yet unidentified distress signal, thereby activating and recruiting helper T cells with trauma-related activity. This might imply that in traumatically injured non-CNS tissues that do not evoke an autoimmune response, the second signal may be insufficient to activate T cells and/or to maintain them in an active form that enables them to become effectors. The specificity of the evoked T cells (in terms of the self-epitopes that activate them and are recognized by them) might, even in the CNS, vary according to the site of the injury. It is conceivable that trauma-related distress signals activate T cells of other relevant self-epitopes for protective purposes.

Another aspect of the nature of the protective autoimmune response concerns the mediators enabling its expression in the context of pathogen-free damage. It is possible that the active molecules produced by the effector helper T cells after trauma-associated damage are neurotrophins and cytokines, and that their secretion by the effector (autoimmune) T cells is antigen-dependent, similar to the documented secretion of cytokines by effector helper T cells after pathogen-induced damage. Alternatively, it is possible that the helper T cells enter into a dialog with resident microglia and/or invading macrophages, thereby making them beneficial rather than destructive to the damaged tissue.

Our results further suggest that non-pathogenic damage to CNS tissue triggers a signal to the immune system to assist in protecting the tissue against the spread of damage. The fact that the spontaneous T cell response does not exert enough protection to cause significant improvement after CNS injury might be attributable to the limited number of endogenous T cells. This view of beneficial autoimmunity in the context of CNS trauma may provide an explanation for the high incidence of autoimmunity in healthy individuals, a phenomenon viewed by some scientists as an indication that autoimmunity may not always be harmful, and may even be useful.

Adoptive transfer of activated autoimmune T cells specific to a CNS antigen is a potential cell therapy that offers some advantages. First, the approach is relatively non-invasive. Second, the activated T cells cross the blood-brain barrier and accumulate specifically at CNS lesions. Third, since T cell accumulation at a site of CNS injury was observed up to day 21 [14, 19] after injury, these T cells would presumably be capable of continuous release of beneficial compounds at the CNS injury site during that period. The timing and dynamics of the release of such compounds might be in accordance with the needs of the tissue. T cells in the injured CNS are eliminated by self-limiting mechanisms involving apoptosis, allowing the response to be extinguished.

This new view, once fully understood, is likely to open up a novel approach to the treatment of chronic and acute injuries by exploiting the adaptive arm of the immune system in the interest of recovery from trauma. This resource, up to now neglected and even shunned by immunologists, might represent a therapeutic gold mine. Its exploration can also be expected to unravel some long-standing enigmas, including the meaning of a danger signal in immunology, and the way in which the immune response is evoked.

The onset of T-cell response to active vaccination is very rapid (3–5 days). Since the therapeutic window is open for at least one week after spinal cord injury, and for an unlimited period in chronic neurodegenerative disorders, the method of passive T-cell transfer could be translated into an active therapeutic vaccination [27, 46, 49].

The use of safe synthetic peptides that resemble and cross-activate myelin-associated self peptides may constitute a strategy for developing anti-self vaccination for neuroprotection. Future studies should seek to identify the specific antigen(s) active in any particular disease, the optimal timing and type of immunization (passive or active), and the most appropriate adjuvant, in order to best exploit the long-neglected immune system for the development of a physiological approach to CNS therapy from degenerative disorders enabling maximal benefit with minimal risk [27, 48, 49].

References

1 Lotan M, Schwartz M (1994) Cross talk between the immune system and the nervous system in response to injury: Implications for regeneration. *FASEB J* 8: 1026–1033

2 Schwartz M, Yoles E, Levin LA (1999) "Axogenic" and "somagenic" neurodegenerative diseases: Definitions and therapeutic implications. *Mol Med Today* 5: 470–473

3 Schwartz M (2000) Autoimmune involvement in CNS trauma is beneficial if well controlled. *Prog Brain Res* 128: 259–263

4 Cserr HF, Knopf PM (1992) Cervical lymphatics, the blood-brain barrier and the immunoreactivity of the brain: A new view. *Immunol Today* 13: 507–512

5 Cserr HF, Harling-Berg CJ, Knopf PM (1992) Drainage of brain extracellular fluid into blood and deep cervical lymph and its immunological significance. *Brain Pathol* 2: 269–276

6 Griffin D, Levine B, Tyor W, Ubol S, Despres P (1997) The role of antibody in recovery from alphavirus encephalitis. *Immunol Rev* 159: 155–161

7 Hickey WF, Hsu BL, Kimura H (1991) T-lymphocyte entry into the central nervous system. *J Neurosci Res* 28: 254–260

8 Shrikant P, Benveniste EN (1996) The central nervous system as an immunocompetent organ: role of glial cells in antigen presentation. *J Immunol* 157: 1819–1822

9 Bell MD, Taub DD, Perry VH (1996) Overriding the brain's intrinsic resistance to leukocyte recruitment with intraparenchymal injections of recombinant chemokines. *Neuroscience* 74: 283–292

10 Goverman J, Brabb T, Paez A, Harrington C, von Dassow P (1997) Initiation and regulation of CNS autoimmunity. *Crit Rev Immunol* 17: 469–480

11 Matyszak MK, Perry VH (1995) Demyelination in the central nervous system following a delayed-type hypersensitivity response to bacillus Calmette-Guerin. *Neuroscience* 64: 967–977

12 Matyszak MK, Townsend MJ, Perry VH (1997) Ultrastructural studies of an immune-mediated inflammatory response in the CNS parenchyma directed against a non-CNS antigen. *Neuroscience* 78: 549–560

13 Perry VH, Brown MC, Gordon S (1987) The macrophage response to central and peripheral nerve injury. A possible role for macrophages in regeneration. *J Exp Med* 165: 1218–1223

14 Moalem G, Monsonego A, Shani Y, Cohen IR, Schwartz M (1999) Differential T cell response in central and peripheral nerve injury: connection with immune privilege. *FASEB J* 13: 1207–1217

15 Flugel A, Schwaiger FW, Neumann H, Medana I, Willem M, Wekerle H, Kreutzberg

GW, Graeber MB (2000) Neuronal FasL induces cell death of encephalitogenic T lymphocytes. *Brain Pathol* 10: 353–364

16 Hirschberg DL, Moalem G, He J, Mor F, Cohen IR, Schwartz M (1998) Accumulation of passively transferred primed T cells independently of their antigen specificity following central nervous system trauma. *J Neuroimmunol* 89: 88–96

17 Schwartz M, Cohen IR, Lazarov-Spiegler O, Moalem G, Yoles E (1999) The remedy may lie in ourselves: Prospects for immune cell therapy in central nervous system protection and repair. *J Mol Med* 77: 713–717

18 Yoles E, Schwartz M (1998) Degeneration of spared axons following partial white matter lesion: Implications for optic nerve neuropathies. *Exp Neurol* 153: 1–7

19 Moalem G, Leibowitz-Amit R, Yoles E, Mor F, Cohen IR, Schwartz M (1999) Autoimmune T cells protect neurons from secondary degeneration after central nervous system axotomy. *Nat Med* 5: 49–55

20 Moalem G, Yoles E, Leibowitz-Amit R, Muller-Gilor S, Mor F, Cohen IR, Schwartz M (2000) Autoimmune T cells retard the loss of function in injured rat optic nerves. *J Neuroimmunol* 106: 189–197

21 Moalem G, Gdalyahu A, Shani Y, Otten U, Lazarovici P, Cohen IR, Schwartz M (2000) Production of neurotrophins by activated T cells: implications for neuroprotective autoimmunity. *J Autoimmun* 15: 331–345

22 Hauben E, Nevo U, Yoles E, Moalem G, Agranov E, Mor F, Akselrod S, Neeman M, Cohen IR, Schwartz M (2000) Autoimmune T cells as potential neuroprotective therapy for spinal cord injury. *Lancet* 355: 286–287

23 Hauben E, Butovsky O, Nevo U, Yoles E, Moalem G, Agranov E, Mor F, Leibowitz-Amit R, Pevsner S, Akselrod S et al (2000) Passive or active immunization with myelin basic protein promotes recovery from spinal cord contusion. *J Neurosci* 20: 6421–6430

24 Nevo U, Hauben U, Yoles E, Agranov E, Akselrod S, Schwartz M, Neeman M (2001) Diffusion anisotropy MRI for quantitative assessment of recovery in injured rat spinal cord. *Magn Reson Med* 45: 1–9

25 Butovsky O, Hauben E, Schwartz M (2001) Morphological aspects of spinal cord autoimmune neuroprotection: Colocalization of T cells with B7.2(CD86) and prevention of cyst formation. *FASEB J* 15: 1065–1067

26 Fisher J, Levkovitch-Verbin H, Schori H, Yoles E, Butovsky O, Kay JF, Ben-Nun A, Schwartz M (2001) Vaccination for neuroprotection in the mouse optic nerve: Implications for optic neuropathies. *J Neurosci* 21: 136–142

27 Hauben E, Agranov E, Gothilf A, Nevo U, Cohen A, Smirnov I, Steinman L, Schwartz M (2001) Vaccination after spinal cord injury prevents complete paralysis: Autoimmunity without risk of autoimmune disease. *J Clin Invest; in press*

28 Besser M, Wank R (1999) Cutting edge: Clonally restricted production of the neurotrophins brain-derived neurotrophic factor and neurotrophin-3 mRNA by human immune cells and Th1/Th2-polarized expression of their receptors. *J Immunol* 162: 6303–6306

29 Ehrhard PB, Erb P, Graumann U, Otten U (1993) Expression of nerve growth factor and

nerve growth factor receptor tyrosine kinase Trk in activated CD4-positive T-cell clones. *Proc Natl Acad Sci USA* 90: 10984–10988

30 Heese K, Hock C, Otten U (1998) Inflammatory signals induce neurotrophin expression in human microglial cells. *J Neurochem* 70: 699–707

31 Kerschensteiner M, Gallmeier E, Behrens L, Leal VV, Misgeld T, Klinkert WE, Kolbeck R, Hoppe E, Oropeza-Wekerle RL, Bartke I et al (1999) Activated human T cells, B cells, and monocytes produce brain-derived neurotrophic factor *in vitro* and in inflammatory brain lesions: a neuroprotective role of inflammation? *J Exp Med* 189: 865–870

32 Artis D, Humphreys NE, Bancroft AJ, Rothwell NJ, Potten CS, Grencis RK (1999) Tumor necrosis factor alpha is a critical component of interleukin 13-mediated protective T helper cell type 2 responses during helminth infection. *J Exp Med* 190:953–962

33 Bethea JR, Castro M, Keane RW, Lee TT, Dietrich WD, Yezierski RP (1998) Traumatic spinal cord injury induces nuclear factor-kappaB activation. *J Neurosci* 18: 3251–3260

34 Loddick SA, Rothwell NJ (1999) Mechanisms of tumor necrosis factor alpha action on neurodegeneration: interaction with insulin-like growth factor-1. *Proc Natl Acad Sci USA* 96: 9449–9451

35 Blesch A, Grill RJ, Tuszynski MH (1998) Neurotrophin gene therapy in CNS models of trauma and degeneration. *Prog Brain Res* 117: 473–484

36 Bregman BS, McAtee M, Dai HN, Kuhn PL (1997) Neurotrophic factors increase axonal growth after spinal cord injury and transplantation in the adult rat. *Exp Neurol* 148: 475–494

37 Davies SJ, Fitch MT, Memberg SP, Hall AK, Raisman G, Silver J (1997) Regeneration of adult axons in white matter tracts of the central nervous system. *Nature* 390: 680–683

38 Yoles E, Hauben E, Palgi O, Agranov E, Gothilf A, Cohen A, Kuchroo VK, Cohen IR, Weiner H, Schwartz M (2001) Protective autoimmunity is a physiological response to CNS trauma. *J Neurosci* 21: 3740–3748

39 Yoles E, Friedmann I, Barouch R, Shani Y, Schwartz M (2001) Self-protective mechanism awakened by glutamate in retinal ganglion cells. *J Neurotrauma* 18: 339–349

40 Gennarelli TA (1993) Mechanisms of brain injury. *J Emerg Med* 1 (Suppl 1): 5–11

41 Mukhin AG, Ivanova SA, Knoblach SM, Faden AI (1997) New *in vitro* model of traumatic neuronal injury: evaluation of secondary injury and glutamate receptor-mediated neurotoxicity. *J Neurotrauma* 14: 651–663

42 Ikonomidou C, Qin Qin Y, Labruyere J, Olney JW (1996) Motor neuron degeneration induced by excitotoxin agonists has features in common with those seen in the SOD-1 transgenic mouse model of amyotrophic lateral sclerosis. *J Neuropathol Exp Neurol* 55: 211–224

43 Yudkoff M, Daikhin Y, Grunstein L, Nissim I, Stern J, Pleasure D, Nissim I (1996) Astrocyte leucine metabolism: significance of branched-chain amino acid transamination. *J Neurochem* 66: 378–385

44 Yudkoff M, Daikhin Y, Nissim I, Grunstein R, Nissim I (1997) Effects of ketone bodies on astrocyte amino acid metabolism. *J Neurochem* 69: 682–692

45 Gritti A, Rosati B, Lecchi M, Vescovi AL, Wanke E (2000) Excitable properties in astrocytes derived from human embryonic CNS stem cells. *Eur J Neurosci* 12: 3549–3459

46 Schwartz M, Kipnis J (2001) Protective autoimmunity: regulation and prospects for vaccination after brain and spinal cord injuries. *Trends Mol Med* 7: 252–258

47 Kipnis J, Yoles E, Schori H, Hauben E, Shaked I, Schwartz M (2001) Neuronal survival after CNS insult is determined by a genetically encoded autoimmune response. *J Neurosci* 21: 4564–4571

48 Kipnis J, Yoles E, Porat Z, Cohen A, Mor F, Sela M, Cohen IR, Schwartz M (2000) T cell immunity to Copolymer-1 confers neuroprotection on the damaged optic nerve: Possible therapy for optic neuropathies. *Proc Natl Acad Sci USA* 97: 7446–7451

49 Schori H, Kipnis J, Yoles E, Wolde Mussie E, Ruiz G, Wheeler LA, Schwartz M (2001) Vaccination for protection of retinal ganglion cells against death from glutamate cytotoxicity and ocular hypertension: Implications for glaucoma. *Proc Nat Acad Sci USA* 98: 3398–3403

50 Burnet FM (1971) "Self-recognition" in colonial marine forms and flowering plants in relation to the evolution of immunity. *Nature* 232: 230–235

51 Bretcher P, Cohn M (1970) A theory of self-nonself discrimination. *Science* 169: 1042–1049

52 Cohen IR (1988) The self, the world and autoimmunity. *Sci Am* 258: 52–60

53 Jameson SC, Hogquist KA, Bevan MJ (1995) Positive selection of thymocytes. *Annu Rev Immunol* 13: 93–126

54 Janeway CA Jr (1992) The immune system evolved to discriminate infectious nonself from noninfectious self. *Immunol Today* 13: 11–16

55 Jerne NK (1984) Idiotypic networks and other preconceived ideas. *Immunol Rev* 79: 5–24

56 Matzinger P (1994) Tolerance, danger, and the extended family. *Annu Rev Immunol* 12: 991–1045

Traumatic brain injury: is head trauma an inflammatory disease?

Philipp M. Lenzlinger[1,2], Thomas Kossmann[2], Tracy K. McIntosh[1] and Maria Cristina Morganti-Kossmann[2]

[1]Department of Neurosurgery, University of Pennsylvania, and Veterans Administration Medical Center, 105 Hayden Hall, 3320 Smith Walk, Philadelphia, PA 19104-6316, USA; [2]Research Division and Trauma Division, Department of Surgery, University Hospital, Rämistrasse 100, CH-8091 Zürich, Switzerland

Introduction

Traumatic brain injury (TBI) remains one of the leading causes of injury related deaths in the industrialized countries, accounting for 26% of all trauma-associated deaths in the USA (between 17 and 25 per 100,000 residents) [1, 2]. Of the 2 million people who sustain TBI in the USA each year, approximately 70,000 to 90,000 will suffer from long-term disability with dramatic impacts on the life of the individuals and their families and enormous socio-economic costs [3]. Traumatic brain damage is a result of direct (immediate mechanical disruption of brain tissue, or primary injury) and indirect (secondary or delayed) mechanisms. These secondary mechanisms involve such diverse pathways as inflammation, calcium associated cytotoxicity, and ischemic events, all of which may lead to acute as well as chronic cell destruction [4].

Inflammatory events following TBI

There is increasing evidence that one aspect of the secondary events following TBI bear the hallmarks of a profound inflammatory response. The central nervous system (CNS) has historically been defined as an "immunologically privileged organ" due to its separation from the systemic circulation by a blood-brain barrier (BBB). By effectively preventing the entry of peripheral blood cells and larger molecules under normal conditions, the BBB maintains the particular environment necessary for normal brain function. The ability of the CNS to counteract pathogenic agents is consequently poor, since immune cells and humoral factors do not have free access to the brain. In addition, minimal expression of histocompatibility antigens, adhesion molecules and immune mediators under normal conditions renders the CNS refractory to immune responses as compared to peripheral organs.

Inflammation and Stroke, edited by Giora Z. Feuerstein

Increasing evidence over the past years, however, suggests the active involvement of resident cells of the nervous system in the intracranial immune defense *via* the release of inflammatory mediators that are able to regulate both immunological and neuronal functions. A cascade of events resulting in activation of leukocytes and glial cells, release of cytokines, chemokines, complement proteins, and upregulation of adhesion molecules, which lead to cellular migration, proliferation and phagocytosis characterizes the inflammatory response evoked in neuropathology. However, in addition to the deleterious effects of these inflammatory processes on injured brain tissue, it appears that the same cascades may also initiate repair and regeneration *via* the induction of neurotrophic factors and the creation of an environment necessary for neuronal recovery. In the following we will address the different aspects of the post-traumatic inflammatory response associated with experimental and clinical TBI.

Breakdown of the BBB and cellular infiltration

TBI leads to a profound but variable swelling of brain tissue, clinically apparent as elevation of intracranial pressure (ICP). This increased ICP and associated reduced cerebral perfusion pressure (CPP) is among the leading causes of unfavorable outcome following TBI [5]. This swelling of the brain is thought to be caused by cellular edema formation due to complex cytotoxic events as well as vascular edema following the breakdown of the BBB [6, 7] which has been observed in a variety of experimental TBI models [7–12], as well as in humans [13–15]. The initial breakdown of the BBB due to trauma has been described to occur within minutes after injury and to last for hours, while secondary hypoxia may lead to a prolonged BBB impairment, which may persist for several days [7–10, 16].

Activation of white blood cells (WBC) may influence cerebral microcirculation and therefore cerebral blood flow (CBF) [17]. The role of WBCs in mediating BBB breakdown, however, is controversial. While some studies suggest that neutrophil infiltration may be involved in damage to the BBB [18, 19], WBCs do not appear to be mediating the early BBB breakdown following TBI [17, 20, 21]. Infiltration and accumulation of polymorphonuclear leukocytes (PMNs) into brain parenchyma have been documented to occur in the acute posttraumatic period, reaching maximal accumulation by 24 h post injury [22]. Zhuang et al. [23] have suggested a relationship between cortical PMN accumulation and secondary brain injury, including lowered CBF, increased edema, and elevated ICP. The migration of leukocytes into damaged tissue typically requires the adhesion of these cells to the endothelium and therefore the expression of the intercellular adhesion molecule (ICAM-1), a member of the immunoglobulin supergene family, that has been reported to be upregulated in several experimental TBI models [24–26]. In a model of stroke, mice deficient of the ICAM-1 gene showed a significant reduction in infarct volume and neurologic deficit as well as increased survival [27]. However, Wahlen and coworkers [28] were unable to observe a difference in accumulation of neutrophils at the injured site, in lesion volume as well as in neurologic motor function and cognitive outcome between ICAM-1 knockout mice and wild-type controls following controlled cortical impact (CCI) brain injury. In humans, soluble ICAM-1 (sICAM-1) in cerebrospinal fluid (CSF) has been associated with the breakdown of the BBB after severe isolated TBI [15].

Immunocytochemical studies have demonstrated the presence of activated macrophages, natural killer (NK) cells, helper T cells, and T-cytotoxic suppressor cells by 2 days post injury, which persists up to 16 days following weight-drop brain injury in rats [29, 30]. The entry of macrophages into brain parenchyma following injury has been shown to be maximal by 24–48 h following lateral FP brain injury in rats and after human TBI [22, 29, 30]. In a recent study in patients with severe TBI, it was reported that the cell population being activated following trauma appeared to be predominantly of the macrophage/microglia lineage, as opposed to the T-cell lineage [31]. Both macrophages and microglia have been proposed as key cellular elements in the progressive tissue necrosis following spinal cord as well as brain trauma, presumably associated with the release of cytotoxic molecules (among them oxygen free radicals and inflammatory cytokines) that may be involved in mediating the local inflammatory response and phagocytosis of debris from dying cells [32–38]. Activated macrophages which cross the BBB may provide a stimulus for changes in extracellular matrix molecules after CNS injury [39]. Some component of the macrophage response may also participate in reparative cascades, including wound healing and regeneration [40, 41], indicating a possible beneficial effect of intrathecal cellular immune activation.

Cytokines

The specific cytokines that have been implicated in posttraumatic neuropathologic damage include tumor necrosis factor (TNF) and the interleukin (IL) family of peptides [42–45]. Increases in systemic and CSF concentrations of cytokines such as IL-1, IL-6, IL-8, IL-10, IL-12 and TNFα have been reported to occur in humans following severe head injury [13, 42, 43, 46–52], and regional brain tissue mRNA and protein concentrations of these factors have been shown to markedly increase in the acute posttraumatic period following experimental brain trauma in the rat [40, 53–58]. Upregulation of gene (mRNA) expression for both IL-1β and TNF has been reported as early as 1–2 h following lateral FP brain injury in the rat [53, 54], suggesting that these cytokines are actually synthesized in the injured brain and may play a role in the pathophysiological sequelae of brain trauma. The increase in IL-1α, IL-1β, and TNFα following stab wound injury to the rat brain has been related to trauma-induced astrogliosis [59]. IL-6 mRNA has been shown to be up-regulated in a weight drop model of TBI in rats in infiltrating macrophages as well as in cortical and thalamic neurons as early as 1 h post-injury, while IL-6 immunoreactivity and protein levels in rat CSF peaked within the first 24 h after the trauma [40]. IL-6 released in the CNS has also been shown to be associated with the systemic acute phase response following severe TBI in humans [46], implying a role for centrally released immune mediators in the systemic reaction to trauma.

The role of posttraumatic immune activation in the CNS remains controversial. While most studies suggest a pathologic function for the cytokines IL-1 and TNFα in the setting of CNS injury, others infer a more beneficial role for IL-1β and IL-6 in neuronal survival [45, 60, 61]. Recent studies documenting the beneficial effects of pharmacological blockade of the complement cascade [62] and the cytokines IL-1β [63, 64] and TNF [65], suggest that the release and/or upregulation of these pathways may be pathogenic in the setting of brain trauma. However, Loddick et al. [66] recently reported that cerebral ischemia produces a marked increase in IL-6 bioactivity in the ischemic hemisphere and intracerebroventricular (ICV) administration of recombinant IL-6 significantly reduced brain damage after permanent focal cerebral ischemia in rats. Work with transgenic brain-injured mice deficient in TNF (TNF$^{-/-}$) also showed that while the neurologic motor scores of these animals were initially better than brain-injured wild-type (WT) controls in the acute posttraumatic period, the trend was reversed from 7–28 days post injury [67]. Moreover, mice deficient in both subtypes of TNF receptors were shown to be more vulnerable to TBI than wild-type animals, further indicating a neuroprotective role for TNFα in the pathological sequelae of head injury [68]. Taken together these results suggest that although the increase of cytokines in the acute post-traumatic period may be deleterious, they may also play a role in facilitating long-term behavioral recovery, thereby underscoring the potential for post-injury cellular and molecular changes to be either pathologic or protective, depending on when they occur during the post-injury cascade.

Complement system

There is increasing evidence that the complement system plays an important role in tissue damage associated with brain trauma [69], and activation of the complement cascade after brain injury may contribute significantly to cerebral inflammation [70]. Clinical studies have demonstrated complement activation in serum [71] and increased levels of proteins belonging to the alternative pathway of complement activation in CSF of head trauma patients [72]. Evidence for intracerebral complement activation was found in an immunohistochemical study detecting activated complement fragments following CCI [73]. A study by Stahel et al. [74] on experimental diffuse axonal injury has demonstrated enhanced posttraumatic expression of the C5a receptor (C5aR) mRNA in cortical neurons, cerebellar Purkinje cells, and intrathecally infiltrating leukocytes. Interestingly, neuronal C5aR expression was attenuated in TNF/LT-$\alpha^{-/-}$ mice by 7 days after closed head injury, suggesting a regulation of intracerebral C5aR expression through a TNF receptor-dependent pathway [75]. Apart from mediating a cellular inflammatory response to CNS trauma, the complement system may also be involved in neuronal programmed cell death as suggested by the ability of the anaphylatoxin C5a to induce apoptosis in a human neuroblastoma cell line *in vitro* [76].

Antiinflammatory therapy in TBI

Only recently has research concerning the possible beneficial effects of cytokine blockade or antiinflammatory compounds been initiated. The soluble human recombinant complement (sCR-1) receptor BRL-55730 has been used with success to inhibit PMN accumulation and improve neurobehavioral recovery following CCI injury in the rat [62]. Post-traumatic ICV administration of IL-1 receptor antagonist (IL-1ra), which competitively binds to the IL 1 receptor and inhibits its physiological function, has been shown to reduce the extent of neuronal death in cortex and hippocampus and to improve cognitive function following lateral FP brain injury in the rat [63, 64]. DeKosky et al. [77] have shown that implantation of fibroblasts transfected with a retroviral vector containing the human IL-1ra gene can significantly reduce microglial proliferation and inhibit IL-1 mediated NGF upregulation following weight-drop injury. Inhibition of TNFα activity in rat brain has been shown to significantly reduce edema and to improve motor function following weight-drop brain injury [65, 78], while antibodies against MAC-1, the leukocyte counterreceptor of ICAM-1, have shown promising effects in reducing the accumulation of PMNs after cortical impact injury in rats [79]. It can be speculated that the recent finding of upregulation of the inflammatory mediator cyclooxygenase-2 (COX2) on neurons [80] may lead to the evaluation of the potent anti-rheumatic drugs of the COX-inhibitor class in attenuating posttraumatic sequelae in the CNS. However, any anti-inflammatory intervention following TBI will have to take into account that posttraumatic inflammation may also pave the road for a regenerative response. Therefore, timing will be crucial for successful anti-inflammatory therapy, and maybe modulation of the response as opposed to a complete blocking of inflammatory mediators will yield better results.

Conclusion

A large body of clinical and experimental evidence exists that associates a major inflammatory response to head trauma. Although immunologically privileged, the brain exhibits many features of inflammation found in other tissues following trauma. This initial posttraumatic inflammation is sustained by infiltrating inflammatory cells and the release of a myriad of soluble inflammatory mediators. Thus, even though many other pathways are involved in the pathophysiological sequelae of TBI, it shares the above characteristics with "classical" inflammatory pathologies of the CNS, such as bacterial meningitis. Traumatic brain injury therefore appears to be, in part, an inflammatory disease.

The role of this inflammatory process in the setting of CNS injury is unclear and the question of whether inflammation is good or bad for the injured brain remains unanswered. The acute response to trauma with its early edema formation is likely to be associated with inflammatory events and, together with the cytotoxic effects of immune mediators, is believed to be deleterious for the injured brain by causing further secondary damage and neurological dysfunction. However, this inflammatory response may also contribute or even may be a prerequisite to the initiation of regeneration and repair in the injured CNS. Several cytokines have been shown to possess either direct neuroprotective effects or to induce growth factor production, which in turn can enhance cell survival and may cause endogenous cells to replicate and differentiate. Other mediators such as TNF appear to have differential effects early on and later in the time-course of TBI pathology. Understanding these differences with regard to timing and extent of release as well as differential effects on different targets may prove to be the key to developing new modalities in antiinflammatory therapies following TBI. Only once we better understand the duality of posttraumatic inflammation in the CNS can we hope to find an effective intervention to modulate this response for the good of the patient suffering from this complex disease.

Acknowledgments
This work was supported, in part, by grants from the Swiss National Science Foundation (SNF) Nos. 31-36375.92, 31-42490.94 and 31-52482.97 and the Hartmann-Müller and Olga-Meyenfisch Foundations Zurich, Switzerland (MC. Morganti-Kossmann and T. Kossmann) as well as by NIH grants NINDS P50-NS08803, NIGMS RO1-GM34690 and a Merit Review Grant from the United States Veterans Administration (T.K. McIntosh). P.M. Lenzlinger was supported in part by a research fellowship from the SNF and NIH NRSA T32 NS07413-04.

References

1   Sosin DM, Sacks JJ, Smith SM (1989) Head injury-associated deaths in the United States from 1979 to 1986. *JAMA* 262: 2251–2255

2   Sosin DM, Sniezek JE, Waxweiler RJ (1995) Trends in death associated with traumatic brain injury, 1979 through 1992: success and failure. *JAMA* 273: 1778–1780

3   NIH Consensus Development Panel on Rehabilitation of Persons With Traumatic Brain Injury (1999) Consensus conference. Rehabilitation of persons with traumatic brain injury. *JAMA* 282: 974–983

4   McIntosh TK, Saatman KE, Raghupathi R, Graham DI, Smith DH, Lee VM, Trojanowski JQ (1998) The Dorothy Russell Memorial Lecture. The molecular and cellular sequelae of experimental traumatic brain injury: pathogenetic mechanisms. *Neuropath Appl Neurobiol* 24: 251–267

5   Marmarou A, Anderson RL, Ward JD, Choi SC, Young HF, Eisenberg HM, Foulkes MA, Marshall LF, Jane JA (1991) Impact of ICP instability and hypotension on outcome in patients with severe head trauma. *J Neurosurg* 75: S59–S66

6   Unterberg AW, Stroop R, Thomale UW, Kiening KL, Pauser S, Vollmann W (1997) Characterisation of brain edema following "controlled cortical impact injury" in rats. *Acta Neurochir* (Supp) 70: 106–108

7   Baskaya MK, Rao AM, Dogan A, Donaldson D, Dempsey RJ (1997) The biphasic opening of the blood-brain barrier in the cortex and hippocampus after traumatic brain injury in rats. *Neurosci Lett* 226: 33–36

8   Hicks RR, Baldwin SA, Scheff SW (1997) Serum extravasation and cytoskeletal alterations following traumatic brain injury in rats. Comparison of lateral fluid percussion and cortical impact models. *Mol Chem Neuropathol* 32: 1–16

9   Barzo P, Marmarou A, Fatouros P, Corwin F, Dunbar J (1996) Magnetic resonance imaging-monitored acute blood-brain barrier changes in experimental traumatic brain injury. *J Neurosurg* 85: 1113–1121

10   Fukuda K, Tanno H, Okimura Y, Nakamura M, Yamaura A (1995) The blood-brain barrier disruption to circulating proteins in the early period after fluid percussion brain injury in rats. *J Neurotrauma* 12: 315–324

11   Soares HD, Thomas M, Cloherty K, McIntosh TK (1992) Development of prolonged focal cerebral edema and regional cation changes following experimental brain injury in the rat. *J Neurochem* 58: 1845–1852

12   Cortez SC, McIntosh TK, Noble LJ (1989) Experimental fluid percussion brain injury: vascular disruption and neuronal and glial alterations. *Brain Res* 482: 271–282

13   Csuka E, Morganti-Kossmann MC, Lenzlinger PM, Joller H, Trentz O, Kossmann T (1999) IL-10 levels in cerebrospinal fluid and serum of patients with severe traumatic brain injury: relationship to IL-6, TNF-alpha, TGF-beta1 and blood-brain barrier function. *J Neuroimmunol* 101: 211–221

14   Morganti-Kossmann MC, Hans VH, Lenzlinger PM, Dubs R, Ludwig E, Trentz O, Kossmann T (1999) TGF-beta is elevated in the CSF of patients with severe traumatic brain injuries and parallels blood-brain barrier function. *J Neurotrauma* 16: 617–628

15   Pleines UE, Stover JF, Kossmann T, Trentz O, Morganti-Kossmann MC (1998) Soluble ICAM-1 in CSF coincides with the extent of cerebral damage in patients with severe traumatic brain injury. *J Neurotrauma* 15: 399–409

16   Tanno H, Nockels RP, Pitts LH, Noble LJ (1992) Breakdown of the blood-brain barri-

er after fluid percussion brain injury in the rat: Part 2: Effect of hypoxia on permeability to plasma proteins. *J Neurotrauma* 9: 335–347

17   Hartl R, Medary MB, Ruge M, Arfors KE, Ghajar J (1997) Early white blood cell dynamics after traumatic brain injury: effects on the cerebral microcirculation. *J Cereb Blood Flow Metab* 17: 1210–1220

18   Bell MD, Taub DD, Perry VH (1996) Overriding the brain's intrinsic resistance to leukocyte recruitment with intraparenchymal injections of recombinant chemokines. *Neuroscience* 74: 283–292

19   Perry VH, Anthony DC, Bolton SJ, Brown HC (1997) The blood-brain barrier and the inflammatory response. *Mol Med Today* 3: 335–341

20   Whalen MJ, Carlos TM, Kochanek PM, Clark RS, Heineman S, Schiding JK, Franicola D, Memarzadeh F, Lo W, Marion DW, DeKosky ST (1999) Neutrophils do not mediate blood-brain barrier permeability early after controlled cortical impact in rats. *J Neurotrauma* 16: 583–594

21   Hartl R, Medary M, Ruge M, Arfors KE, Ghajar J (1997) Blood-brain barrier breakdown occurs early after traumatic brain injury and is not related to white blood cell adherence. *Acta Neurochir* (Supp) 70: 240–242

22   Soares HD, Hicks RR, Smith D, McIntosh TK (1995) Inflammatory leukocytic recruitment and diffuse neuronal degeneration are separate pathological processes resulting from traumatic brain injury. *J Neurosci* 15: 8223–8233

23   Zhuang J, Shackford SR, Schmoker JD, Anderson ML (1993) The association of leukocytes with secondary brain injury. *J Trauma* 35: 415–422

24   Carlos TM, Clark RS, Franicola-Higgins D, Schiding JK, Kochanek PM (1997) Expression of endothelial adhesion molecules and recruitment of neutrophils after traumatic brain injury in rats. *J Leukocyte Biol* 61: 279–285

25   Isaksson J, Lewen A, Hillered L, Olsson Y (1997) Up-regulation of intercellular adhesion molecule 1 in cerebral microvessels after cortical contusion trauma in a rat model. *Acta Neuropathol* 94: 16–20

26   Shibayama M, Kuchiwaki H, Inao S, Yoshida K, Ito M (1996) Intercellular adhesion molecule-1 expression on glia following brain injury: participation of interleukin-1 beta [published erratum appears in *J Neurotrauma* 1997 Feb; 14(2): 119]. *J Neurotrauma* 13: 801–808

27   Connolly ES Jr, Winfree CJ, Springer TA, Naka Y, Liao H, Yan SD, Stern DM, Solomon RA, Gutierrez-Ramos JC, Pinsky DJ (1996) Cerebral protection in homozygous null ICAM-1 mice after middle cerebral artery occlusion. Role of neutrophil adhesion in the pathogenesis of stroke. *J Clin Invest* 97: 209–216

28   Whalen MJ, Carlos TM, Dixon CE, Schiding JK, Clark RS, Baum E, Yan HQ, Marion DW, Kochanek PM (1999) Effect of traumatic brain injury in mice deficient in intercellular adhesion molecule-1: assessment of histopathologic and functional outcome. *J Neurotrauma* 16: 299–309

29   Holmin S, Soderlund J, Biberfeld P, Mathiesen T (1998) Intracerebral inflammation after human brain contusion. *Neurosurgery* 42: 291–298

30 Holmin S, Mathiesen T, Shetye J, Biberfeld P (1995) Intracerebral inflammatory response to experimental brain contusion. *Acta Neurochir* 132: 110–119

31 Lenzlinger PM, Morganti-Kossmann MC, Hans VH, Joller H, Trentz O, Kossmann T (2001) Markers for cell-mediated immune response are elevated in cerebrospinal fluid and serum after severe traumatic brain injury in humans. *J Neurotrauma* 18: 479–489

32 Aihara N, Hall JJ, Pitts LH, Fukuda K, Noble LJ (1995) Altered immunoexpression of microglia and macrophages after mild head injury. *J Neurotrauma* 12: 53–63

33 Korematsu K, Goto S, Nagahiro S, Ushio Y (1994) Microglial response to transient focal cerebral ischemia: an immunocytochemical study on the rat cerebral cortex using anti-phosphotyrosine antibody. *J Cereb Blood Flow Metab* 14: 825–830

34 Kreutzberg GW (1996) Microglia: a sensor for pathological events in the CNS. *TINS* 19: 312–318

35 Popovich PG, Wei P, Stokes BT (1997) Cellular inflammatory response after spinal cord injury in Sprague-Dawley and Lewis rats. *J Comp Neurol* 377: 443–464

36 Spranger M, Fontana A (1996) Activation of microglia: a dangerous interlude in immune function in the brain. *Neuroscientist* 2: 293–299

37 Thomas WE (1992) Brain macrophages: evaluation of microglia and their functions. *Brain Res Rev* 17: 61–74

38 Yamashita K, Niwa M, Kataoka Y, Shigematsu K, Himeno A, Tsutsumi K, Nakano-Nakashima M, Sakurai-Yamashita Y, Shibata S, Taniyama K (1994) Microglia with an endothelin ETB receptor aggregate in rat hippocampus CA1 subfields following transient forebrain ischemia. *J Neurochem* 63: 1042–1051

39 Fitch MT, Silver J (1997) Activated macrophages and the blood-brain barrier: inflammation after CNS injury leads to increases in putative inhibitory molecules. *Exp Neurol* 148: 587–603

40 Hans VH, Kossmann T, Lenzlinger PM, Probstmeier R, Imhof HG, Trentz O, Morganti-Kossmann MC (1999) Experimental axonal injury triggers interleukin-6 mRNA, protein synthesis and release into cerebrospinal fluid. *J Cereb Blood Flow Metab* 19: 184–194

41 Zhang Z, Fujiki M, Guth L, Steward O (1996) Genetic influences on cellular reactions to spinal cord injury: a wound-healing response present in normal mice is impaired in mice carrying a mutation (WldS) that causes delayed Wallerian degeneration. *J Comp Neurol* 371: 485–495

42 Morganti-Kossmann MC, Lenzlinger PM, Hans V, Stahel P, Csuka E, Ammann E, Stocker R, Trentz O, Kossmann T (1997) Production of cytokines following brain injury: beneficial and deleterious for the damaged tissue. *Mol Psychiatr* 2: 133–136

43 Ott L, McClain CJ, Gillespie M, Young B (1994) Cytokines and metabolic dysfunction after severe head injury. *J Neurotrauma* 11: 447–472

44 Hans VH, Kossmann T, Joller H, Otto V, Morganti-Kossmann MC (1999) Interleukin-6 and its soluble receptor in serum and cerebrospinal fluid after cerebral trauma. *Neuroreport* 10: 409–412

45   Rothwell NJ, Hopkins SJ (1995) Cytokines and the nervous system II: Actions and mechanisms of action. *TINS* 18: 130–136

46   Kossmann T, Hans VH, Imhof HG, Stocker R, Grob P, Trentz O, Morganti-Kossmann C (1995) Intrathecal and serum interleukin-6 and the acute-phase response in patients with severe traumatic brain injuries. *Shock* 4: 311–317

47   Kossmann T, Stahel PF, Lenzlinger PM, Redl H, Dubs RW, Trentz O, Schlag G, Morganti-Kossmann MC (1997) Interleukin-8 released into the cerebrospinal fluid after brain injury is associated with blood-brain barrier dysfunction and nerve growth factor production. *J Cereb Blood Flow Metab* 17: 280–289

48   Goodman JC, Robertson CS, Grossman RG, Narayan RK (1990) Elevation of tumor necrosis factor in head injury. *J Neuroimmunol* 30: 213–217

49   Young AB, Ott LG, Beard D, Dempsey RJ, Tibbs PA, McClain CJ (1988) The acute-phase response of the brain-injured patient. *J Neurosurg* 69: 375–380

50   Cohen D, Phillips R, Ott L, Young B (1991) Increased plasma and ventricular fluid interleukin-6 levels in patients with head injury. *J Lab Clin Med* 118: 225–231

51   McClain CJ, Cohen D, Ott L, Dinarello CA, Young B (1987) Ventricular fluid interleukin-1 activity in patients with head injury. *J Lab Clin Med* 110: 48–54

52   Whalen MJ, Carlos TM, Kochanek PM, Wisniewski SR, Bell MJ, Clark RS, DeKosky ST, Marion DW, Adelson PD (2000) Interleukin-8 is increased in cerebrospinal fluid of children with severe head injury. *Crit Care Med* 28: 929–934

53   Fan L, Young PR, Barone FC, Feuerstein GZ, Smith DH, McIntosh TK (1995) Experimental brain injury induces expression of interleukin-1 beta mRNA in the rat brain. *Mol Brain Res* 30: 125–130

54   Fan L, Young PR, Barone FC, Feuerstein GZ, Smith DH, McIntosh TK (1996) Experimental brain injury induces differential expression of tumor necrosis factor-alpha mRNA in the CNS. *Mol Brain Res* 36: 287–291

55   Knoblach SM, Fan L, Faden AI (1999) Early neuronal expression of tumor necrosis factor-alpha after experimental brain injury contributes to neurological impairment. *J Neuroimmunol* 95: 115–125

56   Shohami E, Novikov M, Bass R, Yamin A, Gallily R (1994) Closed head injury triggers early production of TNF alpha and IL-6 by brain tissue. *J Cereb Blood Flow Metab* 14: 615–619

57   Woodroofe MN, Sarna GS, Wadhwa M, Hayes GM, Loughlin AJ, Tinker A, Cuzner ML (1991) Detection of interleukin-1 and interleukin-6 in adult rat brain, following mechanical injury, by *in vivo* microdialysis: evidence of a role for microglia in cytokine production. *J Neuroimmunol* 33: 227–236

58   Taupin V, Toulmond S, Serrano A, Benavides J, Zavala F (1993) Increase in IL-6, IL-1 and TNF levels in rat brain following traumatic lesion. Influence of pre- and post-traumatic treatment with Ro5 4864, a peripheral-type (p site) benzodiazepine ligand. *J Neuroimmunol* 42: 177–185

59   Rostworowski M, Balasingam V, Chabot S, Owens T, Yong VW (1997) Astrogliosis in the neonatal and adult murine brain post-trauma: elevation of inflammatory cytokines

and the lack of requirement for endogenous interferon-gamma. *J Neurosci* 17: 3664–3674

60   Brenneman DE, Schultzberg M, Bartfai T, Gozes I (1992) Cytokine regulation of neuronal survival. *J Neurochem* 58: 454–460

61   Hori O, Matsumoto M, Kuwabara K, Maeda Y, Ueda H, Ohtsuki T, Kinoshita T, Ogawa S, Stern DM, Kamada T (1996) Exposure of astrocytes to hypoxia/reoxygenation enhances expression of glucose-regulated protein 78 facilitating astrocyte release of the neuroprotective cytokine interleukin 6. *J Neurochem* 66: 973–979

62   Kaczorowski SL, Schiding JK, Toth CA, Kochanek PM (1995) Effect of soluble complement receptor-1 on neutrophil accumulation after traumatic brain injury in rats. *J Cereb Blood Flow Metab* 15: 860–864

63   Sanderson KL, Raghupathi R, Saatman KE, Martin D, Miller G, McIntosh TK (1999) Interleukin-1 receptor antagonist attenuates regional neuronal cell death and cognitive dysfunction after experimental brain injury. *J Cereb Blood Flow Metab* 19: 1118–1125

64   Toulmond S, Rothwell NJ (1995) Interleukin-1 receptor antagonist inhibits neuronal damage caused by fluid percussion injury in the rat. *Brain Res* 671: 261–266

65   Shohami E, Bass R, Wallach D, Yamin A, Gallily R (1996) Inhibition of tumor necrosis factor alpha (TNFalpha) activity in rat brain is associated with cerebroprotection after closed head injury. *J Cereb Blood Flow Metab* 16: 378–384

66   Loddick SA, Turnbull AV, Rothwell NJ (1998) Cerebral interleukin-6 is neuroprotective during permanent focal cerebral ischemia in the rat. *J Cereb Blood Flow Metab* 18: 176–179

67   Scherbel U, Raghupathi R, Nakamura M, Saatman KE, Trojanowski JQ, Neugebauer E, Marino MW, McIntosh TK (1999) Differential acute and chronic responses of tumor necrosis factor-deficient mice to experimental brain injury. *Proc Natl Acad Sci USA* 96: 8721–8726

68   Sullivan PG, Bruce-Keller AJ, Rabchevsky AG, Christakos S, Clair DK, Mattson MP, Scheff SW (1999) Exacerbation of damage and altered NF-kappaB activation in mice lacking tumor necrosis factor receptors after traumatic brain injury. *J Neurosci* 19: 6248–6256

69   Mollnes TE, Fosse E (1994) The complement system in trauma-related and ischemic tissue damage: a brief review. *Shock* 2: 301–310

70   Stahel PF, Morganti-Kossmann MC, Kossmann T (1998) The role of the complement system in traumatic brain injury. *Brain Res Rev* 27: 243–256

71   Becker P, Zieger S, Rother U, Lutz H, Osswald PM (1987) Complement activation following head and brain trauma. *Anaesthesist* 36: 301–305

72   Kossmann T, Stahel PF, Morganti-Kossmann MC, Jones JL, Barnum SR (1997) Elevated levels of the complement components C3 and factor B in ventricular cerebrospinal fluid of patients with traumatic brain injury. *J Neuroimmunol* 73: 63–69

73   Bellander BM, von Holst H, Fredman P, Svensson M (1996) Activation of the complement cascade and increase of clusterin in the brain following a cortical contusion in the adult rat. *J Neurosurg* 85: 468–475

74 Stahel PF, Kossmann T, Morganti-Kossmann MC, Hans VH, Barnum SR (1997) Experimental diffuse axonal injury induces enhanced neuronal C5a receptor mRNA expression in rats. *Mol Brain Res* 50: 205–212

75 Stahel PF, Kariya K, Shohami E, Barnum SR, Eugster H, Trentz O, Kossmann T, Morganti-Kossmann MC (2000) Intracerebral complement C5a receptor (CD88) expression is regulated by TNF and lymphotoxin-alpha following closed head injury in mice. *J Neuroimmunol* 109: 164–172

76 Farkas I, Baranyi L, Liposits ZS, Yamamoto T, Okada H (1998) Complement C5a anaphylatoxin fragment causes apoptosis in TGW neuroblastoma cells. *Neuroscience* 86: 903–911

77 DeKosky ST, Styren SD, O'Malley ME, Goss JR, Kochanek P, Marion D, Evans CH, Robbins PD (1996) Interleukin-1 receptor antagonist suppresses neurotrophin response in injured rat brain. *Ann Neurol* 39: 123–127

78 Shohami E, Gallily R, Mechoulam R, Bass R, Ben Hur T (1997) Cytokine production in the brain following closed head injury: dexanabinol (HU-211) is a novel TNF-alpha inhibitor and an effective neuroprotectant. *J Neuroimmunol* 72: 169–177

79 Clark RS, Carlos TM, Schiding JK, Bree M, Fireman LA, DeKosky ST, Kochanek PM (1996) Antibodies against Mac-1 attenuate neutrophil accumulation after traumatic brain injury in rats. *J Neurotrauma* 13: 333–341

80 Strauss KI, Barbe MF, Marshall RM, Raghupathi R, Mehta S, Narayan RK (2000) Prolonged cyclooxygenase-2 induction in neurons and glia following traumatic brain injury in the rat. *J Neurotrauma* 17: 695–711

Cyclic activation and inactivation of brain vessels involving inflammatory mediators – implications for stroke

Christl A. Ruetzler and John M. Hallenbeck

Stroke Branch, National Institute of Neurological Disorders and Stroke, National Institutes of Health, 36 Convent Drive MSC 4128, Building 36, Room 4A03, Bethesda, MD 20892-4128, USA

Endothelium has until recently been viewed by members of the stroke community as a relatively bland tissue that serves as an inert coating for the vascular tubes. Recent studies of endothelial cells in culture systems have proven these simplistic notions untenable and have shed light on the manifold functions of the endotheli um under normal as well as pathological conditions. Endothelium can be characterized as a dynamic, heterogenous, disseminated organ [1] that possesses vital secretory, synthetic, metabolic, and immunologic functions. Endothelial cell surface covers an area of 1 to 7 square meters and weighs about 1 kg [1]. Endothelial cells are heterogeneous [2]. They exhibit organ-specific specialization along with differences in function. It is less well known that endothelial cells express different phenotypes along different segments of the same vascular tree or even within neighboring cells. This variability in phenotype and the existence of subtypes enables endothelial cells to upregulate or downregulate surface proteins in response to local microenvironmental conditions and quickly and efficiently integrate multiple extracellular signals to serve the needs of the underlying tissue.

In health, endothelium controls vasomotor tone, vascular structure, blood fluidity, selective permeability to cells and proteins. It also mediates inflammatory and immunologic responses by maintaining a delicate balance between vascular growth promotion and inhibition, vasoconstriction and vasodilatation, blood cell adherence and nonadherence, and anticoagulation and procoagulation [3]. Under pathological conditions endothelium reacts to activating agonists such as thrombin, endotoxin, IL-1, TNFα, and hypoxia and to physical or chemical perturbation of the vessel wall by trauma, microbes, toxins or other threats to the maintenance of intravascular volume and oxygen delivery by mounting a protective response consisting of rapid transformation of the endothelium to a procoagulant, vasoconstrictive and proinflammatory state that has multiple effects on its structure and behavior [1].

With respect to hemostasis, potent antithrombotic factors that are induced in endothelial cells concurrently with activation of the prothrombotic factors provide the mutual regulation necessary to maintain fluid blood within the circulation (for

Inflammation and Stroke, edited by Giora Z. Feuerstein

review [4, 5]). Systemic fluctuations in thrombogenic potential have been observed as an overall effect of this form of feedback control. For example, tissue plasminogen activator and plasminogen activator inhibitor-1 undergo diurnal fluctuations such that fibrinolysis is at a nadir in the early morning hours and at a peak in the evening [6] and correspondingly, strokes tend to occur preferentially in the early morning [7, 8]. That hemostatic balance can also fluctuate focally within vessel beds is a relatively recent postulate. It owes its origins to the dramatic increase in understanding of endothelial cell biology that has occurred over the last 20 years [9, 10] and to the observation that systemic alterations in hemostatic mechanisms typically give rise to local thrombotic lesions in discrete segments of the vascular tree rather than causing a diffuse thrombotic diathesis with disseminated intravascular coagulation. For example, hypercoagulable states that arise from a general imbalance between procoagulant and anticoagulant forces, such as the congenital deficiencies Factor V Leiden, mutation of the heparin-binding site of antithrombin III, and prothrombin G20210A mutation lead to focal rather than diffuse thrombosis by biasing local endothelial cell control of hemostasis. Some acquired hypercoagulable states also lead to vascular bed specific thrombosis. Patients with antiphospholipid-antibody syndrome develop clots within particular segments of arteries and veins. Patients with thrombotic thrombocytopenic purpura show microthrombotic lesions in all organs except of the liver and the lungs. These and other data as well as data from animal studies have been woven together to support a model for focal development of thrombotic lesions in which signaling pathways specific to a vascular bed are determinate [5].

The mechanisms responsible for generating and maintaining vascular bed-specific phenotypes have been analyzed with regard to extracellular, cell subtype- specific signaling pathways and transcriptional regulation. Local endothelium responds and integrates various extracellular signals residing in the microenvironment. Some of these diverse environmental cues would include cytokines, chemokines, nitric oxide, endothelin, growth factors, hemodynamic forces, components of the extracellular matrix, neighboring cells, cell-to-cell signaling and signaling associated with integrins and other adhesion molecules.

An example of extracellular matrix – cell interaction is the evolving story of the capacity of thrombin which is ordinarily regarded as an intravascular coagulation protein, but has been found in the brain parenchyma to affect the morphology and function of asctrocytes and neurons [11].

The regulation of endothelial cell phenotype by cell – cell interaction can clearly be demonstrated by the ability of astrocytes to induce the blood-brain-barrier phenotype in endothelial cells [12, 13]. How hemodynamic forces can influence the endothelial phenotype is best shown by shear stress effects. Shear stress is higher in arteries than in veins, more pronounced at arterial branchpoints, and varies from one moment to the next. It is higher during systole and lower during diastole. Shear stress can cause rearrangement of the cytoskeleton in endothelial cells as well as changes in gene expression [14, 15]. Shear stress induces expression of thrombo-modulin, tissue type plasminogen activator, tissue factor and nitric oxide synthase. This effect involves modulation of gene transcription. A number of genes contain one or more shear stress responsive elements that include an NF-κB-responsive GAGACC promoter sequence in the 5' upstream region [16].

The extracellular environment varies both in time and space, and so does the endothelial phenotype. Not only do endothelial cells exhibit phenotypes that are vascular bed-specific, they also show different responses to the same signal in different vascular beds. Nitric oxide synthase mRNA is upregulated by increases in blood flow in the aorta but not the pulmonary artery [17]. Endothelial cells from different vascular segments express heterogenous phenotypes when immunohisto-chemically stained by a panel of antibodies [18] and human brain microvessel endothelial cells, compared with other endothelial cells, tend to express a higher level of ICAM-1 in response to cytokine stimulation [19]. Capillary endothelial cells show a strong expression of major histocompatibility complex class I (MHC-I) and class II (MHC-II) antigens and ICAM-1 in contrast with most large-vessel endothe-lial cells, in which these markers are weak to undetectable. Coronary endothelium differs from other large vessels by expressing MHC-II antigens, and VCAM-1 [20]. Endothelial cells harvested from human aortas within 3 h of sudden death revealed heterogeneity in that cells cultured from aortic segments burdened with atheroscle-rotic plaque and considered "high risk" segments had lower surface expression of thrombomodulin and a greater capacity for thrombin generation by prothrombi-nase complex assembly on their surfaces than "low risk" cells from aortic segments free of atherosclerosis [21]. Also the eNOS gene is induced by a variety of extracel-lular signals. In transgenic mice in which the human eNOS promoter was coupled to the coding region of the LacZ gene, transgene expression was detected within the endothelial cells of the brain, heart, skeletal muscle and aorta, but was not expressed in the vascular beds of the liver, kidney and spleen [22].

"Thus the overall expression of a single gene may be mediated by distinct vas-cular-bed-specific signaling pathways that begin in the extracellular milieu and end at separate sites on the promoter region of the gene" [5].

The concept of focal activation of endothelium gained further support from a recent study done in our lab. Immunohistochemical analyses of rat brain sections showed striking patterns of coincident immunoreactive cuffs for manganese super-oxide dismutase (MnSOD), tumor necrosis factor-α (TNFα) and hemoxygenase-1 (HO-1) around scattered vessels throughout the brains of untreated rats. A plausi-ble interpretation of this phenomenon is that the observed halos originate within local endothelium due to cyclic activation and inactivation of vessel segments and spread from there into the surrounding parenchyma.

MnSOD is upregulated by treatments that induce tolerance to ischemia. This phenomenon involves a sublethal stress that after a 1–2 day delay affords a tempo-rary protection against a subsequent ischemic insult in a variety of tissues. Examples of sublethal stresses that can precondition animals and induce tolerance include oxidative stress [23], hypoxia [24], brief ischemia [25, 26] and administration of LPS [27] or TNFα [28]. During a study of MnSOD as a possible mediator of tolerance we found that animals that received preconditioning i.v. injection of LPS expressed MnSOD immunoreactivity around scattered blood vessels and that, to a lesser degree, control animals that only received i.v. saline did as well. Immunohistochemistry in adjacent sections for TNFα and HO-1 showed that these inflammatory markers were expressed as perivascular cuffs around the same vessels as MnSOD. These findings prompted us to look further into the distribution and expression of these three proteins in the brains of untreated rats of different strains to examine spontaneous activation-deactivation cycles in brain vessels.

For the study we used 12 -13 week old rats of the following strains: spontaneously hypertensive rat (SHR), Sprague-Dawley (SD), Wistar, and Wistar-Kyoto (WKY). In addition 18-week old spontaneously hypertensive-stroke prone rats (SHR-SP) were used. Animals from each strain were used in groups of three or four. An additional 10 SHR received bacterial LPS from *Escherichia coli* in a dose of 0.9 mg/kg body weight *via* catheter to the femoral vein. Five control animals received saline only *via* the same route. The animals were divided into five groups and euthanized at different timepoints: 8 h, 24 h, 48 h, 72 h and 168 h. After transcardial perfusion with 4% buffered paraformaldehyde brains were removed, postfixed for another 4 h in the same fixative and embedded in paraffin. Seven micrometer thick sections were stained with Hematoxylin and Eosin for morphological evaluation. Adjacent sections were used for immunohistochemistry.

Enzyme immunohistochemistry was performed by the Avidin-Biotin method (Vector Laboratories Inc., Burlingame, CA) with the following antibodies: Rabbit anti-MnSOD (a gift from Dr. Kato, Department of Biochemistry, Institute for Developmental Research, Aichi, Prefectual Colony, Kamiya. Kaugai. Aichi 480-03, Japan), rabbit anti-HO-1 (StressGen, Victoria, Canada) and goat anti-TNFα (R&D Systems Inc,. Minneapolis, MN). Secondary antibodies were from Jackson Immuno Research Labs. Inc. West Grove, PA). Antigen-antibody binding was visualized with diaminobenzidine. For assessment of nonspecific staining, primary antibodies were omitted or replaced by normal mouse, rabbit or goat IgG.

Enzyme immunohistochemistry for MnSOD showed that it was expressed in the brains of all animals in a striking pattern of clearly defined cuffs and rings around vessels of all sizes. Quantitative analysis of sections revealed that the number of vessels/HPF with perivascular cuffs expressing MnSOD varied among untreated rats of different strains. Wistar rats showed the lowest numbers of vessels with perivascular MnSOD immunoreactivity/high power field (HPF) (51 ± 28, mean ± SD) and SHR-SP showed the highest (184 ± 72) (Fig. 1). S-D, WKY and untreated SHR showed slightly higher values for MnSOD expression than the Wistar and considerable within group variability among the WKY and S-D rats. SHR that received LPS showed increased levels of MnSOD expresssion at all time points (Fig. 1). Mean

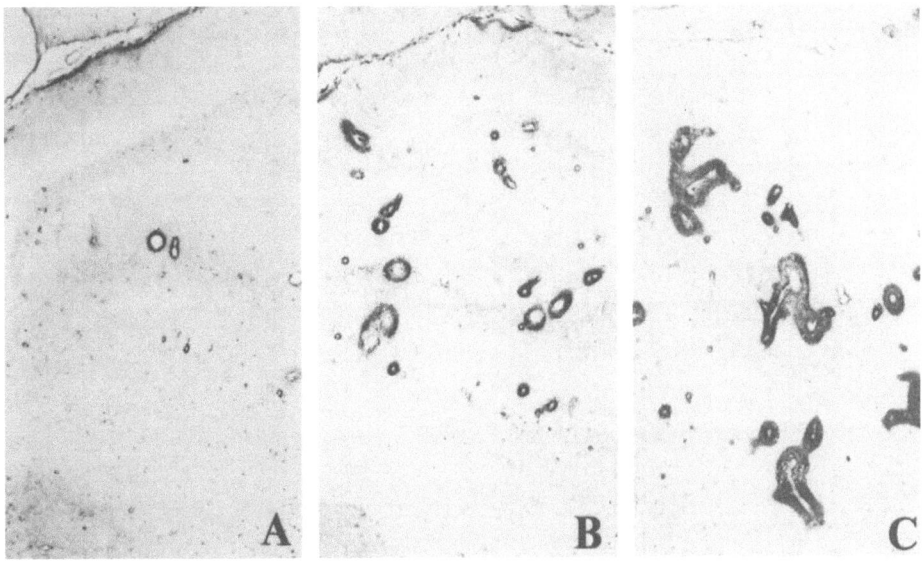

Figure 1
Immunostaining for MnSOD in sections of hippocampus (magnification × 50) of A: naïve Wistar rat; B: LPS-treated SHR, 48 h after treatment; C: naïve SHR-SP.

± SD number of vessels with perivascular MnSOD immunoreactivity/HPF in all SHR exposed to LPS was 131 ± 32 compared to naïve SHR 64 ± 15, $p < 0.02$. SHR that received saline injections at time points corresponding to LPS injections also expressed MnSOD (107 ± 17), but this was not significantly different than the number of cuffs/HPF in naïve SHR ($p < 0.13$).

MnSOD staining was found throughout the brain but was most prominently expressed around vessels of the hippocampus, the striatum and the thalamus. The staining was granular, consistent with the mitochondrial location of MnSOD and followed different staining patterns. Some vessels were surrounded by tightly packed, intensely staining cuffs that did not extend far beyond the vessel wall while others were surrounded by thick cuffs of large diameter and variable staining intensity. Yet other vessels were surrounded by cuffs in which the inner area was completely unstained with only an outer ring staining for MnSOD. These rings could extend to a diameter of 50 μm and in some of them a nascent ring within a ring could be observed (Fig. 2). The striking patterns allow the inference that the enzyme is induced in wave upon wave originating at the vessel wall and spreading radially from there into the surrounding parenchyma. The antioxidant is induced in cells with the morphology of endothelium, pericytes and astrocytes, but is most promi-

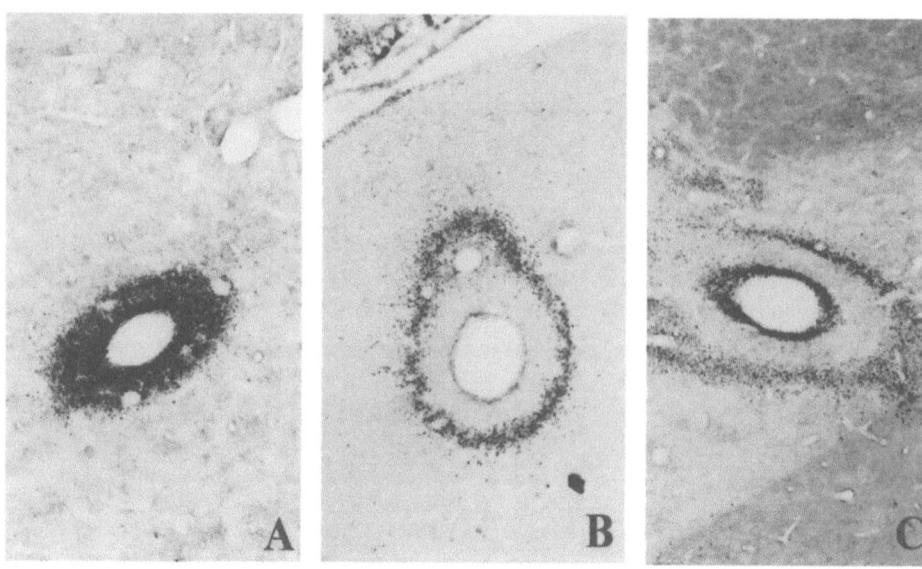

Figure 2
Patterns of MnSOD expression around brain vessels of SHR-SP (magnification × 200)
A: Tightly packed MnSOD perivascular cuff; B: Concentric ring some distance away from vessel lumen with clearing around vessel; C: Second tightly packed ring around vessel appearing within the expanded first ring.

nent in neurons. Double-label immunofluorescence with antibodies against MnSOD, neurofilament-200, glial fibrillary acidic protein, 2',3'-cyclic nucleotide 3'-phosphodiesterase, von Willebrand Factor, monocytes and macrophages (ED-1) confirmed MnSOD expression in neurons, astrocytes, oligodendrocytes, endothelial cells and perivascular macrophages, respectively.

Immunoreactivity for HO-1 in the brains of all experimental animals was coincident with that of MnSOD but not as intense. It showed the same perivascular expression of clearly stained cuffs surrounding scattered blood vessels of all sizes and appeared most frequent in the hippocampus, the striatum and the thalamus. As with MnSOD the staining was most pronounced in the brains of untreated SHR-SP and SHR that had received i.v. injection of LPS.

TNFα showed weak, but clear staining in the same peculiar cuffing pattern around vessels of all sizes as has been described for MnSOD and HO-1 (Fig. 3). Its distribution was less extensive and its intensity was lower, but where it was expressed it matched closely the spatial distribution of the other immunoreactive molecules. The brains of untreated animals of all four strains showed only occa-

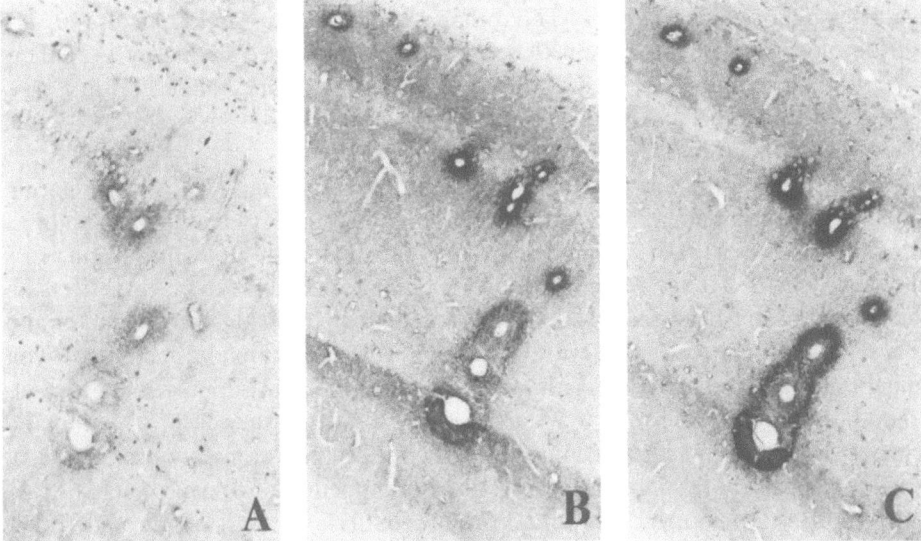

Figure 3
Immunostaining of adjacent vessel segments in adjacent hippocampal sections of naïve SHR-SP (magnification × 200)
A: Cuffs around vessels staining positive for TNFα; B: Coincident cuffs around vessels staining positive for HO-1; C: Coincident cuffs around vessels staining positive for MnSOD

sional cuffed vessels while the brains of SHR-SP and those of LPS-treated SHR showed an increased frequency of vessels with cuffs that stained for TNFα.

Our finding that intraparenchymal brain vessels from normal rats have immunoreactive MnSOD expression surrounding them in the form of cuffs, rings or an occasional ring within a ring suggests that an endogenous stimulus for upregulation of this enzyme originates within the blood vessel and expands centrifugally in cyclic waves.

We have postulated that perivascular cells can release TNFα and convert endothelium in the involved vessel segment from an antithrombotic to a prothrombotic luminal surface [29]. In small vessels, perivascular macrophages [30, 31] and endothelium itself [32] are potential sources of TNFα. Additional cell sources in larger vessels include smooth muscle cells and lymphocytes particularly in atherosclerotic segments [33–35]. Microglia [36], neurons [37, 38] and astrocytes [39] are additional sources of TNFα in brain. In response to a suitably intense LPS stimulus (e.g. 1.8 mg/kg intracisternally), rats with identifiable risk factors for stroke such as streptozotocin-induced diabetes, hypertension, advanced age or genetic stroke-proneness release higher levels of TNFα than stroke risk factor-free controls [40, 41] and develop signs of focal brain ischemia with an increased frequency [42]. This focal vessel activation is viewed as tilting the local hemostatic balance [5] in a pro-thrombotic direction and predisposing to thrombotic occlusion or loss of vessel integrity with hemorrhage.

After a single stimulus such as intravenous LPS injection, TNFα in circulating blood reaches a maximum within 90 min to 2 h and returns to baseline by 6 h [43]. In brain, TNFα peaks at 7 h and returns to baseline 18 h after intravenous LPS injection [36]. TNFα has a number of proinflammatory and procoagulant effects on endothelium (for review see [9, 44, 45]). It stimulates expression of tissue factor and adhesion molecules for leukocytes, release of IL-1, nitric oxide, factor VIII/von Willebrand factor, platelet activating factor and endothelin, suppresses the throm-bomodulin-protein C-protein S system, reduces tissue plasminogen activator and releases plasminogen activator inhibitor-1. TNFα can also stimulate production of reactive oxygen species in endothelium through induction of enzymes such as xan-thine oxidase, cyclooxygenase and NADPH oxidase as well as through other sources [46–48]. In addition, TNFα can directly stimulate production of HO-1 and MnSOD [48, 49]. It does not stimulate expression of other antioxidant enzymes such as copper/zinc SOD, glutathione peroxidase or catalase [50].

Hemoxygenase (HO) has three known isoforms. These isoforms consist of the inducible HO-1, the constitutive HO-2 and a recently identified isoform, HO-3 [51]. Endothelium [52], astrocytes and neurons [53] produce HO-1 in response to stressful stimuli, particularly reactive oxygen species (ROS). Potential mechanisms advanced for TNFα stimulation of HO-1 production include activation of protein kinase C and phospholipase A_2, changes in intracellular calcium and inhibition of protein phosphatase-1 and protein phosphatase-2A [48]. HO-1 reaches a maximum 4 h after stimulation and largely disappears by 6 h [52]. In addition to providing a signal that indicates preceding cellular stress [54, 55], HO-1 also serves as an antioxidant by cleaving the heme molecule, releasing free iron and producing biliverdin, a precursor to bilirubin [56]. HO-1 enzymatic activity makes iron avail-able for sequestration by ferritin, a storage protein that prevents the metal from par-ticipating in redox reactions [57]. The bilirubin that is produced also has antioxi-dant properties [58].

Mammals have three distinct SOD genes that include MnSOD, cytoplasmic cop-per/zinc-SOD and a secreted extracellular (EC-SOD) form of copper/zinc-SOD [59]. The location of MnSOD is mainly in mitochondria. Copper/zinc-SOD and EC-SOD are expressed constitutively and MnSOD is the only antioxidant enzyme that can be induced by cytokines such as TNFα or by ROS [50]. Mitochondria consume 90 % of the oxygen used by cells [60, 61] of which 1–4% is converted to superoxide anions by the electron transfer chain [62, 63]. This renders mitochondria especially vulnerable to oxygen radical attack. MnSOD plays a critical role as a first line of defense against superoxide anions that are produced during normal aerobic respiration in these organelles [63]. In the aged brain and heart it has been shown that mitochondrial mutation frequency increases more than 100-fold [64] and generation of endogenous oxidants (principally by mitochondria) is hypothesized to contribute to aging [65]. In general, oxidative damage to mitochondrial DNA occurs at 16 times the frequency of nuclear DNA [62]. Some of the reasons for this extreme vulnerability are lack of protective histones, limited DNA repair mechanisms and low replication fidelity [61]. These factors render mitochondrial MnSOD a key antioxidant enzyme. The present findings provide a glimpse of the dynamism involved in focal homeostatic balance in the brain. Our interpretation is that intraparenchymal brain vessels undergo an asynchronous cyclic fluctuation in proinflammatory/prothrombotic potential alternating with an anti-inflammatory/antithrombotic potential. These cyclic fluctuations originate within the vessels and spread radially outward to involve parenchymal cells and their processes within a perivascular circumference of about a 50 μm radius. Periodic activation with local release of TNFα and ROS tilt the hemostatic balance of vessel segments in a proinflammatory and prothrombotic direction. In response, vascular and perivascular cells exposed to these stimuli synthesize HO-1 and MnSOD to help restore hemostatic balance. Under normal circumstances, these cyclic fluctuations occur within a hemostatic range and local circulatory disturbances and tissue damage do not supervene. Particularly in the presence of stroke risk factors, larger fluctuations that exceed some threshold could predispose local segments to thrombosis or hemorrhage.

References

1   Cines DB, Pollak ES, Buck CA, Loscalzo J, Zimmerman GA, McEver RP, Pober JS, Wick TM, Konkle BA, Schwartz BS et al (1998) Endothelial cells in physiology and in the pathophysiology of vascular disorders. *Blood* 91: 3527–3561

2   Kumar S, West DC, Ager A (1987) Heterogeneity in endothelial cells from large vessels and microvessels. *Differentiation* 36:57–70

3   Davies MG, Hagen PO (1993) The vascular endothelium. A new horizon. *Ann of Surg* 218: 593–609

4   Stern DM, Esposito C, Gerlach H, Gerlach M, Ryan J, Handley D, Nawroth P (1991) Endothelium and regulation of coagulation. *Diabetes Care* 14 (Suppl 1): 160–166

5   Rosenberg RD, Aird WC (1999) Vascular-bed-specific hemostasis and hypercoagulable states. *New Engl J Med* 340: 1555–1564

6   Angleton P, Chandler WL, Schmer G (1989) Diurnal variation of tissue-type plasminogen activator and its rapid inhibitor (PAI-1). *Circulation* 79: 101–106

7   Marler JR, Price TR, Clark JE, Robertson T, Mohr JP, Hier DB, Wolf PA, Caplan LR, Foulkes MA (1989) Morning increase in onset of ischemic stroke. *Stroke* 20: 473–476

8   Labrecque G, Soulban G (1991) Biological rhythms in the physiology and pharmacology of blood coagulation. *Chronobiol Int* 8: 361–372

9   Pober JS, Cotran RS (1990) Cytokines and endothelial cell biology. *Physiol Rev* 70: 427–451

10   Becker BF, Heindl B, Kupatt C, Zahler S (2000) Endothelial function and hemostasis. *Z Kardiol* 89: 160–167

11   Cunningham DD, Pulliam L, Vaughan PJ (1993) Protease nexin-1 and thrombin: injury–related processes in the brain. *Thromb Haemost* 70: 168–171

12   Kuchler-Bopp S, Delaunoy JP, Artault JC, Zaepfel M, Dietrich JB (1999) Astrocytes induce several blood-brain barrier properties in non-neural endothelial cells. NeuroReport 10: 1347–1353

13   Igarashi Y, Utsumi H, Chiba H, Yamada-Sasamori Y, Tobioka H, Kamimura Y, Furuuchi K, Kokai Y, Nakagawa T, Mori M et al (1999) Glial cell line-derived neurotrophic factor induces barrier function of endothelial cells forming the blood-brain barrier. *Biochem Biophys Res Commun* 261: 108–112

14   Lin M-Ch, Almus-Jacobs F, Chen H-H, Parry GCN, Mackman N, Shyy JY-j, Chien Shu (1997) Shear stress induction of tissue factor gene. *J Clin Invest* 99: 737–744

15   Davies PF (1995) Flow-mediated endothelial mechanotransduction. *Physiol Rev* 75: 519–560

16   Khachigian LM, Resnick N, Gimbrone MA Jr, Collins T (1995) Nuclear factor-kappa B interacts functionally with the platelet-derived growth factor B-chain shear-stress response element in vascular endothelial cells exposed to fluid shear stress. *J Clin Invest* 96: 1169–1175

17   Everett AD, Le Cras TD, Xue C, Johns RA (1998) eNos expression is not altered in pulmonary vascular remodeling due to increased pulmonary blood flow. *Am J Physiol* 274: L1058–1065

18   Turner RR, Beckstead JH, Warnke RA, Wood GS (1987) Endothelial cell phenotypic diversity. *In situ* demonstration of immunologic and enzymatic heterogeneity that correlates with specific morphologic subtypes. *Am J Clin Pathol* 87: 569–575

19   Wong D, Dorovini-Zis K (1992) Upregulation of intercellular adhesion molecule-1 (ICAM-1) expression in primary cultures of human brain microvessel endothelial cells by cytokines and lipopolysaccharide. *J Neuroimmunol* 39: 11–22

20   Page C, Rose M, Yacoub M, Pigott R (1992) Antigenic heterogeneity of vascular endothelium. *Am J Pathol* 141: 673–683

21   Antonov AS, Key NS, Smirnov MD, Jacob HS, Vercellotti GM, Smirnov VN (1992) Prothrombotic phenotype diversity of human aortic endothelial cells in culture. *Thromb Res* 67: 135–145

22   Guillot PV, Guan J, Liu L, Kuivenhoven JA, Rosenberg RD, Sessa WC, Aird WC (1999) A vascular bed-specific pathway regulates cardiac expression of endothelial nitric oxide synthase. *J Clin Invest* 103: 799–805

23   Zahler S, Kupatt C, Becker BF (2000) Endothelial preconditioning by transient oxida-

tive stress reduces inflammatory responses of cultured endothelial cells to TNF-α. *FASEB J* 14: 555–564

24 Liu J, Ginis I, Spatz M, Hallenbeck JM (2000) Hypoxic preconditioning protects cultured neurons against hypoxic stress *via* TNF-alpha and ceramide. *Am J Physiol Cell Physiol* 278: C144–153

25 Barone FC, White RF, Spera PA, Ellison J, Currie RW, Wang X, Feuerstein GZ (1998) Ischemic preconditioning and brain tolerance: temporal histological and functional outcomes, protein synthesis requirement, and interleukin-1 receptor antagonist and early gene expression. *Stroke* 29: 1937–1950

26 Kitagawa K, Matsumoto M, Tagaya M, Hata R, Ueda H, Niinobe M, Handa N, Fukunaga K, Mikoshiba K et al (1990) "Ischemic tolerance" phenomenon found in the brain. *Brain Res* 528: 21–24

27 Tasaki K, Ruetzler CA, Ohtsuki T, Martin D, Nawashiro H, Hallenbeck JM (1997) Lipopolysaccharide pretreatment induces resistance against subsequent focal cerebral ischemic damage in spontaneously hypertensive rats. *Brain Res* 748: 267–270

28 Nawashiro H, Tasaki K, Ruetzler CA, Hallenbeck JM (1997) TNF-alpha pretreatment induces protective effects against focal cerebral ischemia in mice. *J Cereb Blood Flow Metab* 17: 483–490

29 Hallenbeck JM, Dutka AJ, Vogel SN, Heldman E, Doron DA, Feuerstein G (1991) Lipopolysaccharide-induced production of tumor necrosis factor activity in rats with and without risk factors for stroke. *Brain Res* 541: 115–12

30 Woodroofe MN, Cuzner ML (1993) Cytokine mRNA expression in inflammatory multiple sclerosis lesions: detection by non-radioactive *in situ* hybridization. *Cytokine* 5: 583–588

31 Seilhean D, Kobayashi K, He Y, Uchihara T, Rosenblum O, Katlama C, Bricaire F, Dyckaerts C, Hauw J-J (1997) Tumor necrosis factor-α, microglia and astrocytes in AIDS dementia complex. *Acta Neuropathol* 93: 508–517

32 Gourin CG, Shackford SR (1997) Production of tumor necrosis factor-α and interleukin-1β by human cerebral microvascular endothelium after percussive trauma. *J Trauma* 42: 1101–1107

33 Warner SJ, Libby P (1989) Human vascular smooth muscle cells. Target for and source of tumor necrosis factor. *J Immunology* 142: 100–109

34 Barath P, Fishbein MC, Cao J, Berebson J, Helfant RH, Forrester JS (1990) Detection and localization of tumor necrosis factor in human atheroma. *Am J Cardiol* 65: 297–302

35 Kishikawa H, Shimokama T, Watanabe T (1993) Localization of T lymphocytes and macrophages expressing IL-1, IL-2 receptor, IL-6 and TNF in human aortic intima. Role of cell mediated immunity in human atherogenesis. *Virchows Arch A Pathol Anat Histopathol* 423: 433–442

36 Buttini M, Mir A, Appel K, Wiederhold KH, Limonta S, Gebicke-Haerter PJ, Boddeke HWGM (1997) Lipopolysaccharide induces expression of tumor necrosis factor alpha

in rat brain: inhibition by methylprednisolone and by rolipram. *Br J Pharmacol* 122: 1483–1489

37   Breder CD, Hazuka C, Ghayur T, Klug C, Huginin M, Yasuda K, Teng M, Saper CB (1994) Regional induction of tumor necrosis factor alpha expression in the mouse brain after systemic lipopolysaccharide administration. *Proc Natl Acad Sci USA* 91: 11393–11397

38   Liu T, Clark RK, McDonnell PC, Young PR, White RF, Barone FC, Feuerstein GZ (1994) Tumor necrosis factor-alpha expression in ischemic neurons. *Stroke* 25: 1481–1488

39   Benveniste EN, Tang LP, Law RM (1995) Differential regulation of astrocyte TNF-alpha expression by the cytokines TGF-beta, IL-6 and IL-10. *Int J Dev Neurosci* 13: 341–349

40   Siren A-L, Heldman E, Doron D, Lysko PG, Yue T-L, Liu Y, Feuerstein G, Hallenbeck JM (1992) Release of proinflammatory and prothrombotic mediators in the brain and peripheral circulation in spontaneously hypertensive and normotensive Wistar-Kyoto rats. *Stroke* 23: 1643–1651

41   Siren A-L, Feuerstein G, Hallenbeck JM (1993) Increased release of tumor necrosis factor alpha into the cerebrospinal fluid and peripheral circulation of aged rats. *Stroke* 24: 880–888

42   Hallenbeck JM, Dutka AJ, Kochanek PM, Siren A, Pezeshkpour GH, Feuerstein G (1988) Stroke risk factors prepare rat brainstem tissues for modified local Shwartzman reaction. *Stroke* 19: 863–869

43   Feuerstein G, Hallenbeck JM, Vanatta B, Rabinovich R, Perera PY, Vogel SN (1990) Effect of gram-negative endotoxin on levels of serum corticosterone, TNF-α circulating blood cells, and the survival of rats. *Circ Shock* 30: 265–278

44   Hallenbeck JM (1996) Inflammatory reactions at the blood-endothelial interface in acute stroke. In: BK Siesjo, T Wieloch (eds): Adv Neurol 71; *Cellular and molecular mechanisms of ischemic brain damage.* Lippincott-Raven, Philadelphia, 281–300

45   Feuerstein GZ, Liu T, Barone FC (1994 Winter) Cytokines, inflammation, and brain injury: role of tumor necrosis factor-alpha. *Cerebrovasc Brain Metab Rev* 6: 341–360

46   Ishii Y, Partridge CA, Del Vecchio PJ, Malik AB (1992) Tumor necrosis factor-alpha mediated decrease in glutathione increases the sensitivity of pulmonary vascular endothelial cells to H_2O_2. *J Clin Invest* 89: 794–802

47   Weber C, Erl W, Pietsch A, Strobel M, Ziegler-Heitbrock HW, Weber PC (1994) Antioxidants inhibit monocyte adhesion by suppressing nuclear factor-kappa B mobilization and induction of vascular cell adhesion molecule-1 in endothelial cells stimulated to generate radicals. *Arterioscler Thromb* 14: 1665–1673

48   Terry CM, Clikeman JA, Hoidal JR, Callahan KS (1999) TNF-α and IL-1α induce heme oxygenase-1 *via* protein kinase C, Ca^{2+}, and Phospholipase A2 in endothelial cells. *Am J Physiol* 276: H1493–H1501

49   Visner GA, Dougall WC, Wilson JM, Burr IA, Nick HS (1990) Regulation of manganese superoxide dismutase by lipopolysaccharid, interleukin-1, and tumor necrosis factor. *J Biol Chem* 265: 2856–2864

50 Wong GHW, Goeddel DV (1988) Induction of manganous superoxide dismutase by tumor necrosis factor: possible protective mechanism. *Science* 242: 941–944

51 McCoubrey WK Jr, Huang TJ, Maines MD (1997) Isolation and characterization of a cDNA from the rat brain that encodes hemoprotein heme oxygenase-3. *Eur J Biochem* 247: 725–732

52 Terry CM, Clikeman JA, Hoidal JR, Callahan KS (1998) Effect of tumor necrosis factor-α and interleukin-1α on heme oxygenase-1 expression in human endothelial cells. *Am J Physiol* 274: H883–H891

53 Dwyer BE, Nishimura RN, Lu S-Y (1995) Differential expression of heme oxygenase-1 in cultured cortical neurons and astrocytes determined by the aid of a new heme oxygenase antibody. Response to oxidative stress. *Brain Res Mol Brain Res* 30: 37–47

54 Poss DK, Tonegawa S (1997) Reduced stress defense in heme oxygenase 1-deficient cells. *Proc Natl Acad Sci USA* 94: 10925–10930

55 Mautes AEM, Kim DH, Sharp FR, Panter S, Sato M, Maida N, Bergeron M, Guenther K, Noble LJ (1998) Induction of heme oxygenase (HO-1) in the contused spinal cord of the rat. *Brain Res* 795:17–24

56 Tenhunen R, Marver HS, Schmid R (1968) The enzymatic conversion of heme to bilirubin by microsomal heme oxygenase. *Proc Natl Acad Sci USA* 61: 748–755

57 Balla G, Jacob HS, Balla J, Rosenberg M, Nath K, Apple F, Eaton JW, Vercelotti GM (1992) Ferritin: a cytoprotective antioxidant stratagem of endothelium. *J Biol Chem* 267: 18148–18153

58 Stocker R, Yamamoto Y, McDonagh AF, Glazer AN, Ames BN (1987) Bilirubin is an antioxidant of possible physiological importance. *Science* 235: 1043–1046

59 Janssen YMW, Van Houten B, Borm PJA, Mossman BT (1993) Biology of disease. Cell and tissue responses to oxidative damage. *Lab Invest* 69: 261–274

60 Richter C, Park J-W, Ames B (1988) Normal oxidative damage to mitochondrial and nuclear DNA is extensive. *Proc Natl Acad Sci USA* 85: 6465–6467

61 Bandy B, Davison AJ (1990) Mitochondrial mutations may increase oxidative stress: Implications for carcinogenesis and aging. *Free Radic Biol Med* 8: 523–539

62 Wallace DC (1992) Mitochondrial genetics: A paradigm for aging and degenerative diseases? *Science* 256: 628–632

63 Williams MD, Van Remmen H, Conrad CC, Huang TT, Epstein CJ, Richardson A (1998) Increased oxidative damage is correlated to altered mitochondrial function in hetero-zygous manganese superoxide dismutase knockout mice. *J Biol Chem* 273: 28510–28515

64 Cortopassi G, Wang E (1995) Modeling the effects of age-related mtDNA mutation accumulation: Complex I deficiency, superoxide and cell death. *Biochim Biophys Acta* 1271: 171–176

65 Beckman KB, Ames BN (1998) The free radical theory of aging matures. *Physiol Rev* 78: 547–581

Inflammatory cells in stroke

Do leukocytes play a role in focal ischemia in the brain? An objective review of the literature

Dwaine F. Emerich, Reginald L. Dean III and Raymond T. Bartus

Alkermes, Inc., 64 Sidney Street, Cambridge, MA 02139, USA

Introduction

Three general lines of evidence have been put forth to support the role of neutrophil recruitment in ischemic cell death. These include (1) the presence of neutrophils within ischemic tissue at the approximate time that substantial cell death occurs, (2) the reduction of ischemia-induced cell loss following neutropenia, and (3) the observation that treatments which prevent neutrophil trafficking can be neuroprotective. Despite the numerous studies that have been conducted, this hypothesis remains controversial, for an objective assessment of the literature reveals great uncertainty for a pathogenic role of neutrophils in the brain damage associated with ischemia. The present chapter briefly summarizes and critically discusses the available data addressing this hypothesis.

Criteria for a pathogenic role of neutrophils in stroke

At its most basic level, the hypothesis that neutrophils play an active role in ischemic cell death revolves around the observation that neutrophils are often found within infarcted, ischemic tissue. There are, however, at least two distinct interpretations that arise from this observation. In one interpretation, neutrophils participate in the ensuing pathogenesis. In the second interpretation, the recruitment of neutrophils simply occurs in response to the post-ischemic necrosis. In this scenario, the neutrophils do not contribute to the magnitude of the infarct, but rather play a scavenging function for the infarcted tissue. In order to differentiate these two completely different interpretations, the available data must be examined in an objective and indifferent fashion. A number of empirical outcomes can logically be identified that are consistent with a pathogenic role of neutrophils, providing the basis for evaluating the existing literature. Positive support for the pathogenic neutrophil hypothesis requires that: (1) increased accumulation of neutrophils occurs in the area of ischemia *prior to* major, ischemia-induced cell death, (2) brain areas exhibit-

Inflammation and Stroke, edited by Giora Z. Feuerstein
© 2001 Birkhäuser Verlag Basel/Switzerland

ing the greatest cell loss also demonstrate the greatest changes in early neutrophil recruitment, (3) greater numbers of neutrophils reflect greater brain damage (and *vice versa*), and (4) treatments which inhibit neutrophil trafficking or activity produce a corresponding dose-related decrease in neutrophils and ischemic damage.

The presence of neutrophils in ischemic tissue

Table 1 summarizes the published data characterizing neutrophil infiltration following ischemia. Common to all of these studies is the demonstration that neutrophils are present, frequently in large numbers, within ischemic tissue. While often interpreted as support for a pathogenic role of neutrophils in ischemia, these data do not provide the evidence required to justify a pathogenic role, leaving it impossible to conclude what role, if any, neutrophils play in ischemic brain damage. For instance, not all studies have provided a systematic and independent confirmation of neutrophil infiltration and quantification of infarct size [1–7]. In these cases, even though no independent measure of ischemic damage is provided, the visualization of neutrophils within the CNS is used as evidence that they play a role in that same, unmeasured, ischemic damage. Logically, of course, it is impossible to interpret any cause-effect relationship without both variables being measured. An even more common interpretive problem is the universal lack of a demonstration that neutrophils invade the ischemic tissue *prior* to cell death. Indeed, few studies have even attempted to establish a temporal relationship, which would seem to be the minimal evidence required to entertain causal possibilities. Rather, neutrophils are typically observed within the ischemic tissue only after the majority of the infarct has already developed, therefore providing no insight regarding temporal events or causal relationships.

Thus, an objective examination of the literature fails to reveal any data that convincingly shows a clear pathogenic role of neutrophils in ischemia (Tab. 1). Indeed, in some cases a more parsimonious explanation would be just the opposite conclusion: that neutrophil infiltration did not contribute to, but was a result of, the cerebral infarct (e.g., see [8]). Until studies demonstrate, under well-controlled and experimentally blinded conditions, that significant numbers of neutrophils are present in ischemic tissue prior to cell death, it is not logical to conclude that a clear pathogenic role of neutrophils has been established.

Effects of neutropenia on ischemia

A number of pharmacological treatments are used to deplete neutrophils (i.e., induce neutropenia). These studies assume that if neutrophils are important mediators of ischemic damage, their absence would minimize the extent of cell loss fol-

Table 1 - Studies demonstrating the presence of neutrophils in ischemic tissue

Number of studies	% Confirming entrance of neutrophils into ischemic area	% Measuring both variables (neutrophils and infarct)	% Establishing temporal priority for neutrophils	% Support for cause-effect
30	100%	73%	0%	0%

While neutrophils are always found within the area of cerebral infarction, their contribution to the development of the infarct remains uncertain. No study has demonstrated that neutrophils invade the ischemic area in advance of significant brain damage (i.e., the minimal evidence required to demonstrate that neutrophils contribute to the cell death that occurs following ischemia). References comprising table [1–25].

lowing ischemia (Tab. 2). Many times, nearly total depletion of neutrophils (typically > 90%) is seen prior to ischemia and, indeed, decreases in infarct size are often seen following these manipulations. Although these studies appear to support a role of neutrophil trafficking in cell death, a closer examination reveals several interpretive problems and inconsistencies. First, some studies have failed to confirm that a reduction of neutrophils occurred prior to the onset of ischemia [26, 27]. Moreover, the relationship between neutropenia and infarct size is made more obscure because many studies failed to provide any objective histological assessment of the infarct [28–30]. Second, while many studies have demonstrated reductions in neutrophils together with decreases in infarct size, neuroprotection has been reported in the absence of any changes in neutrophils [26], raising the possibility that some mechanism other than altered neutrophil trafficking could be responsible for the beneficial effects. Third, some authors have demonstrated significant neutropenia without any measurable effect on infarct size [8]. Fourth, pharmacologically increasing neutrophils prior to ischemia did not augment the infarct as would be expected if a direct cause-effect relationship existed between neutrophil infiltration and tissue damage [10] .

Finally, a note of caution should be made in that pharmacologically-induced neutropenia produce multiple nonspecific effects on the hemodynamics of the animal. For example, antineoplastic agents cause myelosuppression affecting not only neutrophils, but other white blood cells and platelets [33]. This results in a subsequent decrease in hematocrit [28]. In addition to reducing monocytes, the use of antineutrophil serum to produce neutropenia also activates circulating cells, endothelial cells and tissue macrophages [34]. Thus, these drugs directly or indirectly produce physiological and hemodynamic effects which could affect the outcome of ischemia studies in ways independent of changes in neutrophils. Accordingly, these con-

Table 2 - Neutropenia treatment studies

Number of studies	% Confirming pre-infarct reduction of neutrophils	% Confirming decrease in infarct size	% Establishing relationship between neutrophils and infarct size
9	78%	56%	0%

The induction of neutropenia in animals can produce nearly total decreases in circulating levels of neutrophils which are frequently (though not always) associated with modest decreases in infarct size. However, a clear relationship between neutropenia and neuroprotection is uncertain for several reasons: (1) not all studies have provided independent confirmation that the treatment produced both a pre-infarct reduction in neutrophils and a decrease in infarct size, (2) in some cases, neuroprotection is seen in the absence of changes in neutrophils and vice versa, and (3) the multiple nonspecific effects of neutropenia on the physiology of the animal require numerous control groups to permit definitive conclusions about effects of neutrophil depletion on infarct size. Given these considerations, it is impossible to conclude that neutropenia, per se, is responsible for any reductions in infarct size. References comprising table: [8, 20, 26–32].

founding effects of neutropenic drugs cannot easily be separated from the effects of neutrophil depletion, *per se*. Studies employing them, therefore, require numerous control groups to permit definitive conclusions that neutrophil depletion is solely or even primarily responsible for any change in infarct size. One practical control that has yet to be run would involve replacing neutrophils in neutropenic rats to determine whether the infarct in this group would be restored to its normal (i.e., non-neutropenic size). Since important control groups have not been incorporated into these experimental designs to control for potentially confounding effects, numerous questions exist regarding the interpretation of these experiments. Thus, they fall short of providing definitive support for a cause-effect relationship.

Cell trafficking studies

More sophisticated and presumably more selective means of altering neutrophil trafficking have been used, including the use of anti-ICAM, anti-CD11/CD18, proteasome inhibitors and neutrophil elastase inhibitors. As is the case with the induction of neutropenia, these studies have failed to provide convincing support for a pathogenic role of neutrophils in ischemia (Tab. 3). While reductions in infarct size [20, 35–38] and improvements in neurological outcome [39–41] have been reported in some studies, just as many studies have failed to find any evidence of reduc-

Table 3 - Cell trafficking studies

Number of studies	% Confirming pre-infarct reduction of neutrophils	% Confirming decrease in infarct size	% Establishing relationship between cell trafficking and infarct size
51	2%	78%	0%

A large number of studies have used a variety of methods to alter neutrophil trafficking and/or activity. In the majority of cases, these treatments are associated with decreases in infarct size. However, these studies have not fulfilled several logical criteria for supporting the conclusion that neutrophils, per se, are responsible for the reduction in infarct volume. These include: (1) evidence for a reduction in cell trafficking prior to the development of ischemic brain damage, (2) a relationship between the extent of cell trafficking and the extent of ischemic damage, and (3) a reduction in the size of the infarct. Those studies concluding an important pathogenic role of neutrophils have observed only that last point and assumed the others to be true. References comprising table: [20, 35–38, 40–75].

tions in lesion size following similar treatments [37, 42–47]. Still other studies failed to find any positive benefit of preventing neutrophil trafficking on neurological outcome [48, 49]. No clear explanation yet exists for these disparate findings. What is particularly notable about all of these studies is the virtually complete lack of independent determination of neutrophil levels or activity. Rather, these studies apparently assume that the treatment produces the desired effect on neutrophils with no confirmatory data. Despite that, when reductions in infarct size or improvements in function have been observed, they are attributed to (an undetermined) alteration in neutrophil activity. For all these reasons, while the results from these studies are intriguing, they do not satisfy conventional standards for establishing cause-effect relationships.

Studies using gene knockout animals

An alternative to pharmacologically manipulating neutrophils uses knockout animals that are deficient in specific genes with a purported role in cell trafficking (Tab. 4). Animals deficient in either the CD18 or ICAM-1 genes demonstrate reductions in ischemic infarct size [31, 76–78], improvements in neurological outcome [31], decreased mortality [31] and improved cerebral blood flow within the ischemic penumbra [31], relative to wild-type animals. However, not all results have been as

Table 4 - Knockout mice: neutrophil adhesion genes

Number of studies	% Confirming "knockout" reduced neutrophil infiltration into ischemic area	% Confirming decrease in infarct size	% Establishing relationship between cell trafficking and infarct size
9	0%	89%	0%

Knockout animals lacking specific genes with a suspected role in neutrophil trafficking and/or activity provide a potentially powerful approach for demonstrating a cause-effect relationship between neutrophils and ischemic cell death. Despite confirming significant decreases in infarct size, relative to wild-type animals, no studies to date have confirmed that the genetic manipulation reduces the extent of neutrophil invasion into the ischemic region. Accordingly, no study has provided clear support for a cause-effect relationship between neutrophils and ischemic damage. References comprising table: [31, 76–78].

clear or positive. For instance, Prestigiacomo and colleagues [77] found that CD18 knockouts showed significant reductions in infarct, but did not exhibit improvements in neurological outcome. Moreover, the reductions in infarct size were not apparent when the model was altered to include permanent, rather than, transient ischemia. Others [76] have found that ICAM-I knockouts showed a reduction in infarct size, compared to wild-type animals, without differences in the numbers of neutrophils in the cortex and striatum between the knockout animals and controls (wild-type). This finding raises the logical question of exactly what changes the knockout produced, as well as what role neutrophils might play. More fundamentally, no studies have monitored the infiltration of neutrophils into the ischemic tissue over time. Rather, all studies have examined neutrophils at time points when the majority of the infarct has already developed. While these data have been interpreted as support for a role of neutrophils in ischemic damage, the experimental designs do not allow a definitive cause-effect interpretations to be made. Again, the decreased neutrophil infiltration could simply be the result of, and not a cause of, the decreased ischemic damage.

Synopsis

An extensive literature has developed over the past 10 years that continues to offer intrigue to the hypothesis that neutrophils play a prominent role in the neuropathology of ischemia. Nonetheless, few studies have employed experimental designs required to generate data that fulfills conventional standards for establishing a cause-effect relationship. In this brief review we have attempted to provide an objective assessment of the available data, while at the same time offering an evaluation of the extent to which it supports the neutrophil hypothesis. While the designs of most experiments do not permit definitive conclusions to be drawn, more rigorous and complete experiments could easily be conducted. Along these lines, we offer some explicit suggestions for the type of evidence that needs to be generated to provide more definite evidence for a pathogenic role of neutrophils in ischemic brain damage.

References

1   Barone F, Hillegass L, Tzimas M, Schmidt D, Foley J, White R, Price W, Feuerstein G, Clark R, Griswold D, Sarau H (1995) Time-related changes in myeloperoxidase activity and leukotrine B4 receptor binding reflect leukocyte influx in cerebral focal stroke. *Mol Chem Neuropathol* 24: 13–30

2   Bednar M, Dooley R, Zamani M, Howard D, Gross C (1995) Neutrophil and platelet activity and quantification following delayed tPA therapy in a rabbit model of thromboembolic stroke. *J Thrombosis Thrombolysis* 1: 179–185

3   Zoppo G del, Schmid-Schonbein G, Mori E, Copeland B, Chang C-M (1991) Polymorphonuclear leukocytes occlude capillaries following middle cerebral artery occlusion and reperfusion in baboons. *Stroke* 22: 1276–1283

4   Hallenbeck J, Dutka A, Tanishima T, Kochanek P, Kumaroo K, Thompson C, Obrenovitch T, Contreras T (1986) Polymorphonuclear leukocyte accumulation in brain regions with low blood flow during the early postischemic period. *Stroke* 17: 246–253

5   Jander S, Kraemer M, Schroeter M, Witte O, Stoll G (1995) Lymphocytic infiltration and expression of intercellular adhesion molecule-1 in photochemically induced ischemia of the rat cortex. *J Cereb Blood Flow Metab* 15: 42–51

6   Ritter L, Orozco J, Coull B, McDonagh P (2000) Leukocyte accumulation and hemodynamic changes in the cerebral microcirculation during early reperfusion after stroke. *Stroke* 31: 1153–1161

7   Wang P-Y, Kao C-H, Mui M-Y, Wang S-J (1993) Leukocyte infiltration in acute hemispheric stroke. *Stroke* 24: 236–240

8   Hayward N, Elliott P, Sawyer S, Bronson R, Bartus R (1996) Lack of evidence for neutrophil participation during infarct formation following focal cerebral ischemia in the rat. *Exp Neurol* 139: 188–202

9   Akopov S, Simonian N, Grigorian G (1996) Dynamics of polymorphonuclear leukocyte accumulation in acute cerebral infarction and their correlation with brain tissue damage. *Stroke* 27: 1739–1743

10 Ahmed S-H, He Y, Nassief A, Xu J, Xu X, Hsu C (2000) Effects of lipopolysaccharide priming on acute ischemic brain injury. *Stroke* 31: 193–199

11   Barone F, Schmidt D, Hillegass L, Price W, White R, Feuerstein G, Clark R, Lee E, Griswold D, Sarau H (1992) Reperfusion increases neutrophils and leukotriene B4 receptor binding in rat focal ischemia. *Stroke* 23: 1337–1348

12   Clark R, Lee E, Fish C, White R, Price W, Jonak Z, Feuerstein G, Barone F (1993) Development of tissue damage, inflammation and resolution following stroke: An immunohistochemical and quantitative planimetric study. *Brain Res Bull* 31: 565–572

13   Clark R, Lee E, White R, Jonak Z, Feuerstein Z, Barone F (1994) Reperfusion following focal stroke hastens inflammation and resolution of ischemic injured tissue. *Brain Res Bull* 35: 387–392

14   Dereski M, Chopp M, Knight R, Chen H, Garcia J (1992) Focal cerebral ischemia in the rat: Temporal profile of neutrophil responses. *Neurosci Res Comm* 11: 179–186

15   Garcia J, Kamijyo Y (1974) Cerebral infarction: Evolution of histopathological changes after occlusion of a middle cerebral artery in primates. *J Neuropathol Exp Neurol* 33: 408–421

16   Garcia J, Liu K, Yoshida Y, Lian J, Chen S, Zoppo G del (1994) Influx of leukocytes and platelets in an evolving brain infarct (Wistar rat). *Am J Pathol* 144: 188–199

17   Kato H, Kogure K, Liu X-H, Araki T, Itoyama Y (1996) Progressive expression of immunomolecules on activated microglia and invading leukocytes following focal cerebral ischemia in the rat. *Brain Res* 734: 203–212

18   Lehrmann E, Christensen T, Zimmer J, Diemer N, Finsen B (1997) Microglial and macrophage reactions mark progressive changes and define the penumbra in the rat neocortex and striatum after transient middle cerebral artery occusion. *J Comp Neurol* 386: 461–476

19   Linsdsberg P, Carpen O, Oaetau A, Karjalainen-Lindsberg M-L, Kaste M (1996) Endothelial ICAM-1 expression associated with inflammatory cell response in human ischemic stroke. *Circulation* 94: 939–945

20   Matsuo Y, Onodera H, Shiga Y, Nakamura M, Ninomiya M, Kihara T, Kogure K (1994) Correlation between myeloperoxidase-quantified neutrophil accumulation and ischemic brain injury in the rat: Effects of neutrophil depletion. *Stroke* 25: 1469–1475

21   Matsuo Y, Onodera H, Shiga Y, Shozuhara H, Ninomiya M, Kihara T, Tamatani T, Miyasaka M, Kogure K (1994) Role of cell adhesion molecules in brain injury after transient middle cerebral artery occlusion in the rat. *Brain Res* 656: 344–352

22   Pozzilli C, Lenzi G, Argentino C, Carolei A, Rasura M, Signore A, Bozzao L, Pozzilli P (1985) Imaging of leukocyte infiltration in human cerebral infarcts. *Stroke* 16: 251–255

23   Schroeter M, Jaonder S, Witte O, Stoll G (1994) Local immune responses in the rat cerebral cortex after middle cerebral artery occlusion. *J Neuroimmunol* 55: 195–203

24   Yamasaki Y, Matsuo Y, Matsuura N, Shozuhara H, Onodera H, Itoyama Y, Kogure K (1995) Interleukin-1 as a pathogenic mediator of ischemic brain damage in rats. *Stroke* 26: 676–681

25   Zhang R-L, Chopp M, Chen H, Garcia J (1994) Temporal profile of ischemic tissue damage, neutrophil response, and vascular plugging following permanent and transient (2H) middle cerebral artery occlusion in the rat. *J Neurological Sci* 125: 3–10

26 Lopez O, Lanthorn T (1993) Anti-neutrophil antiserum reduces infarct volume after mouse permanent middle cerebral artery occlusion without producing neutropenia. *Neurosci Res Comm* 13: 45–53

27 Chen H, Chopp M, Bodzin G (1992) Neutropenia reduces the volume of cerebral infarct after transient middle cerebral artery occlusion in the rat. *Neurosci Res Comm* 11: 93–99

28 Dutka A, Kochanek P, Hallenbeck J (1989) Influence of granulocytopenia on canine cerebral ischemia induced by air embolism. *Stroke* 20: 390–395

29 Helps S, Gorman D (1991) Air embolism of the brain in rabbits pretreated with mechlorethamine. *Stroke* 22: 351–354

30 Shiga Y, Onodera Y, Kogure K, Yamasaki Y, Yashima Y, Syozuhara H, Sendo F (1991) Neutrophil as a mediator of ischemic edema formation in the brain. *Neurosci Letts* 125: 110–112

31 Connolly E, Winfree C, Springer T, Naka Y, Liao H, Yan D, Stern D, Solomon R, Gutierrez-Ramos J-C, Pinsky D (1996) Cerebral protection in homozygous null ICAM-1 mice after middle cerebral artery occlusion: Role of neutrophil adhesion in the pathogenesis of stroke. *J Clin Invest* 97: 209–216

32 Bednar M, Raymond S, McAuliffe T, Lodge P, Gross C (1991) The role of neutrophils and platelets in a rabbit model of thromboembolic stroke. *Stroke* 22: 44–50

33 Chabner B, Allegra C, Curt G, Calabresi P (1996) Antineoplastic agents. In: J Jardman et al (eds): *Goodman and Gilman's the pharmacological basis of therapeutics*. McGraw Hill, 1233–1287

34 Härtl R, Schurer L, Schmid-Schonbein GW, Zoppo G del (1996) Experimental anti-leukocyte interventions in cerebral ischemia. *J Cereb Blood Flow Metab* 16: 1108–1119

35 Chopp M, Li Y, Jiang N, Zhang R, Prostak J (1996) Antibodies against adhesion molecules reduce apoptosis after transient middle cerebral artery occlusion in rat brain. *J Cereb Blood Flow Metab* 16: 578–584

36 Shiga Y, Onodera H, Matsuo Y, Kogure K (1992) Cyclosporin A protects against ischemia-reperfusion injury in the brain. *Brain Res* 595: 145–148

37 Zhang R, Chopp M, Jiang N, Tang W, Prostak J, Manning A, Anderson D (1995) Anti-intercellular adhesion molecule-1 antibody reduces ischemic call damage after transient but not permanent middle cerebral artery occlusion in the Wistar rat. *Stroke* 26: 1438–1443

38 Zhang R, Chopp M, Tang W, Zhang Z, Putney S, Starzyk R (1996) Synthetic peptide derived from the *Bordetella pertussis* bacterium reduces infarct volume after transient middle cerebral artery occlusion in the rat. *Neurol* 46: 1437–1441

39 Kochanek P, Dutka A, Kumaroo K, Hallenbeck J (1987) Platelet activating factor receptor blockade enhances recovery after multifocal brain ischemia. *Life Sci* 41: 2639–2644

40 Bowes M, Zivin J, Rothlein R (1993) Monoclonal antibody to the ICAM-1 adhesion site reduces neurological damage in a rabbit cerebral embolism stroke model. *Exp Neurol* 119: 215–219

41 Bowes M, Rothlein R, Fagans S, Zivin J (1995) Monolconal antibodies preventing

leukocyte activation reduce experimental neurologic injury and enhance efficacy of thrombolytic therapy. *Neurol* 45: 815–819

42 Gross C, Howard D, Dooley R, Raymond S, Fuller S, Bednar M (1994) TGF-b1 post-treatment in a rabbit model of cerebral ischaemia. *Neurological Res* 16: 465–470

43 Garcia J, Liu K-F, Bree M (1995) Effects of CD11b/18 monoclonal antibody on rats with permanent middle cerebral artery occlusion. *Am J Pathol* 148: 241–248

44 Garcia J, Liu K-F, Relton J (1995) Interleukin-1 receptor antagonist decreases the number of necrotic neurons in rats with middle cerebral artery occlusion. *Am J Pathol* 147: 1477–1486

45 Jiang N, Zhang R, Chen H, Chopp M (1994) Anti-CD11B monoclonal antibody reduces ischemic cell damage after transient (2h) but not after permanent MCA occlusion in the rat. *Neurosci Res Comm* 15: 85–93

46 Jiang N, Chopp M, Chahwala S (1998) Neutrophil inhibitory factor treatment of focal cerebral ischemia in the rat. *Brain Res* 788: 25–34

47 Takeshima R, Kirsch J, Koehler R, Gomoll A, Traystman R (1992) Monoclonal leukocyte antibody does not decrease the injury of transient focal cerebral ischemia in cats. *Stroke* 23: 247–252

48 Clark W, Madden K, Rothlein R, Zivin J (1991) Reduction of central nervous system ischemic injury by monoclonal antibody to intracellular adhesion molecule. *J Neurosurg* 75: 623–627

49 Clark W, Madden K, Rothlein R, Zivin J (1991) Reduction of central nervous system ischemic injury in rabbits using leukocyte adhesion antibody treatment. *Stroke* 22: 877–883

50 Zhang R, Chopp M, Li Y, Zaloga C, Jiang N, Jones M, Miyasaka M, Ward P (1994) Anti-ICAM-1 antibody reduces ischemic cell damage after transient middle cerebral artery occlusion in the rat. *Neurol* 44: 1747–1751

51 Zhang R, Zhang Z, Chopp M (1999) Increased therapeutic efficacy with rt-PA and anti-CD18 antibody treatment of stroke in the rat. *Neurol* 52: 273–279

52 Yanaka K, Camarata P, Spellman S, Skubitz A, Furcht L, Low W (1997) Laminin peptide ameliorates brain injury by inhibiting leukocyte accumulation in a rat model of transient focal cerebral ischemia. *J Cereb Blood Flow Metab* 17: 605–611

53 Yanaka K, Camarata P, Spellman S, McCarthy J, Furcht L, Low W (1997) Antagonism of leukocyte adherence by synthetic fibronectin peptide V in a rat model of transient focal cerebral ischemia. *Neurosurg* 40: 557–564

54 Yanaka K, Spellman S, McCarthy J, Low W, Camarata P (1996) Reduction of brain injury using heparin to inhibit leukocyte accuulation in a rat model of transient focal cerebral ischemia I: Protective mechanism. *J Neurosurg* 85: 1102–1107

55 Yanaka K, Spellman S, McCarthy J, Low W, Camarata P (1996) Reduction of brain injury using heparin to inhibit leukocyte accumulation in a rat model of transient focal cerebral ischemia II: Dose-response effect and the therapeutic window. *J Neurosurg* 85: 1108–1112

56 Toyoda T, Suzuki S, Kassell N, Lee K (1996) Intraischemic hypothermia attenuates neu-

trophil infiltration in the rat neocortex after focal ischemia-reperfusion injury. *Neurosurg* 39: 1200–1205

57   Spera P, Ellison J, Feuerstein G, Barone F (1998) IL-10 reduces rat brain injury following focal stroke. *Neurosci Lett* 251: 189–192

58   Shimakura A, Kamanaka Y, Ikeda Y, Kondo K, Suzuki Y, Umemura K (2000) Neutrophil elastase inhibition reduces cerebral ischemic damage in the middle cerebral artery occlusion. *Brain Res* 858: 55–60

59   Relton J, Martin D, Thompson R, Russell D (1996) Peripheral administration of interleukin-1 receptor antagonist inhibits brain damage after focal cerebral ischemia in the rat. *Exp Neurol* 138: 206–213

60   Relton J, Rothwell N (1992) Interleukin-1 receptor antagonist inhibits ischaemic and excitotoxic neuronal damage in the rat. *Brain Res Bull* 29: 243–246

61   Prehn J, Backhauss C, Krieglstein J (1993) Transforming growth factor-B1 prevents gluatmate neurotoxicity in rat neocortical cultures and protects mouse neocortex from ischemic injury *in vivo*. *J Cereb Blood Flow Metab* 13: 521–525

62   Phillips J, Williams A, Adams J, Elliott P, Tortella F (2000) Proteasome inhibitor PS 519 reduces infarction and attenuates leukocyte infiltration in a rat model of focal cerebral ischemia. *Stroke* 31: 1686–1693

63   Nawashiro H, Martin D, Hallenbeck J (1997) Neuroprotective effects of TNF binding protein in focal cerebral ischemia. *Brain Res* 778: 265–271

64   Nawashiro H, Martin D, Hallenbeck J (1997) Inhibition of tumor necrosis factor and amelioration of brain infarction in mice. *J Cereb Blood Flow Metab* 17: 229–232

65   Mori E, Zoppo G del, Chambers J, Copeland B, Arfors K (1992) Inhibition of polymorphonuclear leukocyte adherence suppresses no-reflow after focal cerebral ischemia. *Stroke* 23: 712–718

66   Matsumoto T, Ikeda K, Mukaida N, Harada A, Matsumoto Y, Yamashita J, Matsushima K (1997) Prevention of cerebral edema and infarct in cerebral reperfusion injury by an antibody to interleukin-8. *Lab Invest* 77: 119–125

67   Loddick S, Rothwell N (1996) Neuroprotective effects of human recombinant interleukin-1 receptor antagonist in focal cerebral ischaemia in the rat. *J Cereb Blood Flow Metab* 16: 932–940

68   Kochanek P, Dutka A, Hallenbeck J (1987) Indomethacin, prostacyclin, and heparin improve postischemic cerebral blood flow without affecting early postischemic granulocyte accumulation. *Stroke* 18: 634–637

69   Jiang N, Moyle M, Soule H, Rote W, Chopp M (1995) Neutrophil inhibitory factor after focal ischemia in rats. Ann Neurol 38: 935–942

70   Gross C, Bednar M, Howard D, Sporn M (1993) Transforming growth factor-β1 reduced infarct size after experimental cerebral ischemia in a rabbit model. *Stroke* 24: 558–562

71   Dawson D, Martin D, Hallenbeck J (1996) Inhibition of tumor necrosis factor-alpha reduces focal cerebral ischemic injury in the spontaneously hypertensive rat. *Neurosci Lett* 218: 41–44

72 Chopp M, Zhang R, Chen H, Li Y, Jiang N, Rusche J (1994) Postischemic administration of an anti-Mac-1 antibody reduces ischemic cell damage after transient middle cerebral artery occlusion in rats. *Stroke* 25: 869–876

73 Chen H, Chopp M, Zhang R, Bodzin G, Chen Q, Rusche J, Todd R (1994) Anti-CD11b monoclonal antibody reduces ischemic cell damage after transient focal cerebral ischemia in rat. *Ann Neurol* 35: 458–463

74 Bielenberg G, Wagener G, Beck T (1992) Infarct reduction by the platelet activating factor antagonist apafant in rats. *Stroke* 23: 98–103

75 Barone F, Arvin B, White R, Miller A, Webb C, Willette R, Lysko P, Feuerstein G (1997) Tumor necrosis factor-α: A mediator of focal ischemic brain injury. *Stroke* 28: 1233–1244

76 Kitagawa K, Matsumoto M, Mabuchi T, Yagita Y, Ohtsuki T, Hori M, Yanagihara T (1998) Deficiency of intercellular adhesion molecule-1 attenuates microcirculatory disturbance and infarction size in focal cerebral ischemia. *J Cereb Blood Flow Metab* 18: 1336–1345

77 Prestigiacomo C, Kim S, Connolly E, Liao H, Yan S, Pinsky D (1999) CD18-mediated neutrophil recruitment contributes to the pathogenesis of reperfused but not nonreperfused stroke. *Stroke* 30: 1110–1117

78 Soriano S, Lipton S, Wang Y, Xiao M, Springer T, Guiterrez-Ramos J-C, Hickey P (1996) Intercellular adhesion molecule-1-deficient mice are less susceptible to cerebral ischemia-reperfusion injury. *Ann Neurol* 39: 618–624

A more thorough review of this literature and discussion can be found in:
Emerich DF, Dean RL, Bartus RT (2001) A critical evaluation of experimental data addressing a pathogenic role of neutrophils in ischemia. *Exp Neurol; submitted*

The role of microglia in ischemic brain injury

Hiroyuki Kato

Departments of Neurology and Neuroendovascular Therapy, Field of Neuroscience, Tohoku University Graduate School of Medicine, 1-1 Seiryo-machi, Aoba-ku, Sendai 980-8574, Japan

Introduction

Microglia are ubiquitously distributed through the normal adult brain. They form 5–12% of the total number of cells in the mouse brain [1], and constitute about 13% of the glial population in human white matter [2]. Resting microglia are thought to be in a down-regulated form of the cells of the mononuclear phagocyte system. They represent a stable cell pool, and are replenished only rarely by hematogenous cells [3]. Microglia are activated under various pathological conditions, and may develop into brain macrophages when neurons are severely damaged. Studies *in vitro* have shown that microglia, when stimulated, release a variety of cytotoxic agents that may be important mediators of neuronal injury, such as certain kinds of cytokines, reactive oxygen radicals, proteases, and glutamate [4], and that fully activated microglia are phagocytes [5]. Thus, a pathogenic role for microglia has been emphasized. However, microglial effects of tissue damage *in vivo* appear to be under strict control. There are various levels of microglial activation, and microglial activation per se is not always pathogenic.

The normal brain has long been believed to be an immunologically privileged site since it is isolated from the systemic circulation and is able to exclude components of the immune system by the blood-brain barrier (BBB) [6]. Immune cells such as polymorphonuclear leukocytes (PMNs) and monocytes migrate only in response to tissue damage of the brain, and infiltration of these hematogenous leukocytes is added to the local inflammatory response composed of activation of resident microglia. Perivascular cells are the third component of inflammatory cells in the brain. They can be distinguished from resident microglia by their unique localization, being part of vascular wall, and by constitutive expression of immunomolecules such as major histocompatibility complex (MHC) class II antigen and ED2, which are not expressed in resting microglia [7, 8]. Perivascular cells are thought to be the only population of constitutive macrophage-like cells in the brain.

The inflammatory response in the ischemic brain may recruit these subclasses of inflammatory cells, both intrinsic and extrinsic, depending on the nature of injury.

Inflammation and Stroke, edited by Giora Z. Feuerstein

Largely, microglia are the first cells to respond to pathological stimuli, and may be the sole source of inflammatory cells; when the brain is severely damaged, migration of circulating leukocytes may aid or override the lesion. This chapter will provide an overview of the inflammatory response, especially microglial activation, in experimental cerebral ischemia, and discuss the role for microglia in the pathogenesis of ischemic brain damage.

Microglial activation

It has been well documented that microglia are a source of brain macrophages in cerebral ischemia and infarction [9]. However, little is known about the pathogenic role of microglia during the development of ischemic brain damage and the functional characteristics of microglia before undergoing phagocytic transformation. The microglial activation occurs in a stepwise manner, and consists of characteristic events regarding cellular morphology, size and number, the expression of immunomolecules on cell surface, and the production of cytokines and growth factors. Obviously, microglial activation is accompanied by altered gene expression, but we have just begun to understand the detailed mechanisms. We use the following classification for describing the stage of microglial activation [10]. Microglia at different stages of activation appear to have different roles in supporting and damaging neurons in cerebral ischemia.

1. Resting microglia, which are highly ramified cells present in normal adult brain.
2. Activated microglia, which are cells responding to ischemia with morphological and immunophenotypic changes, but are not phagocytic. Morphological changes include enlarged cell bodies and contraction of their processes to show a more stout morphology. The number of immunomolecules expressed is limited.
3. Phagocytic microglia, which are full-blown brain macrophages with an amoeboid morphology and expression of a number of immunomolecules that is shared with cells of the mononuclear phagocyte lineage.

Microglial activation in cerebral ischemia

This section describes the morphological and immunological features of reactive glial and inflammatory cells following cerebral ischemia in the rat. Special attention is paid to the relation between the severity of ischemic brain damage and the induced inflammatory response (Tab. 1). Two cerebral ischemia models, i.e., global and focal cerebral ischemia, are described separately. Three stages of brain injury can be classified in these ischemia models: (1) sublethal injury, (2) selective neuronal damage sparing glial cells, and (3) infarction damaging all the cellular components

Table 1 - Stepwise microglial responses to different severity of ischemic brain injury

Ischemic injury	Microglial activation	Immunomolecules expressed by microglia
1. Normal brain	Resting microglia	CR3
2. Sublethal injury	Activated microglia (transient)	CR3, MHC class I
3. Selective neuronal damage (Global ischemia or peri-infarct regions)	Early activation (activated microglia) followed by neuronal death-induced full activation to phagocytic microglia	CR3, MHC class I CR3, MHC class I and II, LCA, CD4, ED1
4 Infarction (core)	Early destruction of microglia (Invasion of leukocytes)	(The same molecules are expressed on invading monocytes)

of the tissue including glial cells. The latter two settings are extreme forms of brain damage, so that any changes that stand in between may occur, such as those that may be called incomplete infarction or unsalvaged penumbra.

Global cerebral ischemia

The vulnerability of brain cells to brief periods of transient global ischemia is particularly evident in the hippocampus where selective neuronal damage to CA1 neurons is prominent, whereas CA3 neurons and dentate granule neurons are resistant (sublethal injury). The CA1 neuronal damage takes a characteristic time-course called delayed neuronal death, which becomes apparent 2–4 days after 10 min of ischemia [11], and is accompanied by remarkable glial reactions involving both astroglia and microglia [12, 13]. The reactive astrocytes are characterized by hypertrophy and enhanced expression of glial fibrillary acidic protein (GFAP), starting within 1–2 days, reaching a peak by 7 days and maintained for several weeks [14].

The microglial response in the hippocampus is of very early onset occurring within minutes after reperfusion [12, 15]. This early microglial activation occurs rather generally in the entire hippocampus, and is not confined to CA1. This initial phase is characterized by the presence of activated microglia, which is demonstrated by characteristic morphological changes (hypertrophy) as well as increased staining of microglial markers, such as isolectin-B4 from *Griffonia simplicifolia* [16], complement receptor type 3 (CR3 or OX42) [12], and microglial response factor-1 (MRF-1) [13, 17]. This initial activation is followed by an expression of a limited number of immunomolecules within a day, such as the up-regulation of constitutively expressed CR3 and *de novo* synthesis of the MHC class I antigen [12, 18, 19]. These changes may return toward normal by 7 days in brain regions where no neuronal damage follows.

Microglia are further activated when neuronal damage becomes apparent in CA1 by 2–4 days. This neuronal death-induced reaction is protracted, and microglia may remain in an activated state for up to 1 month [18, 19]. The morphology of the fully activated microglia is of amoeboid form, suggesting that they are phagocytes. These phagocytic microglia now express a number of immunomolecules that are shared with cells of the macrophage lineage, such as the MHC class I and class II antigens, the leukocyte common antigen (LCA), CD4, and ED1 [12, 18, 19]. In addition, microglia can proliferate and adapt their morphology to the shape of damaged structures. The microglial processes may extend star-like in all directions, or microglia in the CA1 stratum radiatum may exhibit a polarity in the direction of the proximal dendrites of CA1 neurons, showing the classic pattern of rod cells. Interestingly, the immunomolecules expressed during microglial activation are required for antigen presentation in the T-cell-mediated immune process. However, the upregulation of the MHC antigens by microglia can occur in the absence of T-lymphocyte infiltration [12, 18, 19]. Their activation may not imply that they are truly antigen-presenting cells within the context of a T-cell-mediated immune process. Thus, the sequential expression of imunomolecules appears to reflect a programmed cellular response during microglial activation that occurs as a result of ischemia and subsequent neuronal injury. Infiltration of blood-borne leukocytes and the activation of perivascular cells are not observed in this lesion paradigm.

Focal cerebral ischemia

Focal ischemia contains differently damaged areas. One is the ischemic core where infarction develops and all constituents of the tissue are destroyed. Microglia as well as astroglia may be killed in this densely ischemic region, and blood-borne leukocytes readily infiltrate the region and monocytes constitute the major source of macrophages in this necrotic region. The other is the penumbra, which is a marginally perfused, metabolically unstable zone and is ultimately involved in infarction unless reperfusion or treatment is provided. The transitional or peri-infarct zone is the location of striking microglial as well as astroglial activation. Since phagocytic microglia share many marker antigens with the circulating monocytes, the marker antigens alone do not allow differentiation between microglia-derived and blood-borne macrophages.

The findings in a rat model of transient focal ischemia, in which 1 h of middle cerebral artery occlusion followed by reperfusion is achieved by an intraluminal occlusion of the artery [20], are described below (Fig. 1). The microglial activation in the penumbra is similar in two regards to the microglial reaction to transient

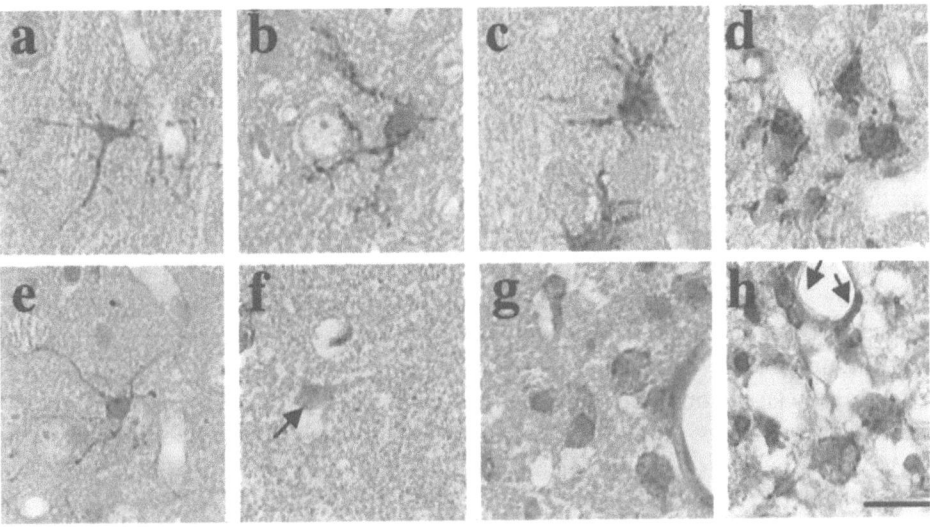

Figure 1

Microglial response following 1 h of middle cerebral artery occlusion in the rat visualized with immunohistochemistry for microglial response factor-1, a microglia/macrophage marker, counterstained with hematoxylin and eosin. a–d: Changes in the penumbra (neocortex). a: Resting microglia in normal cortex. b,c: Activated microglia encircle cortical neurons, which are not morphologically compromised, after 4 h (b) and 1 day (c). d: After 7 days, amoeboid, phagocytic microglia exhibit neuronophagia. e–h: Changes in the ischemic core (striatum). e: Resting microglia in normal striatum. f: After 1 day, all tissue constituents appear damaged. Damaged neurons (arrow) appear eosinophilic without nuclear stainability. No microglia are seen. g: After 3 days, round cells (monocytes) infiltrate the area of infarction. h: After 7 days, infarction further develops and macrophages cover the lesion. The arrows in h indicate hypertrophied perivascular cells. Bar in h is 20 µm and applies to all.

global ischemia [20]. First, early activation of microglia is seen in this area. Activated microglia, as identified by their enlarged size, stout processes, and intense staining characteristics, are observed starting within a few hours and becoming conspicuous by 1 day. Activated microglia are found very close to neurons and microglial processes encircle neurons in the penumbra. Similar, but transient, microglial reaction is also seen in outer areas of the hemisphere where no neurons are damaged. The microglial activation becomes striking by 3 days and reaches a peak by 7 days in the transitional, peri-infarct zone. Second, the expression of immunomolecules, such as MHC antigens, occurs in a sequential and progressive manner. The peri-infarct microglia express various immunomolecules and macrophage-like antigens including the MHC class II antigen and ED1, suggesting a recruitment of microglia-derived macrophages from this transitional zone into the infarction.

Most remarkable changes occur in the ischemic core where infarction develops [20]. All constituents of the tissue including astroglia and microglia are destroyed rapidly (pan-necrosis), the BBB is breached, and the invasion of leukocytes predominates in the inflammatory reaction [21, 22]. PMNs (neutrophils) begin to infiltrate into ischemic tissue 12 h after ischemia, reach a peak after 1-3 days, and disappear by 7 days. Monocytes invade massively as the second wave after 2 to 3 days and cover the entire lesion by 7 days. Both PMNs and monocytes express a number of immunomolecules and adhesion molecules on their cell surface. They express CR3, MHC class I and II antigens, and ED1, which are also expressed on microglia-derived macrophages. Within the infarction, the third component perivascular cells are also activated morphologically and phenotypically, and transform into macrophages [9, 13]. T cells are also seen within the infarct [20, 23].

There are three major steps for the infiltration of leukocytes: (1) rolling, (2) adhesion, and (3) transendothelial migration [24, 25]. All the processes are facilitated by an interaction of specific ligands that are constitutively expressed on leukocytes and receptors on the surface of endothelial cells that are inducible by ischemic stimuli. The first stage (rolling) is mediated by a family of adhesion molecules called selectins. Selectins consist of P-selectin and E-selectin on endothelial cells and L-selectin on leukocytes, and are upregulated by ischemia [26]. The binding of leukocytes to the vasculature is strengthened under the influence of chemokines that are released from the site of injury: interleukin (IL)-8 provokes PMN recruitment [27] and monocyte chemoattractant protein-1 is specific for monocytes [28]. On activation, firm adherence of leukocytes to the endothelial cells is mediated by the binding of a leukocyte membrane glycoprotein receptor complex termed integrin to its endothelial ligand intercellular adhesion molecule (ICAM)-1, ICAM-2, and vascular cell adhesion molecule (VCAM)-1 [29, 30]. ICAM-1 is inducible by proinflammatory cytokines such as IL-1 and tumor necrosis factor-α (TNFα) [31]. The integrin complex consists of three heterodimers. All three share a common β-subunit (CD18) and are distinguished from each other by distinct α-subunits. They are termed leukocyte function associated antigen-1 (LFA-1 or CD11a, present on all leukocytes), Mac-1 (CD11b, present mostly on PMNs and monocytes), and p150,95 (CD11c, present on neutrophils and monocytes). In the final stage, the leukocyte adhering to the endothelium migrates between endothelial cells into the brain tissue. The infiltration of PMNs and monocytes may not only be associated with tissue repair processes, but also may result in injury to potentially viable tissue. The secondary damage may be produced by (1) a reduction of blood flow by capillary plugging or vasoconstrictive mediator release [21], and (2) release of cytotoxic substances such as proteases, oxygen free radicals, nitric oxide, and lipid-derived mediators [21, 32, 33].

The role of microglia in ischemic neuronal damage

These observations allow us to summarize different microglial responses to varying degrees of ischemic neuronal injury ranging from sublethal injury to selective neuronal damage to infarction (Tab. 1). The inflammatory response and recruitment of macrophages are very different among these brain lesions. Even sublethal ischemia activates microglia and astroglia. Microglia in this setting are morphologically activated but do not express macrophage antigens. Selective neuronal damage induces strong, protracted activation of both microglia and astroglia. Microglia are the sole source of brain macrophages here, and express the full panel of immunomolecules that are seen in macrophages. In contrast, the inflammatory response in an area of infarction is complicated by the invasion of blood-borne inflammatory cells. Three classes of mononuclear phagocytes/macrophages are seen: phagocytic microglia (brain macrophages) in peri-infarct regions and blood-borne monocytes/macrophages and perivascular cells within the infarction. The relative importance of each source may be determined by the nature of the specific lesion. Probably, monocytes invade the center of ischemia through the compromised BBB, and microglia-derived macrophages are recruited from the peri-infarct zones during the periods in which the penumbra is involved in infarction. These macrophages may respond to tissue injury by secretion of cytotoxic agents and phagocytosis of damaged neurons, as well as by release of growth factors to promote wound healing.

Microglia are the first non-neuronal cell to respond to acute cerebral ischemia, and the activation is induced within minutes. Microglia are an extremely sensitive indicator of subtle, morphologically non-apparent neuronal injury during the early stage of cerebral ischemia and even after sublethal ischemia. These findings emphasize that stimuli other than neuronal death initiate the early activation of microglia. The stimuli might be ischemia-induced changes in metabolism, or changes in ion and acid-base balances in microenvironment. High extracellular potassium concentration could activate microglia because of their high sensitivity to depolarization due to unique characteristics of their potassium channels [34], and in fact, cortical spreading depression elicits microglial activation [35]. Another hypothesis is that injured neurons release ATP, which activates microglial purinoreceptors and induces Ca^{2+} fluxes, leading to microglial activation [36]. When neuronal death develops later, microglia transform into true brain macrophages phagocytosing neuronal debris [37]. Microglia are capable of recognizing damaged neurons, and therefore it is reasonable to assume the presence of neuronal injury signals. Identification of such signals for microglial activation remains to be shown, but the signals may become a great clue for understanding the mechanism of ischemic neuronal death.

Microglia *in vitro* can be induced to proliferate in response to cytokines, such as ILs and colony-stimulating factors (CSFs). Microglia, on the other hand, express macrophage-derived cytokines such as IL-1 and IL-6, TNFα, and macrophage CSF [38]. The time-dependent manner of immunomolecule expression after ischemia suggests that the microglial activation program is initiated and maintained by some stimulatory factors including certain cytokines. Although the precise functions of microglia are not yet fully understood, fully activated microglia could then be capable of cell killing either by mechanisms involving direct cell-to-cell contacts, or by release of potentially cytotoxic substances, and then phagocytose dead neurons [37]. *In vitro* studies clearly suggest that microglia kill neurons by secreting nitric oxide, oxygen free radicals, glutamate, and other cytotoxic substances [4, 39, 40].

The functional significance of activated microglia that are seen in areas without neuronal damage is little understood, and a supportive role of activated microglia might be postulated [41]. Of particular interest in this regard is the phenomenon called synaptic stripping [42]. Activated microglia induced after facial nerve axotomy encircle closely the axotomized motoneurons and displace afferent synaptic terminals from the surface of regenerating motoneurons. If such deafferentation occurs following ischemic insults, it may protect the neurons against ischemic damage since excitotoxicity caused by exposure to glutamate is blocked. This close position of microglia may be essential for the detection of neuronal injury signals and for microglial intervention to neurons. The hypothesis that activated microglia promote neuronal regeneration is supported by the *in vitro* findings of microglial production of neurotrophins [43, 44]. The encirclement of injured neurons by activated microglia could be viewed simply as preparation for neurotoxicity and phagocytosis, but it is also likely that microglia detect neuronal signals to determine whether the neuron is still viable or not and whether they produce neurotrophic or neurotoxic factors. Such stepwise microglial activation is likely since activated microglia attached to normal-appearing neurons do not express macrophage antigens, but phagocytic microglia encircling dying or dead neurons do, although histopathological observations have not elucidated the functional significance of this process.

Conclusion

It appears clear that microglia have profound influences in determining neuronal survival and death following cerebral ischemia. Generally, the activation of microglia is thought to indicate certain neuronal damage, but there is evidence that the microglial activation is not always pathogenic. Microglial activation is stepwise and strictly controlled, and microglial response reflects the severity of injury. Microglia may exert both neurotoxic and neuroprotective actions depending on the specific circumstances that elicit microglial activation. Although some of the ideas are still hypothetical, uncovering the molecular mechanisms underlying the microglial activation and function remains a great challenge and will provide better understanding of the pathogenesis of cerebral ischemia and a clue for the development of novel strategies for the treatment of stroke.

References

1   Lawson LJ, Perry VH, Dri P, Gordon S (1990) Heterogeneity in the distribution and morphology of microglia in the normal adult mouse brain. *Neuroscience* 39: 151–170

2   Hayes GM, Woodroofe MN, Cuzner ML (1987) Microglia are the major cell type expressing MHC class II in human white matter. *J Neurol Sci* 80: 25–37

3   Lawson LJ, Perry VH, Gordon S (1992) Turnover of resident microglia in the normal adult mouse brain. *Neuroscience* 48: 405–415

4   Banati RB, Gehrmann J, Schubert P, Kreutzberg GW (1993) Cytotoxicity of microglia. *Glia* 7: 111–118

5   Giulian D (1987) Ameboid microglia as effectors of inflammation in the central nervous system. *J Neurosci Res* 18: 155–171

6   Fabry Z, Raine CS, Hart MN (1994) Nervous tissue as an immune compartment: the dialect of the immune response in the CNS. *Immunol Today* 15: 218–224

7   Graeber MB, Streit WJ, Kreutzberg GW (1989) Identity of ED2-positive perivascular cells in rat brain. *J Neurosci Res* 22: 103–106.

8   Mato M, Ookawara S, Sakamoto A, Aikawa E, Ogawa T, Mitsuhashı U, Masuzawa T, Suzuki H, Honda M, Yazaki Y et al (1996) Involvement of specific macrophage-like lineage cells surrounding arterioles in barrier and scavenger function in brain cortex. *Proc Natl Acad Sci USA* 93: 3269–374

9   Brierley JB, Brown AW (1982) The origin of lipid phagocytes in the central nervous system: I. The intrinsic microglia. *J Comp Neurol* 211: 397–406

10 Kato H, Walz W (2000) The initiation of the microglial response. *Brain Pathol* 10: 137–143

11 Kirino T, Tamura A, Sano K (1984) Delayed neuronal death in the rat hippocampus following transient forebrain ischemia. *Acta Neuropathol* 64: 139–147

12 Kato H, Kogure K, Araki T, Itoyama Y (1995) Graded expression of immunomolecules on activated microglia in the hippocampus following ischemia in a rat model of ischemic tolerance. *Brain Res* 694: 85–93

13 Kato H, Tanaka S, Oikawa T, Koike T, Takahashi A, Itoyama Y (2000) Expression of microglial response factor-1 in microglia and macrophages following cerebral ischemia in the rat. *Brain Res* 882: 206–211

14 Schmidt-Kastner R, Szymas J, Hossmann K-A (1990) Immunohistochemical study of glial reaction and serum protein extravasation in relation to neuronal damage in rat hippocampus after ischemia. *Neuroscience* 38: 527–540

15 Morioka T, Kalehua AN, Streit WJ (1991) The microglial reaction in the rat dorsal hippocampus following transient forebrain ischemia. *J Cereb Blood Flow Metab* 11: 966–973

16 Streit WJ (1990) An improved staining method for rat microglial cells using the lectin from *Griffonia simplicifolia* (GSA I-B4). *J Histochem Cytochem* 38: 1683–1686

17 Tanaka S, Suzuki K, Watanabe M, Matsuda A, Tone S, Koike T (1998) Upregulation of

a new microglial gene, mrf-1, in response to programmed neuronal cell death and degeneration. *J Neurosci* 18: 6358–6369

18 Morioka T, Kalehua AN, Streit WJ (1992) Progressive expression of immunomolecules on microglial cells in rat dorsal hippocampus following transient forebrain ischemia. *Acta Neuropathol* 83: 149–157

19 Gehrmann J, Bonnekoh P, Miyazawa T, Hossmann K-A (1992) Immunohistochemical study of an early microglial activation in ischemia. *J Cereb Blood Flow Metab* 12: 257–269

20 Kato H, Kogure K, Liu X-H, Araki T, Itoyama Y (1996) Progressive expression of immunomolecules on activated microglia and invading leukocytes following focal cerebral ischemia in the rat. *Brain Res* 734: 203–212

21 Kochaneck PM, Hallenbeck JM (1992) Polymorphonuclear leukocytes and monocytes/macrophages in the pathogenesis of cerebral ischemia and stroke. *Stroke* 23: 1367–1379

22 Matsuo Y, Onodera H, Shiga Y, Nakamura M, Kihara T, Kogure K (1994) Correlation between myeloperoxidase-quantified neutrophil accumulation and ischemic brain injury in the rat. Effect of neutrophil depletion. *Stroke* 25: 1469–1475

23 Schroeter M, Jander S, Witte OW, Stoll G (1994) Local immune responses in the rat cerebral cortex after middle cerebral artery occlusion. *J Neuroimmunol* 55: 195–203

24 Kishimoto TK, Rothlein R (1994) Integrins, ICAMs and selectins: role and regulation of adhesion molecules in neutrophil recruitment to inflammatory sites. *Adv Pharmacol* 25: 117–169

25 Clark WM, Zivin JA (1997) Antileukocyte adhesion therapy: preclinical trials and combination therapy. *Neurology* 49 (Suppl 4): S32–S38

26 Zhang R, Chopp M, Zhang Z, Jiang N, Powers C (1998) The expression of P-and E-selectins in three models of middle cerebral artery occlusion. *Brain Res* 785: 207–214

27 Liu T, Young PR, McDonnell PC, White RF, Barone FC, Feuerstein GZ (1993) Cytokine-induced neutrophil chemoattractant mRNA expressed in cerebral ischemia. *Neurosci Lett* 164: 125–128

28 Wang X, Yue TL, Barone FC, Feuerstein GZ (1995) Monocyte chemoattractant protein-1 messenger RNA expression in rat ischemic cortex. *Stroke* 26: 661–665

29 Zhang RL, Chopp M, Zalonga C, Zhang ZG, Jiang N, Gautam SC, Tang WX, Tsang W, Anderson DC, Manning AM (1995) The temporal profiles of ICAM-1 protein and mRNA expression after transient MCA occlusion in the rat. *Brain Res* 682: 182–188

30 Jander S, Pohl J, Gillen C, Schroeter M, Stoll G (1996) Vascular cell adhesion molecule-1 mRNA is expressed in immune-mediated and ischemic injury of the rat nervous system. *J Neuroimmunol* 70: 75–80

31 Matsuo Y, Onodera H, Shiga Y, Shozuhara H, Ninomiya M, Kihara T, Tamatani T, Miyasaka M, Kogure K (1994) Role of cell adhesion molecules in brain injury after transient middle cerebral artery occlusion in the rat. *Brain Res* 656: 344–352

32 Matsuo Y, Kihara T, Ikeda M, Ninomiya M, Onodera H, Kogure K (1995) Role of neutrophils in radical production during ischemia and reperfusion of the rat brain: effect of

neutrophil depletion on extracellular ascorbyl radical formation. *J Cereb Blood Flow Metab* 15: 941–947

33   Iadecola C, Zhang F, Xu S, Casey R, Ross E (1995) Inducible nitric oxide synthase gene expression in brain following cerebral ischemia. *J Cereb Blood Flow Metab* 15: 378–384

34   Kettenmann H, Hoppe D, Gottmann K, Banati R, Kreutzberg GW (1990) Cultured microglial cells have a distinct pattern of membrane channels different from peritoneal macrophages. *J Neurosci Res* 26: 278–287

35   Gehrmann J, Mies G, Bonnekoh P, Banati R, Iijima T, Kreutzberg GW, Hossmann K-A (1993) Microglial reaction in the rat cerebral cortex induced by cortical spreading depression. *Brain Pathol* 3: 11–17

36   Walz W, Ilschner S, Ohlemeyer C, Banati R, Kettenmann H (1993) Extracellular ATP activates a cation conductance and a K+ conductance in cultured microglial cells from mouse brain. *J Neurosci* 13: 4403–4411

37   Gehrmann J, Bonnekoh P, Miyazawa T, Oschlies U, Dux E, Hossmann K-A (1992) The microglial reaction in the rat hippocampus following global ischemia: immuno-electron microscopy. *Acta Neuropathol* 84: 588–595

38   Dickson DW, Mattiace LA, Kure K, Hutchuns K, Lyman WD, Brosnan CF (1991) Microglia in human disease, with an emphasis on acquired immune deficiency syndrome. *Lab Invest* 64: 135–156

39   Colton AC, Gilbert DL (1987) Production of superoxide by a CNS macrophage, the microglia. *FEBS Lett* 223: 284–288

40   Boje KM, Arora PK (1992) Microglial-produced nitric oxide and reactive nitrogen oxides mediate neuronal cell death. *Brain Res* 587: 250–256

41   Banati RB, Graeber MB (1994) Surveillance, intervention and cytotoxicity: Is there a protective role of microglia? *Dev Neurosci* 16: 114–127

42   Blinzinger K, Kreutzberg GW (1968) Displacement of synaptic terminals from regenerating motoneurons by microglial cells. *Z Zellforsch* 85: 145–157

43   Elkabes S, DiCicco-Bloom EM, Black IB (1996) Brain microglia/macrophages express neurotrophins that selectively regulate microglial proliferation and function. *J Neurosci* 16: 2508–2521

44   Mallat M, Houlgatte R, Brachet P, Prochiantz A (1989) Lipopolysaccharide-stimulated rat brain macrophages release NGF *in vitro*. *Dev Biol* 133: 309–311

Inflammatory activation of brain cells by hypoxia: transcription factors and signaling pathways

Danica B. Stanimirovic

Institute for Biological Sciences, National Research Council of Canada, Montreal Road Campus, Bldg. M-54, Ottawa, ON, K1A 0R6, Canada

Preamble

Cytokines play a major role in the initiation, propagation, regulation and suppression of inflammatory responses [1–3]. Most cells do not constitutively express cytokines, but rather an activation event results in cytokine gene transcription. The major intrinsic sources of cytokines in the brain are glial cells [1]. However, elements of the brain vasculature including cerebral endothelial cells (CEC), pericytes, and perivascular macrophages, as well as peripheral immune cells that infiltrate the brain in pathological states, are significant sources of cytokines [1–4].

Inflammatory cytokines are induced in the ischemic brain [4, 5] and stimulate CEC, granulocyte and platelet activation thus linking pathophysiological mechanisms of inflammation and ischemia [4, 5]. The mechanisms by which hypoxia triggers inflammatory cytokine expression and molecular consequences of cytokine receptor activation in brain cells will be discussed in this section.

Transcription factor activation by hypoxia

Immediate early genes (IEGs) represent the first wave of gene expression in cells exposed to an environmental stress, and their induction occurs in a protein synthesis-independent manner. IEGs encode for many functionally different products such as secreted pro-inflammatory proteins including cytokines and chemokines, cytoplasmic enzymes such as COX-2, and inducible transcription factors (ITFs) [6, 7]. Whereas ITFs are not expressed by brain cells in the basal state [7], transcription factors such as calcium/cyclic AMP responsive-element binding protein (CREB), activating transcription factor-2 (ATF-2), and nuclear factor-κB (NF-κB) are constitutively expressed in cells in latent form and are activated *via* post-translational modification (usually phosphorylation) [6, 7]. These constitutive transcription factors initiate the transcription of target genes, including ITFs. The expression of ITFs occurs rapidly and transiently [6], and ITFs then go on to regulate a delayed, but

Inflammation and Stroke, edited by Giora Z. Feuerstein
© 2001 Birkhäuser Verlag Basel/Switzerland

generally more prolonged expression of effector genes by interacting with the AP-1 sites in the regulatory regions of these genes [6]. Hypoxia-inducible factor-1 (HIF-1) is a transcription factor that is specifically activated by hypoxia [8, 9]. HIF-1 can be activated by both modifications in protein processing and by the transcriptional induction [8]. The specific effector genes induced will depend upon the combination of transcription factors expressed in neurons and non-neuronal brain cells in response to any particular stimulus.

Cerebral ischemia has been shown to cause activation and/or induction of HIF-1 [10], constitutive transcription factors including NF-κB [11–13] and CREB [12], and inducible transcription factors including c-Fos, c-Jun, JunD, Krox-24, etc. [12]. Induced expression of the immediate-early genes c-jun, c-fos, and junB in the penumbra and the peri-infarct tissue has been seen as early as 1 h after vascular occlusion [7, 12] in parallel with increases in AP-1 binding activity. Increases in HIF-1α mRNA and protein were detected in the cerebral cortex as early as 4–7 h [10], whereas NF-κB and CREB binding activities were up-regulated 1–7 days after stroke [11, 12].

Inflammatory cytokines in brain ischemia can be "turned on" by the activation of either constitutive or inducible transcription factors, or both. Inflammatory gene activation *via* NF-κB in response to different stimuli has been repeatedly described in various cell types [13]. Inflammatory genes, including IL-1β, TNFα, ICAM-1 and COX-2 also contain AP-1 site(s) in their regulatory and promoter regions and can be induced by ITFs including various complexes of c-fos, c-jun, junD, ATF2, etc. [13, 14]. Since the observed temporal patterns of transcription factor activation and inflammatory cytokine expression largely overlap in models of cerebral ischemia [5], the "transactivation" event that sets off the initial transcription of inflammatory cytokines remains an enigma. Potential roles of two transcription factors, NF-κB and HIF-1, both readily activated by changes in cellular redox state, will be discussed in more detail.

NF-κB

NF-κB is a key transcription factor required for the expression of many inflammatory genes, including IL-1β [13, 15, 16]. NF-κB is composed of homo- and heterodimeric complexes of members of the Rel protein family comprising p50, p65 (RelA), c-Rel, p52, and RelB [16]. In quiescent cells, NF-κB resides in the cytosol in latent form bound to an inhibitory protein κB (IκB), which masks the nuclear localization sequences of the most common p50/p65 heterodimer [13, 16]. Stimulation of cells with cytokines, LPS, viruses or oxidants triggers a series of signaling events (see below) that lead to the phosphorylation and proteolytic degradation of IκB, and subsequent activation of NF-κB [13, 16]. NF-κB then translocates into the nucleus and stimulates the transcription of target genes including cytokines, chemokines and cell adhesion molecules [13, 16]. The regulated proteolysis of IκB is mediated by the ubiquitin-proteasome pathway of protein degradation [16, 17]. Phosphorylation is generally believed to target IκB for ubiquitination and ubiquitinated IκB is then selectively degraded by the 26S proteasome [16, 17]. However, recent evidence suggests that tyrosine phosphorylation of IκB can activate NF-κB in the absence of proteolytic degradation of IκB [18]. Inhibitors of enzymes of the ubiquitin-proteaosome pathway are believed to suppress the activation of NF-κB by stabilizing the inhibitor IκB, thereby potentially acting as anti-inflammatory agents. NF-κB activation in cerebral ischemia has been linked to both neuroprotective and cell death-promoting pathways [15] suggesting that NF-κB may be a new pharmacological target in stroke.

Hypoxia-inducible factor-1

HIF-1 was originally identified as a nuclear factor required for transcriptional regulation of the human erythropoietin (EPO) gene, and has subsequently been shown to regulate more than 30 genes involved in cellular adaptation to hypoxia [8]. A recent study [16] describes an induction of HIF-1α and HIF-1-regulated genes including glucose transporter-1 and several glycolytic enzymes in tissues surrounding ischemic brain infarct [16].

HIF-1 is a heterodimeric protein composed of HIF-1α and HIF-1β (ARNT) subunits [8]. In most cell types, both HIF-1α and ARNT are consitutively expressed and are not significantly affected by hypoxia at mRNA level [8]. However, hypoxia has been shown to markedly increase HIF-1α protein levels [8].

The activation of HIF-1 by hypoxia depends on a sensing and signaling process that likely involves a heme protein since cobalt chloride ($CoCl_2$) and the iron chelator, desfferioxamine, strongly induce both HIF-1 and hypoxia-regulated genes [19], whereas carbon monoxide and nitric oxide inhibit HIF-1 activation [9, 19]. Incidentally, changes in oxygen tension are also important in regulating NF-κB activation [20]. HIF-1α is extremely unstable and undergoes a rapid oxygen-dependent degradation *via* the ubiquitin-proteasome pathway [21]. Therefore, inhibitors of the ubiquitin-proteasome pathway are expected to reduce the transcription of NF-κB regulated genes, but are likely to increase the transcription of HIF-1 regulated genes.

HIF-1-mediated induction of hypoxia sensitive genes takes place *via* HIF-1 binding to hypoxia response elements, DNA sequences containing a core 5'-[A/G]CGTG-3' motif at functionally essential HIF-1 binding sites [8]. All genes regulated by HIF-1 share the following properties: (1) transcription is induced by hypoxia, $CoCl_2$ or desferrioxamine and can be blocked by cycloheximide, and (2) the promoter or enhancer region of these genes contains a hypoxia-response element of < 100 bp that has one or more HIF-1 binding sites [8]. Mutation of these sites results in a loss of transcriptional response to hypoxia [8].

Triggers of inflammatory gene expression in ischemic brain cells

In an effort to discover which transcriptional event triggers inflammatory gene expression during hypoxia, we measured nuclear binding and transcriptional activity of NF-κB and HIF-1α in human astrocyte cultures exposed to hypoxia *in vitro*. NF-κB nuclear binding and transcriptional activity were increaased during reoxygenation, but not by hypoxia alone [22]. The NF-κB activation during reoxygenation was found to be dependent on the release of IL-1β [23] from hypoxic cells, since it was blocked by the IL-1 receptor antagonist (IL-1Ra) [22]. In another experiment, the proteasome inhibitor, MG-132, completely suppressed NF-κB activation during reoxygenation, but caused a parallel increase in hypoxia/reoxygenation-stimulated IL-1β expression [22]. These observations suggested that NF-κB in human astrocytes is activated *via* a IL-1β-mediated autocrine loop and that, in the absence of this loop, hypoxia-induced up-regulation of IL-1β is not critically dependent on NF-κB activation [22, 23].

A synergistic effect of the proteasome inhibitor and hypoxia on the IL-1β expression in astrocytes, suggested that hypoxia induces IL-1β *via* a transcription factor degraded by proteasome, such as HIF-1α. In fact, gene alignment analyses of promoter regions of IL-1β and interleukin-converting enzyme (ICE) revealed that both genes have multiple HIF-1α binding sites (5'-RCGTG-3') resembling hypoxia response elements of "classical" HIF-1-induced genes such as VEGF [24]. Both HIF-1α mRNA and HIF-1α nuclear binding and transcriptional activities were found to increase in human astrocytes subjected to hypoxia [24]. Furthermore, the exposure of both human astrocytes and human CEC to the known HIF-1 inducer, $CoCl_2$, resulted in a simultaneous up-regulation of HIF-1α, IL-1β, and ICE mRNAs, and increased secretion of immunoreactive IL-1β into cell media [24]. Finally, astrocyte cultures derived from Hif1α[+/−] mice demonstrated reduced HIF-1α stimulation by hypoxia in parallel with lower release of immunoreactive VEGF and IL-1β than astrocytes derived from wild Hif1α[+/+] mice [24]. These findings support the notion that at least some inflammatory cytokines belong to the battery of genes regulated by HIF-1α during brain hypoxia/ischemia.

Inflammatory circulus viciosus

The cytokine system in the brain, as in other organs, displays pleiotropism and redundancy. These properties of cytokines underlie the known ability of inflammation to spread in time and space by mobilizing a variety of secondary inflammatory mediators in surrounding tissues. Two major routes employed in amplifying inflammation are propagation through receptor signaling and autocrine/paracrine recruitment of neighboring cells.

Propagation through signaling

Cytokines initiate their actions by binding to specific cell surface receptors on target cells; these receptors generally show high affinities, with dissociation constants in the range of 10^{-10}–10^{-12} M [1]. Inflammatory cytokines and their receptors are engaged in exceptionally sensitive loop mechanisms that cause fast amplification of the inflammatory response.

Signaling through IL-1R1

The IL-1 cytokine family consists of IL-1α, IL-1β, two IL-1 receptors, and IL-1 receptor antagonist (IL-1Ra) [2]. IL-1β is cleaved from the inactive precursor, pro-IL-1β, by ICE [2]. IL-1β binds two types of receptors, a signaling type I (IL-1RI) receptor, and type II (IL-1RII) receptor, a decoy that inhibits IL-1 activity [2]. The IL-1R1 signal transduction system is amazingly efficient in that fewer than 10 ligand-occupied receptors are required to induce a strong signaling response, as compared to 10–100-fold greater occupancy required for most other receptor systems [25].

Signaling through IL-1R1 (Fig. 1) is initiated by the association of the receptor with IL-1 (α or β) and the IL-1R1 accessory protein (IL-1R1AcP). IL-1R1AcP is a protein capable of cross-linking with IL-1 and increasing IL-1 avidity to IL-1R1, and is essential for IL-1-dependent NF-κB activation [25]. IL-1R1 and IL-1RAcP form a functional heterodimer in the presence of the ligand by recruiting IL-1R-associated kinase (IRAK) [25]. A cytoplasmic domain of IL-1R1 contains a sequence that is required for the coupling to IκB kinase (IKK) *via* IRAK [25]. Although the mechanism of IκB kinase activation is not fully understood, it appears that two other proteins, TRAF6 and NIK (a MAP kinase kinase), physically couple IRAK to IκB kinase [25, 26]. IKK-mediated phosphorylation of IκB targets IκB for degradation by proteasome resulting in NF-κB activation.

However, recent evidence suggests that only about half of the NF-κB activity induced by IL-1 is due to IKK-mediated IκB phosphorylation [25]. It has been shown that cytoplasmic domain of IL-1R1 is also capable of recruiting phosphatydylinositol-3 kinase (PI3K), an enzyme that can activate PKC and Akt kinases [25] and appears to be responsible for NF-κB activation independent of IκB kinase [25, 27] (Fig. 1).

The activation of MAP kinases is another well-known consequence of IL-1R1 stimulation [28] (Fig. 1). The IL-1 responsive MAP kinase pathways are those that activate JNK, SAP/p38 and ERK2 kinase pathways [28]. While the mechanisms of activation of p38 and ERK kinase pathways are unknown, JNK kinases appear to be directly activated by the action of TRAF6, an adapter molecule that binds to the IL-1R1 *via* IRAK [25, 26]. One of the functions of MAP kinases is to activate transcription factors required for the expression of target genes, including those binding to AP-1 sites [28] (Fig. 1).

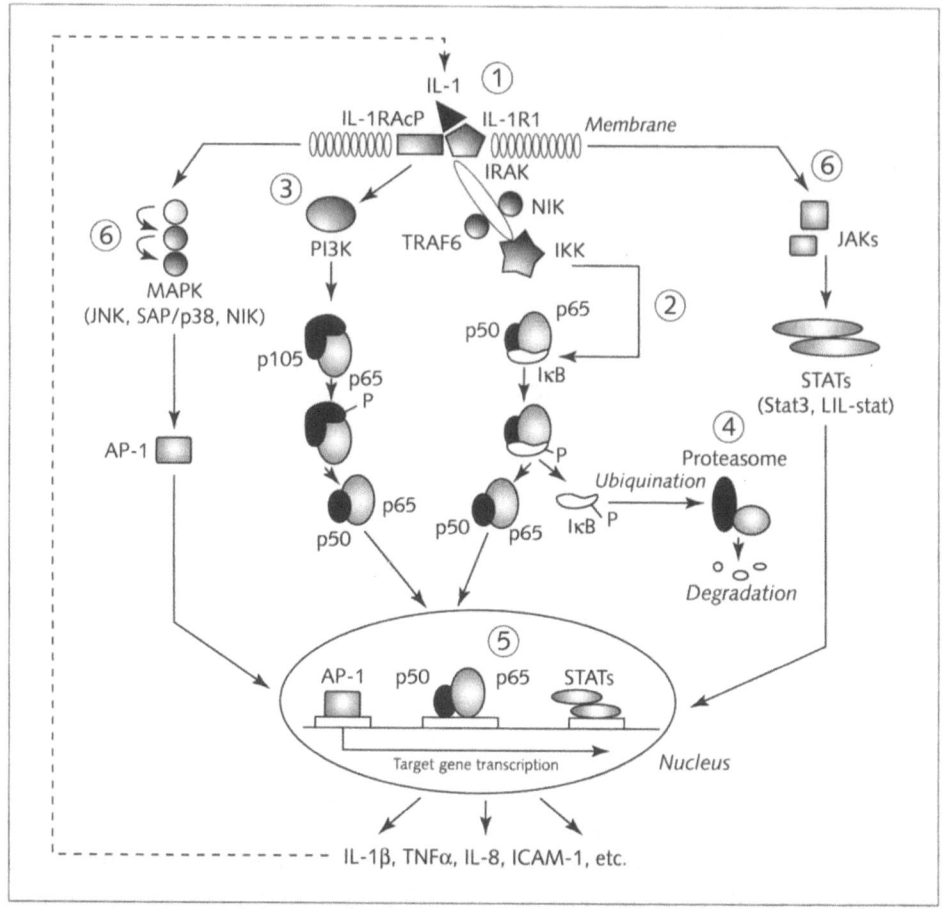

Figure 1
Signaling cascades initiated through IL-1RI and potential sites for pharmacological interven-
tion (see description in the text).

At least three other transcription factors are activated by IL-1, including c-Jun, c-Fos and C/EBPβ [25]. IL-1β is also capable of an immediate induction of two members of STAT family of transcription factors, Stat3 and LIL-Stat, recruited by Janus kinases (JAK) [25] (Fig. 1).

Even though IL-1R1 receptor signaling described above appears to be tissue dependent, it is likely that brain cells expressing IL-1R1 will propagate IL-1-triggered signals using one or more of the described pathways. For example, human CEC and human astrocytes in culture express IL-1R1 [23] and are likely cellular targets of IL-1 produced in ischemic brain.

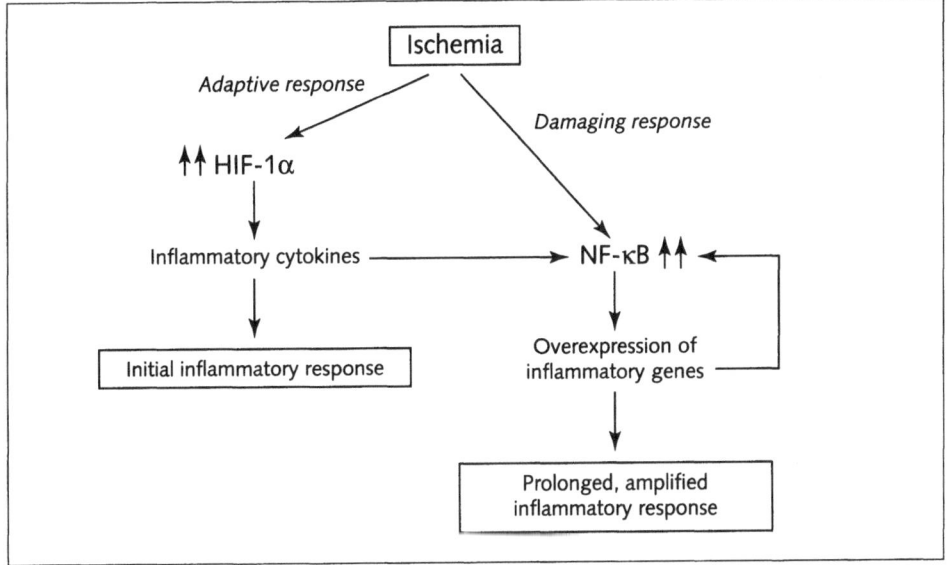

Figure 2

Roles of HIF-1α and NF-κB in ischemic brain inflammation. HIF-1α triggers initial transcription of inflammatory cytokines that then amplify inflammation by the receptor-mediated NF-κB activation.

Multiple pathways initiated through IL-1R1 activation result in the activation of numerous transcription factors and the expression of a myriad of target genes. Since NF-κB activation appears to be a mandatory result of IL-1R1 stimulation, many of the target genes induced by IL-1 will belong to the NF-κB-regulated inflammatory gene cluster (Fig. 1). Given the exquisite sensitivity of the IL-1 receptor-signal transduction system, it is easy to envisage how initial increases of IL-1 induced by hypoxia in NF-κB-independent manner can promptly result in an excessive NF-κB-dependent enhancement of inflammation (Fig. 2).

Several intrinsic checkpoints are activated within this cascade that act to suppress inflammatory propagation. Probably the most important "controller" of the cascade is IL-1Ra, the naturally occurring ligand to IL-1R1 that binds the receptor without inducing any known signal responses [2, 25]. The role of IL-1Ra as an endogenous neuroprotectant in cerebral ischemia has been shown by experiments in which the blockade of IL-1Ra function resulted in marked exacerbation of ischemic brain damage, while brain injection or systemic infusion of IL-1Ra reduced infarct lesion and neurological deficits in focal brain ischemia [29].

The other process that limits inflammatory propagation is IL-1R1 downregulation triggered by the IL-1 receptor occupancy [23, 30]. A dose-dependent downregulation of IL-1R1 mRNA and IL-1R1 surface expression by IL-1 has been observed in various cell types including CEC and astrocytes [23, 30]. IL-1R1 downregulation requires *de novo* protein synthesis and appears to be the consequence of a rapid receptor mRNA destabilization [30]. Since IL-1R1 is the receptor that mediates all biological activities of IL-1α and β [1, 2], IL-1R1 downregulation is essential for limiting inflammatory propagation.

Autocrine/paracrine cell recruitment

A variety of brain cells respond to cytokines by producing cytokines. For example, IL-1 stimulation of rat astrocytes induces TNFα, IL-6 and TGFβ [1], whereas in human astrocytes IL-1 stimulates expression of TNFα, and expression/secretion of chemokines IL-8 and MCP-1 [31]. IL-1β is the principal paracrine effector secreted from human astrocytes that induces pro-inflammatory phenotype in CEC [23]. In human CEC both IL-1β and TNFα stimulate the expression of adhesion molecules, and IL-1β induces the release of IL-8 and MCP-1 [31]. Therefore, cytokines can induce other inflammatory mediators in autocrine and paracrine manner leading to spatial spreading of inflammation through the mobilization of neighboring cells.

Therapeutic targets in transcription and signaling cascades

Two major approaches to control postischemic inflammation in the brain have been (i) to inhibit singular inflammatory mediator by blocking its interaction with the receptor (Fig. 1, site 1), and (ii) to reduce overall immune responses by immuno-suppressant drugs [32]. Since inflammation develops as a cascade, the inhibition of any singular mediator is easily circumvented by alternate pathways and is likely to be ineffective in the clinical setting. Immunomodulation strategies on the other hand are highly non-selective.

Novel approaches to treat ischemic brain inflammation may arise from a better understanding of the transcriptional regulation of inflammatory genes. These genes are often transcribed as clusters and many genes are regulated through the same transcription pathway. Targeting key transcription elements responsible for the expression of inflammatory gene clusters may provide both selectivity and simultaneous inhibition of multiple inflammatory mediators.

For example, NF-κB activation can be prevented by the simultaneous targeting of various signaling molecules including IκB kinase (Fig. 1, site 2) and/or PI3 kinase (Fig. 1, site 3). Proteasome inhibitors that prevent IκB degradation (Fig. 1, site 4) proved to be effective in reducing infarct size after focal brain ischemia [33]. A NF-κB "decoy" approach (Fig. 1, site 5) has been shown to suppress the induction of inflammatory genes in endothelial cells *in vitro* [34]. Other potential targets in cytokine-induced signaling cascades include pathways linked to NF-κB-independent target-gene transcription such as MAP and JAK kinases (Fig. 1, site 6). However, it appears that until new strategies are developed, NF-κB cascade remains a realistic target to pharmacologically regulate inflammatory responses in cerebral ischemia.

Acknowledgement

Studies on NF-κB and HIF-1 roles in inflammatory gene transcription are supported in part by a grant (#T3509) from the Heart and Stroke Foundation of Ontario.

References

1   Benveniste ET (1997) Cytokine expression in the nervous system. In: RW Keane, WF Hickey (eds): *Immunology of the nervous system*. Oxford University Press, New York, Oxford, 419–460

2   Dinarello CA (1998) Interleukin-1, interleukin-1 receptors and interleukin-1 receptor antagonist. *Int Rev Immunol* 16: 457–499

3   Stanimirovic D and Satoh K (2000) Inflammatory mediators of cerebral endothelium: A role in ischemic brain inflammation. *Brain Pathol* 10: 113–126

4   Feuerstein GZ, Wang X, Barone FC (1998) The role of cytokines in the neuropathology of stroke and neurotrauma. *Neuroimmunomodulation* 5: 143–159

5   Hill JK, Gunion-Rinker L, Kulhanek D, Lessov N, Kim S, Clark WM, Dixon MP, Nishi R, Stenzel-Poore MP, Eckenstein FP (1999) Temporal modulation of cytokine expression following focal cerebral ischemia in mice. *Brain Res* 820: 45–54

6   Herdegen T, Leah JD (1998) Inducible and constitutive transcription factors in the mammalian nervous system: control of gene expression by Jun, Fos and Krox, and CREB/ATF proteins. *Brain Res Rev* 28: 370–490

7   Hughes PE, Alexi T, Walton M, Williams CE, Dragunow M, Clark RG, Gluckman PD (1999) Activity and injury-dependent expression of inducible transcription factors, growth factors and apoptosis-related genes within the central nervous system. *Prog Neurobiol* 57: 421–450

8   Semenza GL (2000) Expression of hypoxia-inducible factor 1: mechanisms and consequences. *Biochem Pharmacol* 59: 47–53

9   Ratcliffe PJ, O'Rourke JF, Maxwell PH, Pugh CW (1998) Oxygen sensing, hypoxia-inducible factor-1 and the regulation of mammalian gene expression. *J Exp Biol* 201: 1153–1162

10 Bergeron M, Yu AY, Solway KE, Semenza GL, Sharp FR (1999) Induction of hypoxia-inducible factor-1 (HIF-1) and its target genes following focal ischemia in rat brain. *Eur J Neurosci* 11: 4159–4170

11 Stephenson D, Yin T, Smalstig EB, Hsu MA, Panetta J, Little S, Clemens J (2000) Tran-

scription factor nuclear factor-kappa B is activated in neurons after focal cerebral ischemia. *J Cereb Blood Flow Metab* 20: 592–603

12   Salminen A, Liu PK, Hsu CY (1995) Alteration of transcription factor binding activities in the ischemic rat brain. *Biochem Biophys Res Comm* 212: 932–944

13   Collins T, Read MA, Neish AS, Whitley MZ, Thanos D, Maniatis T (1995) Transcriptional regulation of endothelial cell adhesion molecules: NF-κB and cytokine-inducible enhancers. *FASEB J* 9: 899–909

14   Novotny V, Prieschl EE, Csonga R, Fabjani G, Baumruker T (1998) Nrf1 in a complex with fosB, c-jun, junD and ATF2 forms the AP1 component at the TNF alpha promoter in stimulated mast cells. *Nucleic Acids Res* 26: 5480–5485

15   Grilli M, Memo M (1999) Nuclear factor-kappaB/Rel proteins: a point of convergence of signalling pathways relevant in neuronal function and dysfunction. *Biochem Pharmacol* 57: 1–7

16   Baldwin Jr AS (1996) The NF-κB and IκB proteins: New discoveries and insights. *Ann Rev Immunol* 14: 649–681

17   Grisham MB, Palombella VJ, Elliott PJ, Conner EM, Brand S, Wong HL, Pien C, Mazzola LM, Destree A, Parent L, Adams J (1997) Inhibition of NF-κB activation *in vitro* and *in vivo*: role of 26S proteasome. *Methods in Enzymology* 300: 345–363

18   Imbert V, Rupec RA, Livolsi A, Pahl HL, Traenckner EBM, Mueller-Diekmann C, Farahifar D, Baeuerle PA, Peyron J-F (1996) Tyrosine phosphorylation of IκB-α activates NF-κB without proteolytic degradation of IκB-α. *Cell* 86: 787–798

19   Wenger RH (2000) Mammalian oxygen sensing, signalling and gene regulation. *J Exp Biol* 203: 1253–1263

20   Haddad JJ, Olver RE, Land SC (2000) Antioxidant/pro-oxidant equilibrium regulates HIF-1(alpha) and NF-(kappa)B redox sensitivity: Evidence for inhibition by glutathione oxidation in alveolar epithelial cells. *J Biol Chem* 275: 21130–21139.

21   Kallio PJ, Wilson WJ, O'Brien S, Makino Y, Poellinger L (1999) Regulation of the hypoxia-inducible transcription factor 1a by the ubiquitin-proteasome pathway. *J Biol Chem* 274: 6519–6525

22   Stanimirovic D, Zhang W, Howlett C, Lemieux P, Smith C (2000) Inflammatory gene transcription in human astrocytes exposed to hypoxia: Role of NF-κB and autocrine stimulation. *J Neuroimmunol; in press*

23   Zhang W, Smith C, Stanimirovic DB (2000) Inflammatory activation of human brain endothelial cells by hypoxic astrocytes *in vitro* is mediated by IL-1β. *J Cerebral Blood Flow Metab* 20: 967–978

24   Zhang W, Howlett C, Mojsilovic-Petrovic J, Carmeliet P, Stanimirovic D (2000) Evidence that interleukin converting enzyme (ICE) and interleukin-1β (IL-1β) are transcriptionally regulated by the hypoxia-inducible factor-1 (HIF-1) in human astrocytes and brain endothelial cells exposed to hypoxia. *J Biol Chem; submitted*

25   Auron PE (1998) The interleukin-1 receptor: Ligand interactions and signal transduction. *Cytokine and Growth Factors Reviews* 9: 221–237

26   Baud V, Liu ZG, Bennett B, Suzuki N, Xia Y, Karin M (1999) Signaling by proinflam-

matory cytokines: oligomerization of TRAF2 and TRAF6 is sufficient for JNK and IKK activation and target gene induction *via* an amino-terminal effector domain. *Genes Dev* 13: 1297–308

27   Sizemore N, Leung S, Stark GR (1999) Activation of phosphatidylinositol 3-kinase in response to interleukin-1 leads to phosphorylation and activation of the NF-kappaB p65/RelA subunit. *Mol Cell Biol* 19: 4798–4805

28   Clerk A, Harrison JG, Long CS, Sugden PH (1999) Pro-inflammatory cytokines stimulate mitogen-activated protein kinase subfamilies, increase phosphorylation of c-Jun and ATF2 and upregulate c-Jun protein in neonatal rat ventricular myocytes. *J Mol Cell Cardiol* 31: 2087–1099

29   Loddick SA, Wong ML, Bongiorno PB, Gold PW, Licinio J, Rothwell NJ (1997) Endogenous interleukin-1 receptor antagonist is neuroprotective. *Biochem Biophys Res Commun* 234: 211–215

30   Ye K, Koch KC, Clark BD, Dinarello CA (1992) Interleukin-1 down-regulates gene and surface expression of interleukin-1 receptor type I by destabilising mRNA whereas interleukin-2 increases its expression. *Immunology* 75: 427–434

31   Zhang W, Smith C, Monette R, Shapiro A, Hutchison J, Stanimirovic D (1999) Increased expression of bioactive chemokines in human cerebromicrovascular endothelial cells and astrocytes subjected to simulated ischemia *in vitro*. *J Neuroimmunol* 101: 148–160

32   Young P (1998) Pharmacological modulation of cytokine action and production through signaling pathways. *Cytokine and Growth Factors Reviews* 9: 239–257

33   Buchan AM, Li H, Blackburn B (2000) Neuroprotection achieved with a novel proteasome inhibitor which blocks NF-kappaB activation. *Neuroreport* 11: 427–430

34   Tomita N, Morishita R, Tomita S, Yamamoto K, Aoki M, Matsushita H, Hayashi S, Higaki J, Ogihara T (1998) Transcription factor decoy for nuclear factor-κB inhibits tumor-necrosis factor-a-induced expression of interleukin-6 and intracellular adhesion molecule-1 in endothelial cells. *J Hypertension* 16: 993–1000

Inflammatory cytokines, interleukins and chemokines in stroke and CNS trauma

Cytokine effects on CNS cells: implications for the pathogenesis and prevention of stroke

Mark F. Mehler[1] and John A. Kessler[2]

[1]Departments of Neurology, Neuroscience and Psychiatry, Albert Einstein College of Medicine, Rose F. Kennedy Center for Research in Mental Retardation and Developmental Disabilities, Room 401, 1410 Pelham Parkway South, Bronx, NY 10461, USA; [2]Davee Department of Neurology and Clinical Neurological Sciences, Northwestern University School of Medicine, Abbott Hall, Room 1120, 710 North Lake Shore Drive, Chicago, IL 60611, USA

Introduction

After a stroke, cytokines in the brain mediate a variety of injury responses, some of which may be beneficial and some detrimental to clinical outcome. This suggests that it may be possible to enhance functional outcome through therapeutic intervention with specific cytokine agonists and/or antagonists. Further, knowledge of cytokine actions in the nervous system is essential for the design of therapeutic strategies for actually repairing brains damaged by stroke.

During ontogeny cytokines and growth factors are essential for neural induction, patterning of the neural tube, neural lineage restriction and commitment, and progressive progenitor cell proliferation, survival and terminal neuronal and glial differentiation. Stem and progenitor cells that persist even in the adult brain remain responsive to these signals, and cytokine actions are essential for directing the differentiation of cultured stem cells that could potentially be used therapeutically. Thus knowledge of cytokine actions in the developing and adult brain is necessary both for understanding the pathophysiologic processes underlying injury responses and for potential regenerative strategies. This chapter will first review the role of different cytokine families in neural development, their actions on stem and progenitor cells, and their potential applications to regenerative strategies. We will then discuss the role of cytokines in injury responses of specific cellular elements, the mechanisms underlying these actions, and potential avenues for therapeutic intervention in these processes.

Inflammation and Stroke, edited by Giora Z. Feuerstein
© 2001 Birkhäuser Verlag Basel/Switzerland

Role of cytokines in neural induction and anteroposterior and dorsoventral patterning

Bone morphogenetic proteins (BMPs), a rapidly expanding subclass of the TGFβ superfamily, play an important role in orchestrating neural induction [1, 2]. BMP4 and BMP7, both expressed within the embryonic ectoderm, inhibit neurulation while concurrently acting to promote epidermal induction [3, 4]. Activins, a distinct subclass of the TGFβ superfamily, prevent neurulation through a different developmental mechanism by induction of mesoderm instead of epidermis [4]. Several BMP antagonists within the vertebrate organizer, including noggin, chordin and follistatin, differentially bind to and selectively inhibit individual BMP ligands to establish the elaborate morphogenetic gradients required for later neural tube patterning [5–8]. Follistatin is expressed within the organizer and the notochord, and exhibits direct neural inductive potential [9]. These overall studies suggest that inhibition of BMP signaling is necessary for the conversion of ectoderm to neuroectoderm, and that the epidermal fate represents an active BMP-induced state. Additional genetic analysis further suggests that several BMP ligands may be involved in inhibiting neural induction by acting through multiple developmental pathways [10]. Anterior neurulation appears to be mediated solely by inhibition of BMP signaling. By contrast, induction of neural tissue within more caudal regions may require additional soluble cues, including fibroblast growth factor (FGF), noggin and Wnt signaling [11]. BMPs are also essential for proper dorsoventral patterning of the neural tube. Non-neural cells adjacent to the dorsal neural tube secrete inductive signals that enhance the elaboration of neural crest stem/progenitor cells, sensory neurons and roof plate cells [3, 10]. The BMP-related protein, dorsalin-1 is expressed within the dorsal neural tube, and is capable of inducing regional neuronal subtypes [10].

Closure of the neural tube in murine tissues is associated with downregulation of BMP ligands in neighboring epidermal cells, and the incipient expression of BMP2 within the anterior neural folds [10, 12]. After neural tube closure, BMP4 is expressed in the anterior dorsal midline region, BMP5 and BMP7 in partially overlapping areas of the dorsal midline and BMP6 throughout the entire length of the evolving neural tube [3, 10]. BMP developmental actions are mediated through both local and long-range signaling interactions. Long-range signals are modulated through the expression of different classes of BMP-binding proteins that inhibit BMP signaling, and complementary zinc metalloproteases, such as BMP1, that potentiate BMP actions by releasing BMP ligands previously sequestered by the various BMP-binding molecules [1, 3, 6–8, 10, 13].

Conversely, sonic hedgehog (Shh), a secreted morphogen of the notochord and floorplate, induces ventral cell types, including motor neurons and other ventral interneurons and oligodendrocytes (OLs), cooperates with BMP ligands to induce the elaboration of intermediate cell types with distinct phenotypic properties and antagonizes the "dorsalizing" effects of the BMPs within ventral neural tube domains [14]. Different concentrations of Shh signals are required to establish appropriate progenitor species, to refine progenitor cell boundaries, to preserve the integrity of uncommitted cells and to thereafter orchestrate the expression of different classes of transcription factors that confer neuronal subtype identity [15, 16].

Cytokines and regional neural stem cell populations

Anteroposterior, mediolateral and dorsoventral patterning are essential for the concurrent establishment of neural stem cell (NSC) and more lineage-restricted progenitor populations within paramedian generative zones that are elaborated from the inner lining of the neural tube [3, 11]. These specialized regional microdomains, extending from the forebrain anlage to the spinal cord, consist of an initial ventricular zone (VZ), composed of pseudostratified epithelium, that during mid-embryonic life gives rise to secondary subventricular zones (SVZs) that continue in abbreviated form during mature stages of life [17–20]. Early embryonic NSCs of the VZ give rise to neurons and radial glia, whereas later embryonic and perinatal SVZ-derived NSCs preferentially generate astrocytes and oligodendrocytes [17–22].

NSCs are defined by their ability to undergo constitutive proliferation, to exhibit self-maintenance (self-renewal), and to elaborate large numbers of more lineage-restricted progenitor species and differentiated neurons and glia during specific neurodevelopmental stages and in response to specific injury cues [17–19]. Phenotypic maintenance of NSCs is orchestrated by both daughter cells during the initial phase of rapid stem cell pool expansion (symmetric cell divisions), and by one daughter cell of each pair during later phases of neurogenesis and gliogenesis (asymmetric cell divisions) [18, 23]. NSC proliferation, survival, self-renewal and early stages of cellular differentiation are mediated by specific cytokines, such as basic FGF (bFGF) and epidermal growth factor (EGF), and by other cell-associated and transcriptional regulatory signals [24–27].

Early embryonic forebrain VZ-derived NSCs are multipotent and exhibit cellular responsiveness to bFGF, although they are predisposed to undergo radial glial and neuronal lineage commitment and differentiation [24–26, 28]. In addition, recent studies have shown that graded FGF signals are instrumental in modulating neural fate decisions within these early embryonic NSC species: application of low concentrations of bFGF favors neuronal lineage commitment, whereas higher concentrations promote oligodendroglial or astroglial differentiation [26]. SVZ-derived NSCs that exhibit EGF/TGFα cellular responsiveness appear to be derived from FGF-responsive VZ-derived NSCs [29–31].

Although these SVZ progenitor species retain the potential to generate all major neural phenotypes, they are predisposed toward glial cell differentiation during the perinatal period. Along the adult neuraxis, the biological properties of NSCs are modulated by differing profiles of cellular responsiveness to bFGF and to EGF receptor signaling [20]. In addition, noggin production by mature ependymal cells inhibits BMP signaling within the adjacent SVZ to promote specific patterns of adult neurogenesis [32].

Cytokine effects on neural lineage restriction and commitment during brain development

Neural lineage restriction and commitment is a progressive regional CNS process that requires the concerted actions of a broad array of environmental and cell intrinsic signaling molecules. Shh is expressed within ventral regions from the embryonic spinal cord to the forebrain [14]. This gradient morphogen appears to collaborate with bFGF to potentiate the initial expansion of uncommitted progenitor species and to assist in the sequential generation of neurons and OLs. BMP ligands, by contrast, promote progenitor cell cycle exit and incipient neuronal differentiation, while concurrently suppressing the generation of OLs [33–35].

Continuous progenitor cell exposure to Shh signaling may be required to potentiate the elaboration of neurons and later OLs by regulating the early context-dependent induction of BMP ligands and the later induction of the BMP antagonist, noggin [36, 37]. Subsequent progenitor cell exposure to oligotrophins, including platelet-derived growth factor (PDGF) or leukemia inhibitory factor (LIF), may be required for the efficient elaboration of a robust complement of OL lineage species following relief of the BMP-sanctioned OL inhibitory signal by the developmental actions of noggin [36, 38, 39].

Profiles of neural lineage elaboration are also orchestrated by changes in the patterns of NSC environmental responsiveness and by the pleiotropic actions of specific cytokines. BMP ligands potentiate the elaboration of neurons and concurrently actively suppress the generation of radial glial and oligodendrocytes from NSCs present within the early embryonic forebrain VZ [28]. Conversely, BMP ligands promote the generation of astrocytes, then suppress the elaboration of neurons and continue to inhibit the generation of radial glia and OLs from NSCs located within the late embryonic SVZ [28, 40].

BMP developmental actions can also be modified by interactions with associated transduction pathways. In this regard, the profiles of neural lineage elaboration during seminal developmental stages may represent, in large part, the composite actions of multiple environmental signaling pathways. Thus, the elaboration of radial glia from NSCs during cerebral cortical neurogenesis, and the generation of oligodendrocytes from glial-restricted progenitors during perinatal gliogenesis represent the cooperative modulation of developmental stage-specific BMP inhibitory cues by the positive glial-lineage specific actions of LIF [28]. Conversely, the presence of unopposed BMP inhibitory signals serves to prevent the ectopic elaboration of specific neuronal and glial species at specific developmental stages during which their presence could result in various morphogenetic errors that could seriously impair the physiological efficacy and integrity of evolving neural network connections [28].

Lineage restriction of different species of NSCs is also orchestrated by the actions of hematopoietic (gp 130 homodimeric receptors: interleukin, IL, 6; IL 11) and neuropoietic (gp 130/ LIFβ receptor: ciliary neurotrophic factor, CNTF; LIF; oncostatin-M, OM) gp 130-associated cytokines, by additional hemopoietin subclasses (IL-5, -7, -9, -11) and by the tyrosine kinase receptor-associated hemopoietin, stem cell factor (SCF) [41–44]. Additional studies suggest that a novel developmental transduction module composed of a secreted cardiotrophin-like cytokine (CLC) and a soluble receptor cytokine-like-factor-1 (CLF) may represent the long sought after signaling cassette for modulating early neuropoietic gp 130-associated cytokine signals involved in regulating nascent stages of embryonic NSC lineage commitment and early cellular differentiation [45]. Further, recent studies documenting the broad profiles of expression of erythropoietin and its cognate receptor within embryonic and perinatal generative zones and within progressive regional neural maturational pathways suggest that this hemopoietin may orchestrate an interrelated series of developmental processes that govern the sequential elaboration of neurons and glia from both VZ- and SVZ-derived neural stem and progenitor species [46].

Cytokine actions during central nervous system neurogenesis

Neurons and radial glia are the initial cell types to be elaborated within more rostral brain regions. LIF sanctions the generation of radial glia from early embryonic forebrain NSCs by promoting the commitment of this lineage at the expense of alternate lineages (instructive mechanism), and by selectively enhancing their mitogenic potential [28]. Further, radial glial differentiation is favored by the cooperative effects of the neuregulin, glial growth factor and by Notch receptor activation [47, 48]. Developmental interconversion of radial glia to astrocytes is promoted by exposure to different BMP ligands [28]. Recent observations suggest that radial glia may exhibit even broader lineage potential, such as the ability to generate neuronal precursor species during early embryogenesis [49, 50]. Additional investigations have suggested that neural species with phenotypic similarities to astrocytes may represent a population of NSCs within the adult CNS [51]. These developmental findings are particularly important because of the observation that adult astrocytes can undergo transformation into transitional radial glia to support the migration of immature neurons transplanted into areas of experimental brain injury [52]. Nascent neuroblasts respond to distinct profiles of region-specific cytokines that promote cellular survival and proliferation prior to cell cycle exit and terminal differentiation. The cellular survival of cultured early embryonic regional mouse and rat neuroblasts is enhanced by exposure to IL-3, -4, -5, -7, -10, -13, LIF, SCF, flt3 ligand, colony stimulating factor-1 (CSF 1), granulocyte-macrophage (GM)-CSF (GM-CSF), erythropoietin and tumor necrosis factor-α (TNFα) [53–59]. These cellular effects are region-selective, dose-dependent, orchestrated by direct (e.g., IL-7), paracrine (e.g., CSF-1 effects on microglia) or cooperative (e.g., GM-CSF) growth factor signaling, linked to concurrent actions on axodendritic outgrowth (e.g., IL-10) or partially mediated by the induction of additional cytokine effectors (e.g., SCF). Regional neuronal survival is also potentiated by BMP subclass ligands, either alone (e.g., growth and differentiation factor-15 for midbrain dopaminergic neurons) or in association with individual neurotrophins or members of the glial-cell derived neurotrophic factor (GDNF) family (e.g., BMP7 for spinal cord neuroblasts) [60, 61]. Similarly, the early proliferation of nascent regional cultured embryonic neuroblasts is enhanced by an array of hemopoietins that include IL-3, -4, -7, -15 and GM-CSF [53, 54, 56].

The terminal differentiation of various regional neuronal subpopulations is defined by the evolution of an interrelated spectrum of maturational processes that include the expression of neurotransmitters, neuropeptides, and biosynthetic enzymes; neuronal polarity and axodendritic process outgrowth; sequential viability of neuronal lineage species; synaptogenesis; modulation of cellular excitability and synaptic plasticity. The expression of distinct neuromodulatory molecules and signaling pathways is mediated by the actions of CNTF, LIF, IL-1β, IL 3, CSF-1, GM-CSF and erythropoietin [62–68]. Other facets of neuronal maturation, including the expression of neurofilament proteins, cellular excitability, survival of later developmental and mature lineage species, neurite outgrowth and synaptogenesis are orchestrated by a different profile of hematolymphopoietic growth factors, including IL-1, -2, -3, -4, -6, -7, -8, -9, -11, -12, -13, -15, -16, GM-CSF, granulocyte-CSF, erythropoietin, thrombopoietin, SCF, interferon-(IFN) α/β and γ [68–73]. A subset of these cytokines, including IL-1β, -2, -6, IFNα/β, negatively modulate higher order parameters of synaptic plasticity during terminal neuronal differentiation [70]. Very recent investigations of the potential negative CNS immunomodulatory effects of higher-order interleukins, including IL-17 and -18, have demonstrated the intricate and precarious balance that may exist between the actions of inflammatory and positive immunomodulatory cytokines during normal developmental processes and particularly in the setting of specific injury responses [74–77].

Cytokine actions during central nervous system gliogenesis

Within the developing central nervous system, gliogenesis encompasses a complex spectrum of developmental processes that involve multipotent, oligopotent and unipotent progenitor species [22]. The elaboration of astrocytes from multipotent progenitor species is promoted by TGFβ superfamily factors, including TGFβ and BMP ligands, and by neuropoietic gp 130-associated factors, including CNTF, LIF and OM [39–41, 78–80]. By contrast, both CNTF and LIF promote astrocyte elaboration from uncommitted rat embryonic forebrain progenitor species, whereas BMP ligands potentiate the generation of astrocytes from perinatal SVZ-derived NSCs and from a distinct pool of cerebral cortical NSCs through an instructive mechanism [41, 81–84]. Further, although earlier embryonic forebrain multipotent progenitors express functional LIFβ receptors, application of CNTF or LIF to these developmental species do not promote the elaboration of the astroglial lineage [85]. These experimental observations demonstrate that progenitor cell responsiveness to these classes of cytokines change during ontogeny.

Another TGFβ subclass factor (e.g., activin A) further enhances the LIF-mediated generation of astrocytes from multipotent progenitors [86]. The generation of astrocytes from both radial glia and from perinatal glial-restricted progenitors is also enhanced by exposure to BMP ligands [28]. Although OLs are preferentially elaborated during perinatal developmental stages in more rostral brain regions, OLs can also be generated from embryonic forebrain NSCs by increasing concentrations of bFGF or by brief exposure to thyroid hormone [26, 81]. During perinatal developmental phases, OL progenitors are elaborated from multipotent progenitors under the influence of tyrosine kinase receptor-associated hematolymphopoietic factors that include PDGF, bFGF and insulin-like growth factor-1 (IGF1) [38, 39]. Limited survival of OL progenitors *in vitro* is promoted by CNTF, LIF, OM and glial growth factor, whereas more long-term cellular viability is afforded by the concerted actions of these growth factors, in concert with cytokines such as IGF1 and neurotrophin-3 [38, 39, 80]. The OL lineage has recently been shown to possess a remarkable degrees developmental plasticity that translates into a myriad of potential therapeutic applications for reactive OL progenitor and more mature OL lineage pools. For example, OL progenitors can be re-programmed under the cooperative influence of bFGF and BMP ligands to exhibit properties of NSCs, including the potential to differentiate into neuronal and glial species when exposed to members of specific classes of differentiating cytokines [87]. Further, myelinating OLs are capable of undergoing dedifferentiation and de novo proliferation in response to application of bFGF and glial growth factor [88 ,89].

Profiles of expression of cytokine signaling molecules during neural development

Examination of the profiles of spatiotemporal expression of selected hemopoietin and TGFβ superfamily ligands, receptor subunits and associated signaling molecules have helped to define the cellular and developmental actions of these broad classes of environmental cues. The early embryonic expression of IL-3 transcripts reflects the preferential effects of this growth factor on early progenitor cell proliferation and survival [53, 54]. The more intermediate developmental patterns of expression of transcripts for IL-4 are compatible with the actions of this cytokine on bipotent OL-type II astrocyte progenitor cells [53, 54, 90]. By contrast, the later embryonic and early postnatal expression profiles of IL-5 and IL-7 transcripts correlate with the known actions of these hemopoietins on intermediate stages of neuronal maturation [43, 53, 54]. Further, IL-12 transcripts display maximal expression during late postnatal life, a profile consist with the established regulatory effects of this gp 130-associated cytokine on terminal phases of neuronal differentiation, including axodendritic process outgrowth and neurotransmitter expression [43, 54].

A close correspondence also exists between expression of transcripts for ligands and for their cognate receptor subunits. These complementary expression profiles are best exemplified by the spatiotemporal patterns of SCF and the c-kit protooncogene receptor, reflecting the multiple roles of SCF during both initial stages of neural crest maturation and more terminal phases of neuronal differentiation within the developing brain [44, 91, 92]. More detailed analysis of the patterns of cytokine cellular transcript and protein expression have revealed the complex nature of autocrine, paracrine and cooperative signaling events, as mediated by extracellular, receptor-associated, cytoplasmic transduction and transcriptional regulatory molecules. For example, single cell analysis has demonstrated that IL-7 exerts direct cellular actions on nascent embryonic neuroblasts *in vitro* [53, 59]. In addition, the selective presence of IL-7α receptor subunits on regional neuroblast populations and IL-7 ligands exclusively within glial cell subpopulations suggests the presence of a glial-neuronal paracrine signaling loop [59]. More detailed analysis of early IL-7 signaling interactions has revealed the rapid phosphorylation of the src family member, p59^{fyn}, and the preferential expression of c-myc transcripts, indicating that within the developing brain hemopoietin receptors that do not contain intrinsic kinase activity represent versatile transduction modules capable of recruiting and activating multiple intracellular pathways for mediating context-specific effector events [59].

The constitutive and activated developmental profiles of expression of seminal hemopoietin-associated intracellular signaling molecules (e.g., JAK-STAT and src-family kinases) are now in the process of being mapped at a fine level of regional, cellular and subcellular detail. These preliminary investigations reveal a complex and elaborate network of interrelated signaling pathways that will eventually allow the construction of functional maps of cytokine actions during progressive stages of neural development and also during adult maintenance functions. JAK-STAT signaling molecules represent combinatorial codes of latent transcriptional regulators that integrate and regulate the ligand, cellular and developmental contextual specificity of various hemopoietins and associated cytokines [93]. During mammalian forebrain development, JAK2 displays high levels of expression during embryonic life, with progressive reductions in levels of expression during postnatal and adult development and maintenance [93]. By contrast, JAK1 exhibits relatively low levels of constitutive expression as compared to JAK2, with no evidence of significant modulation during forebrain maturation [93].

Analysis of various STAT proteins also reveal differential patterns of expression during neural development. STAT3 does not display changes in patterns of expression, STAT1 and 5 exhibits complex expression profiles and STAT6 shows progressive decline in levels of expression during important developmental transitions [93]. Regional patterns of cellular expression of src family transcripts also provide important clues concerning hemopoietin developmental functions. For example, fyn transcripts are expressed within growth cones of nascent neuroblasts and at mature synapses [94]. These expression profiles may relate to the potential dual roles of fyn in cellular proliferation and in calcium homeostasis [94, 95]. Consistent with these context-specific cellular functions, fyn homozygous null mice display developmentally-mediated abnormalities in regional hippocampal organization and in synaptic plasticity [95].

By contrast, src kinase may represent one of several signaling pathways that regulate axodendritic process outgrowth [96]. Src knockout mice display minimal neuropathological deficits, but selective impairments in regional neurite outgrowth of nascent neuroblasts when assayed *in vitro* using L1-containing substrates [94, 96]. The intricate and partially redundant patterns of expression of individual src family members within the developing brain suggest important roles for these cytoplasmic tyrosine kinase signaling molecules in multiple, progressive hemopoietin-mediated and associated cellular regulatory events.

Additional investigations of the profiles of expression of TGFβ superfamily factors and binding proteins, receptor subunits and intracellular signaling molecules (e.g., Smad latent transcription factors) have already confirmed the complex and diverse cellular effects of individual TGFβ subclass factors on multiple neural stem, progenitor and more differentiated lineage species throughout progressive stages of brain development [97]. TGFβ ligand and receptor subunit transcripts are present throughout neural development [98, 99]. Transcripts for TGFβ1 are expressed in cultured CNS macrophages and in the developing neural crest [54]. TGFβ2 and 3 transcripts are preferentially upregulated during early embryogenesis and during later maturational stages in the brain and spinal cord [100].

Whereas TGFβ2 is selectively expressed within the cerebral cortex, TGFβ3 is preferentially expressed in the olfactory bulb [69]. TGFβ isoforms are also differentially expressed during embryonic development. OLs produce TGFβ1 and undergo proliferation in response to factor application, whereas all three of these TGFβ isoforms are expressed in cultured brain astrocytes, with TGFβ2 secreted in latent form [54]. Transcripts for BMP2–7 are expressed throughout CNS development with complex and partially overlapping ligand profiles [40, 54, 101, 102]. BMP2 and 7 transcripts are predominantly localized to cultured neurons, astrocytes and microglia, whereas those for BMP4 are localized to OL lineage species [33, 54, 103, 104]. Transcripts for BMP6 are localized to neurons and radial glia during the perinatal periods, suggesting a role for this cytokine in modulating the cessation of neurogenesis and in mediating the transition of radial glia to postnatal astrocytes [105,

106]. Transcripts for BMP type I (BMPRIA, BMPRIB) and type II (BMPRII) receptor subunits are expressed within the early embryonic cortical VZ, with persistence within the late embryonic and the early postnatal SVZ [101, 107]. Maximal expression within the SVZ occurs during the peak period of perinatal cerebral cortical gliogenesis [107]. BMP receptor expression (predominantly BMPRIA) is also apparent within the superficial region of the cortical plate during late embryogenesis, with continued expression within the supragranular portion of the neocortex in the first 2 postnatal weeks [107]. In the adult, there is persistence of BMP receptor transcripts within all cortical layers, with predominantly non-overlapping regional cellular profiles of expression of individual BMP receptor subunits, particularly BMPRII [107]. These latter observations suggest that individual BMP receptor subunits may be capable of mediating adult maintenance functions as opposed to the composite signaling requirements thought to be necessary for optimal modulation of BMP-mediated developmental actions. Transcripts for ACTRI and ACTRII, receptor subunits that can mediate both BMP and activin signals, are also expressed preferentially during important early neurodevelopmental transitions [101]. Dramatic advances in our understanding of the levels of regulatory control of signal modulation present within TGFβ superfamily transduction pathways will help to promote the development of sophisticated functional assays to help define the detailed cellular actions of these versatile cytokine subclass factors.

Effects of progenitor cells on recovery from cerebrovascular injury

There are both global and focal models of cerebrovascular injury [108]. Global ischemia, due to cardiac arrest, coronary artery occlusion or coronary bypass surgery, usually results in selective profiles of neuronal death within vulnerable brain regions (i.e., CA1 region of the hippocampus). By contrast, loss of blow flow to specific cerebral arteries frequently causes irreversible cellular injury within a characteristic focal brain region, and the presence of a surrounding "penumbra" consisting of potentially reversible neuronal and glial cell injury. In global ischemic injury models, limited structural and functional recovery have been achieved by the use of homotypic fetal cell transplants that have led to the reestablishment of neural network connectivity between donor and recipient cell types [109]. In the global ischemic model, functional recovery has also been achieved by implantation of a mouse hippocampal neuroepithelial cell line into regions of the damaged host hippocampus [110]. However, analysis of the CA1 region of the hippocampus following implementation of the embryonic cell transplantation paradigm revealed that only a small proportion of the engrafted cells differentiated into neuronal or glial cell types. Thus, the basis for functional recovery could not be firmly established using this regenerative strategy. In focal stroke models (middle cerebral artery occlusion, MCAO), the introduction of embryonic cortical grafts into areas of irreversible cerebral cortical injury have resulted in preferential functional recovery in the setting of an enriched host environment that may foster *de novo* neurogenesis [111–113]. The cortical grafts receive prodigious afferent inputs from cortical, subcortical and thalamic host regions, but display sparse efferent projections [114].

Functional recovery in focal ischemic rat models has been observed following intrastriatal introduction of neurons derived from a human teratocarcinoma cell line [115, 116]. However, there is no evidence that the transplanted cells developed appropriate phenotypic properties of striatal neurons. Additional studies suggest that transplantation protocols can be significantly improved by the use of earlier region-selective neural tissue and contiguous germ layers.

Using a hypertensive rat model of focal ischemia (MCAO), implantation of embryonic rat mesencephalic neural plate and adjacent ventral mesenchyme into the ischemic striatum resulted in significant behavioral recovery [117]. Histological examination revealed the presence of multiple areas of revascularization and engrafted cells with mature neuronal properties. These observations suggest that neurobehavioral recovery is dependent upon the ability of immature engrafted cells to survive and differentiate into adult CNS structural and functional elements within the mature ischemic brain under the influence of multiple inductive and neurotrophic signals.

In another experimental paradigm, the introduction of bFGF-generated rat embryonic cortical NSCs into different regions of adult rats following focal ischemic damage resulted in early (1–7 days) progenitor cell proliferation and differentiation into astrocytes, OLs and microglia, and delayed (21–45 days) maturation into cells of the neuronal lineage [118]. In addition, transplantation into areas of the SVZ resulted in greater cellular proliferation and neuronal and glial differentiation than direct introduction into regions of ischemic damage within the cerebral cortex.

A further investigation has demonstated that the combined introduction of neonatal murine NSCs and bFGF in transplantation paradigms using a rat focal ischemia model resulted in enhanced behavioral recovery and the presence of smaller areas of cortical infarction [119]. Interestingly, recent observations suggest that human bone marrow cells also have the capacity to differentiate into mature neurons, OLs and astrocytes and to ameliorate the characteristic neurological deficits present in rats with focal ischemia following transplantation into areas of cerebrovascular damage [120].

Following the induction of transient forebrain ischemia, affected mice also displayed enhanced proliferation of endogenous neural precursors within areas of the dentate gyrus, suggesting the presence of intrinsic adaptive responses to cerebrovascular injury [121]. In fact, neuroimaging studies have shown that significant functional reorganization can occur after ischemic strokes [122]. Clinical stroke trials are already in progress using both teratocarcinoma and porcine fetal CNS cells [108]. Finally, transplantation of human neuronal cellular preparations into targeted regions of patients with basal ganglia strokes and chronic fixed motor deficits resulted in both significant functional improvements and additional PET evidence of enhanced fluorodeoxyglucose uptake at the site of transplantation [123].

Effects of cytokines on cerebrovascular injury responses

Factors from each of the major cytokine superfamilies have been shown to exhibit neuroprotective and/or neural regenerative responses when administered prior to or following episodes of cerebrovascular injury. Application of TGFα has been shown to reduce the infarction volume in rodent MCAO models, with cellular survival effects mediated directly by the EGF receptor [124]. After focal ischemia, infarct volume is also reduced in a blood flow-independent manner by exposure to bFGF [125]. Interestingly, the neuroprotective actions of bFGF after acute excitotoxic brain injury are mediated by the induction of activin A, and these secondary trophic effects can be effectively blocked by application of follistatin [126]. TGFβ1 displays neuroprotective actions, in part, by exerting a negative modulatory effect on N-methyl-D-aspartate (NMDA) receptor-mediated excitotoxicity [127]. Intracisternal injection of BMP7 at early (1–5 days), but not later (7–9 days) intervals after cerebrovascular injury enhances behavioral recovery, suggesting the existence of a critical period of cellular responsiveness to cytokine signals following acute ischemic injury [128].

Furthermore, BMP7 also displays prospective neuroprotective actions, defined by the ability of the cytokine to ameliorate the effects of ischemia-induced cerebral cortical injury when administered 24 h prior to experimental induction of focal (MCAO) ischemia [129]. Perivascular injury results in the early (6 h) upregulation and activation of Stat6, a prominent intracellular transducer of IL-4 and IL-13 signals, with later (7 days) downregulation of expression of the latent transcription factor [130]. Analysis of the differential profiles of regulation of CNTR and the CNTFα receptor following focal cerebral ischemia suggest a significant role for this neuropoietic cytokine in modulating the effects of cerebrovascular injury [131]. Transcripts for CNTF are elevated in the acute phase after cerebral ischemia, and also in areas adjacent to those undergoing parenchymal necrosis [131]. By contrast, CNTRα receptor transcripts display delayed induction profiles following focal ischemia and layer-specific patterns of cortical modulation [131].

Infusion of erythropoietin prevents the behavioral deficits and reduces the severity of cerebral cortical infarction in rats with permanent focal (MCAO) ischemic lesions [132]. The erythropoietin receptor is upregulated on neurons at the periphery of MCAO ischemic lesion sites, suggesting that cytokine signaling may be facilitated by neuronal lineage recruitment, increased cytokine receptor density and by positive feedback regulation [132]. TNF binding protein, a dimeric form of the soluble type I TNF receptor that inhibits TNFα signaling, also exhibits neuroprotective actions following acute focal (MCAO) cerebral ischemia, and these trophic effects are sustained for at least 2 weeks [133]. These observations suggest that continuous blockade of TNFα signaling results in prolonged protection from the pathological sequelae of cerebrovascular injury.

Vascular endothelial growth factor (VEGF) may also participate in cellular repair in association with partial stroke recovery [134]. VEGF and the VEGF receptor are induced by hypoxia and this cytokine signaling pathway can promote the growth of new blood vessels following cerebral ischemia [135]. Intraventricular administration of IL-10 has also been shown to reduce the size of the infarction following focal cerebral ischemia [136]. Conversely, induction of focal (MCAO) ischemia in IL-10 homozygous null mice significantly increases the cortical infarction volume [137]. These complementary observations suggest that both endogenous and exogenous sources of IL-10 exhibit neuroprotective actions in response to cerebral ischemia. However, IL-6 may epitomize the biological complexity of cytokine actions in response to neural cell injury in general, and following cerebral ischemia in particular. As an inflammatory cytokine, IL-6 is released predominantly by activated astrocytes during early injury responses and may, therefore, contribute to propagation of the pathogenic cascade of adverse signaling events [138]. Thus, elevated level of IL-6 in plasma samples is an important marker associated with early worsening in ischemic strokes [139].

By contrast, IL-6 is also known to exhibit neuroprotective, neurotrophic and neuromodulatory actions [138, 140]. Further, some of the effects of IL-6 may be mediated by the induction of accessory molecules, such as the classical neurotrophins that can furnish a local supply of effector signals to potentiate neuronal survival and additional adaptive injury responses [141]. Further, different inflammatory cytokines (e.g., IL-1, IL-6, TNFα) appear to exert their positive modulatory responses to excitotoxic injury by activation of distinct signaling molecules and pathways, perhaps offering a glimpse into the spectrum of potential complementary neuroprotective mechanisms that can be recruited in response to cerebrovascular injury [142].

Potential mechanisms of cytokine actions in stroke

During the evolution of cerebral ischemic lesions, inflammatory and immunomodulatory cytokines participate actively in the initiation of cellular and matrix-associated forms of parenchymal injury and in the subsequent profiles of reparative responses, respectively [143, 144]. However, the precise patterns of expression of effector cytokines and the requisite profiles of targeted neural progenitor and differentiated cellular species that comprise the pathogenic cascades are still poorly defined. Innovative neuroprotective and neural regenerative strategies for stroke prevention and rehabilitation will require harnessing the developmental potential of cytokines and neural stem and progenitor species to promote the reconstitution of functional neural circuits from residual reactive progenitor cell pools and associated differentiated neuronal and glial lineage elements located both within regional paramedian generative zones and also adjacent to the sites of ischemic injury. Numerous cytokines and progenitor and more mature neural cell lineage preparations have already been shown to be effective in ameliorating the clinicopathological sequelae of global and focal cerebral ischemia. However, the precise mechanisms of action underlying these neuroprotective and neural regenerative responses have remained elusive.

The therapeutic effects of TGFα can be mediated by direct cytokine actions on the survival, proliferation, self-renewal, migration and incipient differentiation of neural stem and progenitor cells located within regional paramedian generative zones and surrounding the lesion site, or by local enhancement of the viability of post-mitotic neurons [145]. A complementary spectrum of cellular actions can be orchestrated by application of bFGF [24–27]. However, bFGF also participates in the secondary induction of bioactive cytokines (e.g., activin A) and the dedifferentiation of myelinating OLs to reactive glial progenitor species [88, 126]. Further, this early CNS cytokine can exhibit cooperative signaling when co-applied with gradient morphogens, such as Shh to promote the sequential elaboration of targeted neuronal subtypes and associated OL species [146]. BMP ligands can promote neuronal and glial lineage elaboration from NSCs and from more lineage-restricted progeny, enhance regional neuronal dendritic process outgrowth and also potentiate neuronal survival, either alone or in concert with additional cytokines (e.g., neurotrophin-3 and GDNF) through BMPRII-mediated signaling pathways [28, 33, 34, 40, 82, 97, 102, 104, 147–150]. BMPs can also promote the dedifferentiation of reactive OL progenitor pools to NSCs that are thereafter capable of undergoing lineage-specific differentiation to allow the precise cell-cell matching needed to facilitate the efficient cellular reconstitution of ischemic lesion sites [87]. Finally, cooperative and antagonistic signaling interactions between BMP and other cytokine pathways can either promote the elaboration of specific neural lineages or accelerate the transition between individual neural progenitor species that exhibit changing profiles of neural lineage potential or different degrees of developmental maturation. For example, BMP2 and LIF display the developmental context-specific cooperative signaling interactions required to potentiate the generation of astrocytes from NSCs, through recruitment of the transcriptional co-regulator, p300/CBP that respectively links seminal transcriptional regulatory elements (Smads, STAT3) for these cardinal developmental pathways [151]. Conversely, the sequential elaboration and coordinate maturation of neurons and OLs from NSCs appears to be mediated by sequential antagonistic signaling interactions between EGF-BMP-Shh pathways that are orchestrated by MAP kinase-mediated Smad suppression and Smad-associated release of Shh-mediated transcriptional inhibitory signals (i.e., N-terminal forms of Gli3), respectively [152, 153].

Another TGFβ subclass factor, TGFβ1, displays an additional neuroprotective mechanism through the ability of this cytokine to block NMDA receptor-induced excitotoxicity [127]. Members of the neuropoietic gp130-associated cytokines, including CNTF and LIF, can promote neuronal and glial specification from regional NSCs, enhance the generation of radial glia that contribute to the fidelity of neuronal migration, potentiate the elaboration of OLs from glial-restricted progenitors and also regulate neuronal phenotype switching in post-mitotic cells (respecification) [28, 38, 39, 81, 150, 154, 155]. Erythropoietin can enhance neuronal survival, neurite outgrowth and the expression of distinct neuromodulatory molecules [46, 156, 157]. Neuronal survival and axodendritic process outgrowth can also be potentiated by application of IL-10 [157]. The early STAT 6-mediated neuroprotective actions of IL-4 and IL-13 are likely due to direct trophic effects of these γ-receptor subunit hemopoietin subclass factors on neuroblast proliferation and survival [157]. Conversely, the neuroprotective actions of the pleiotropic factor, IL6 are preferentially mediated by the secondary induction of neurotrophins that can actively participate in neuronal survival and in other adaptive injury responses [141].

The ultimate challenge in developing new cytokine, gene and stem cell therapeutic approaches to various forms of cerebrovascular injury will be to selectively activate the specific integrated cytokine signaling pathways required to optimize the reconstitution of functional regional neural network connections. The achievement of this goal will require a better understanding of: (i) the developmental hierarchy of cytokine regulation of regional neural progenitor species, (ii) the role of non-neural tissues and associated germ layers in the induction and specification of regional neural cellular elements, (iii) the cross-modulatory actions of lesion-associated and therapeutically-targeted cytokine subgroup factors, (iv) the critical periods governing progenitor cell responsiveness to specific cytokines, (v) the interrelationships between and the associated environmental regulation of neural stem and progenitor populations present in generative zones and adjacent to ischemic lesion sites, and (vi) the cellular source, spatiotemporal profiles and signaling routes of different classes of cytokines.

Acknowledgements
Experimental studies cited from the authors laboratories were supported by grants from the National Institute of Neurological Disorders and Stroke, National Institutes of Health and the F.M. Kirby Foundation. We are grateful to Ms. Anne Barnecott for her expert assistance in the preparation of this manuscript.

References

1   Weinstein DC, Hemmati-Brivanlou A (1999) Neural induction. *Annu Rev Cell Dev Biol* 15: 411–433
2   Massague J, Blain SW, Lo RS (2000) TGFbeta signaling in growth control, cancer, and heritable disorders. *Cell* 103: 295–309

3   Tanabe Y, Jessell TM (1996) Diversity and pattern in the developing spinal cord. *Science* 274: 1115–1123

4   Hemmati-Brivanlou A, Melton D (1997) Vertebrate embryonic cells will become nerve cells unless told otherwise. *Cell* 88: 13–17

5   Lemaire P, Kodjabachian L (1996) The vertebrate organizer: structure and molecules. *Trends Genet* 12: 525–531

6   Piccolo S, Sasai Y, Lu B, De Robertis EM (1996) Dorsoventral patterning in *Xenopus*: inhibition of ventral signals by direct binding of chordin to BMP4. *Cell* 86: 589–598

7   Zimmerman LB, DeJesus-Escobar JM, Harland RM (19960 The Spemann organizer signal noggin binds and inactivates bone morphogenetic protein 4. *Cell* 86: 599–606

8   Holley SA, Neul JL, Attisano L, Wrana JL, Sasai Y, O'Connor MB, De Robertis EM, Ferguson EL (1996) The Xenopus dorsalizing factor noggin ventralizes *Drosophila* embryos by preventing Dpp from activating its receptor. *Cell* 86: 607–617

9   Hemmati-Brivanlou A, Kelley OG, Melton DA (1994) Follistatin, an antagonist of activin, is expressed in the Spemann organizer and displays direct neuralizing activity. *Cell* 77: 283–295

10   Hogan BLM (1996) Bone morphogenetic proteins: multifunctional regulators of vertebrate development. *Genes Develop* 10: 1580–1984

11   Lumsden A, Krumlau FR (1996) Patterning the vertebrate axis. *Science* 274: 1109–1115

12   Winnier G, Blessing M, Labosky PA, Hogan BL (1995) Bone morphogenetic protein 4 is required for mesoderm formation and patterning in the mouse. *Genes Develop* 9: 2105–2116

13   Biehs B, Francois V, Bier E (1996)The Drosophila short gastrulation gene prevents Dpp from autoactivating and suppressing neurogenesis in the neuroectoderm. *Genes Develop* 10: 2922–2934

14   Litingtung Y, Chiang C (2000) Control of Shh activity and signaling in the neural tube. *Dev Dyn* 219: 143–154

15   Briscoe J, Ericson J (1999) The specification of neuronal identity by graded sonic hedgehog signalling. *Cell Dev Biol* 10: 353–362

16   Briscoe J, Pierani A, Jessell TM, Ericson J (2000) A homeodomain code specifies progenitor cell identity and neuronal fate in the ventral neural tube. *Cell* 101: 435–445

17   Gage FH, Ray J, Fisher, LJ (1995) Isolation, characterization, and use of stem cells from the CNS. *Annu Rev Neurosci* 18: 159–192

18   McKay R (1997) Stem cells in the central nervous system. *Science* 276: 66–71

19   Weiss S, Reynolds BA, Vescovi AL, Morshead C, Craig CG , van der Kooy D (1996) Is there a neural stem cell in the mammalian forebrain? *Trends Neurosci* 9: 387–393

20   Weiss S, Dunne C, Hewson J, Wohl C, Wheatley M, Peterson AC , Reynolds BA (1996) Multipotent CNS stem cells are present in the adult mammalian spinal cord and ventricular neuroaxis. *J Neurosci* 16: 7599–7609

21   Cameron RS, Rakic P (1991) Glial cell lineage in the cerebral cortex: a review and synthesis. *GLIA* 4: 124–137

22 Goldman JE, Zerlin M, Newman S, Zhang L, Gensert J (1997) Fate determination and migration of progenitors in the postnatal mammalian CNS. *Dev Neurosci* 19: 42–48

23 Caviness VS Jr, Takahashi T (1995) Proliferative events in the cerebral ventricular zone. *Brain Dev* 17: 159–163

24 Qian X, Goderie S, Shen Q, Stern J, Temple S (1998) Intrinsic programs of patterned cell lineage in isolated vertebrate CNS ventricular zone cells. *Development* 125: 3143–3152

25 Burrows RC, Wancio D, Levitt P, Lillien L (1997) Response diversity and the timing of progenitor cell maturation are regulated by developmental changes in EGFR expression in the cortex. *Neuron* 19: 251–267

26 Qian X, Davis AD, Goderie SK, Temple S (1997) FGF2 concentration regulates the generation of neurons and glia from multipotent cortical stem cells. *Neuron* 18: 81–93

27 Shen Q, Qian X, Capela A, Temple S (1998) Stem cells in the embryonic cerebral cortex: their role in histogenesis and patterning. *J Neurobiol* 36: 162–174

28 Gokhan S, Yung SY, Kessler JA, Mehler MF (2000) Cerebral cortical neurogenesis and gliogenesis require transcriptional activation of inhibitor of differentiation (ID) 2 and 4 in neural stem cells by bone morphogenetic proteins. *Ann Neurol* 48: 415–416

29 Martens DJ, Tropepe V, van der Kooy D (2000) Separate proliferation kinetics of fibroblast growth factor-responsive and epidermal growth factor-responsive neural stem cells within the embryonic forebrain germinal zone. *J Neurosci* 20: 1085–1095

30 Ciccolini F, Svendsen CN (1998) Fibroblast growth factor 2 (FGF-2) promotes acquisition of epidermal growth factor (EGF) responsiveness in mouse striatal precursor cells: identification of neural precursors responding to both EGF and FGF-2. *J Neurosci* 18: 7869–7880

31 Vescovi AL, Reynolds BA, Fraser DD, Weiss S (1993) bFGF regulates the proliferative fate of unipotent (neuronal) and bipotent (neuronal/astroglial) EGF-generated CNS progenitor cells. *Neuron* 11: 951–966

32 Lim DA, Tramontin AD, Trevejo JM, Herrera DG, Garcia-Verdugo JM, Alvarez-Buylla A (2000) Noggin antagonizes BMP signaling to create a niche for adult neurogenesis. *Neuron* 28: 713–726

33 Mabie PC, Mehler MF, Kessler JA (1999) Multiple roles of bone morphogenetic protein signaling in the regulation of cortical cell number and phenotype. *J Neurosci* 19: 7077–7088

34 Mehler MF, Mabie PC, Zhu G, Gokhan S, Kessler JA (2000) Developmental changes in progenitor cell responsiveness to bone morphogenetic proteins differentially modulate progressive CNS lineage fate. *Dev Neurosci* 22: 74–85

35 Zhu G, Mehler MF, Zhao J, Yung SY, Kessler JA (1999) Sonic hedgehog and BMP2 exert opposing actions on proliferation and differentiation of embryonic neural progenitor cells. *Dev Biol* 215: 118–129

36 Hirsinger E, Duprez D, Jouve C, Malapert P, Cooke J, Pourquie O (1997) Noggin acts downstream of Wnt and Sonic Hedgehog to antagonize BMP4 in avian somite patterning. *Development* 124: 4605–4614

37 Drossopoulou G, Lewis KE, Sanz-Ezquerro JJ, Nikbakht N, McMahon AP, Hofmann C, Tickle C (2000) A model for anteroposterior patterning of the vertebrate limb based on sequential long- and short-range Shh signalling and Bmp signalling. *Development* 127: 1337–1348

38 Miller RH (1996) Oligodendrocyte origins. *Trends Neurosci* 19: 92–96.

39 Pfeiffer SE, Warrington AE, Bansal R (1993) Oligodendrocyte and its many cellular processes. *Trends Cell Biol* 3: 191–198

40 Gross RE, Mehler MF, Mabie PC, Zang Z, Santschi L, Kessler JA (1996) Bone morphogenetic proteins promote astroglial lineage commitment by mammalian subventricular zone progenitor cells. *Neuron* 17: 595–606

41 Richards LJ, Kilpatrick TJ, Dutton R, Tan S.-S, Gearing DP, Bartlett PF, Murphy M (1996) Leukemia inhibitory factor or related factors promote the differentiation of neuronal and astrocytic precursors within the developing murine spinal cord. *Eur J Neurosci* 2: 291–299

42 Mehler MF, Mabie PC, Marmur R, Kessler JA (1996) Differential regulation of radial glia and astroglial lineage elaboration from subventricular zone (SVZ) progenitor cells by leukemia inhibitory factor β (LIFβR) receptor activation and bone morphogenetic proteins (BMPs). *Soc Neurosci Abstr* 22: 285

43 Mehler MF, Rozental R, Dougherty MJ, Spray DC, Kessler JA (1993) Cytokine regulation of neuronal differentiation in immortalized hippocampal progenitor cells. *Nature* 362: 62–65

44 Langtimim-Sediak CJ, Schroeder B, Saskowski JL, Carnahan JF, Sieber-Blum M (1996) Multiple actions of stem cell factor in neural crest cell differentiation *in vitro*. *Develop Biol* 174: 345–359

45 Elson GC, Lelievre E, Guillet C, Chevalier S, Plun-Favreau H, Froger J, Suard I, de Coignac AB, Delneste Y, Bonnefoy JY et al (2000) CLF associates with CLC to form a functional heteromeric ligand for the CNTF receptor complex. *Nat Neurosci* 3: 867–872

46 Juul SE, Yachnis AT, Rojiani AM, Christensen RD (1999) Immunohistochemical localization of erythropoietin and its receptor in the developing human brain. *Pediatr Dev Pathol* 2: 148–158

47 Gaiano N, Nye JS, Fishell G (2000) Radial glial identity is promoted by notch1 signaling in the murine forebrain. *Neuron* 26: 395–404

48 Mehler MF, Gokhan S, Mabie PC, Kessler JA (2000) Embryonic cerebral cortical astrocytes are generated from multipotent neural precursor pools under the influence of distinct environmental signals. *Soc Neurosci Abstr* 26: 1069

49 Gray GE, Sanes JR (1992) Lineage of radial glia in the chicken optic tectum. *Development* 114: 271–283

50 Malatesta P, Hartfuss E, Gotz M (2000) Isolation of radial glial cells by fluorescent-activated cell sorting reveals a neuronal lineage. *Development* 127: 5253–5263

51 Doetsch F, Caille I, Lim DA, Garcia-verdugo JM, Alvarez-Buylla A (1999) Subventricular zone astrocytes are neural stem cells in the adult mammalian brain. *Cell* 97: 703–716

52   Leavitt BR, Hernit-Grant CS, Macklis JD (1999) Mature astrocytes transform into transitional radial glia within adult mouse neocortex that supports directed migration of transplanted immature neurons. *Exp Neurol* 157: 43–57

53   Mehler MF, Kessler JA (1994) Growth factor regulation of neuronal development. *Develop Neurosci* 16: 180–196

54   Mehler MF, Kessler JA (1995) Cytokines and neuronal differentiation. *Crit Rev Neurobiol* 9: 419–446

55   Keegan AD, Nelms K, Wang L-M, Pierce JH, Paul WE (1994) Interleukin 4 receptor: signalling mechanisms. *Immunol Today* 14: 423–432

56   Mabie PC, Mehler MF, Marmur R, Papavasiliou A, Kessler JA (1995) The developmental neurotrophic potential of an interleukin subset that regulates hematolymphoid development and signals through a common gamma receptor subunit. *Neurology* 45: A335

57   Motro B, Van Der Kooy D, Rossant J, Reith A, Bernstein A (1991) Contiguous patterns of c-kit and steel expression: analysis of mutations at the W and SI loci. *Development* 113: 1207–1221

58   Michaelson MD, Bieri PL, Mehler MF, Xu H, Arezzo JC, Pollard JW, Kessler JA (1996) CSF1 deficiency in mice results in abnormal brain development. *Development* 122: 2661–2672

59   Michaelson MD, Mehler MF, Xu H, Gross RE, Kessler JA (1996) Interleukin 7 is a neuronal growth factor. *Develop Biol* 179: 251–263

60   Strelau J, Unsicker K (1999) GDNF family members and their receptors: expression and functions in two oligodendroglial cell lines representing distinct stages of oligodendroglial development. *GLIA* 26: 291–301

61   Baloh RH, Enomoto H, Johnson EM Jr, Milbrandt J (2000) The GDNF family ligands and receptors – implications for neural development. *Curr Opin Neurobiol* 10: 103–110

62. Du X, Stull ND, Iacovitti L (1995) Brain-derived neurotrophic factor works coordinately with partner molecules to initiate tyrosine hydroxylase expression in striatal neurons. *Brain Res* 680: 229–233

63   Kato AC, Lindsay RM (1994) Overlapping and additive effects of neurotrophins and CNTF on cultured human spinal cord neurons. *Exp Neurol* 130: 196–210

64   Michikawa M, Kikuchi S, Kim SU (1992) Leukemia inhibitory factor (LIF) mediated increases of choline acetyltransferase activity in mouse spinal cord neurons in culture. *Neurosci Lett* 140: 75–77

65   Kamegai, M, Niijima K, Kunishita T, Nishizawa M, Ogawa M, Araki M, Ueki A, Konishi Y, Tabira T (1990) Interleukin 3 as a trophic factor for central cholinergic neurons *in vitro* and *in vivo*. *Neuron* 2: 429–436

66   Konishi Y, Chui D-H, Hirose H, Kunishita T, Tabira T (1993) Trophic effects of erythropoietin and other hematopoietic factors on central cholinergic neurons *in vitro* and *in vivo*. *Brain Res* 609: 29–35

67   Tabira T, Konishi Y, Gallyas F Jr (1995) Neurotrophic effects of hematopoietic cytokines on cholinergic and other neurons *in vitro*. *Int J Dev Neurosci* 13: 241–252

68 Erkman L, Wuarin L, Cadelli D, Kato AC (1989) Interferon induces astrocyte maturation causing an increase in cholinergic properties of cultured human spinal cord cells. *Develop Biol* 132: 375–388

69 Henderson CE (1996) Role of neurotrophic factors in neuronal development. *Curr Opin Neurobiol* 6: 64–70

70 Plata-Salaman CR (1991) Immunoregulators in the nervous system. *Neurosci Biobehav Rev* 15: 185–215

71 Patterson PH (1992) The emerging neuropoietic cytokine family: first CDF/LIF, CNTF and IL-6; next ONC, MGF, GCSF? *Curr Opin Neurobiol* 2: 94–97

72 Plioplys AV (1988) Expression of the 210 kDa neurofilament subunit in cultured central nervous system from normal and trisomy 16 mice: regulation by interferon. *J Neurol Sci* 85: 209–222

73 Barish M, Mansdorf NB, Raissdana SS (1991) Gamma-interferon promotes differentiation of cultured cortical and hippocampal neurons. *Develop Biol* 144: 412–423

74 Pelidou SH, Zou LP, Deretzi G, Oniding C, Mix E, Zhu J (2000) Enhancement of acute phase and inhibition of chromic phase of experimental autoimmune neuritis in Lewis rats by intranasal administration of recombinant mouse interleukin 17: potential immunoregulatory role. *Exp Neurol* 163: 165–172

75 Wheeler RD, Culhane AC, Hall MD, Pickering-Brown S, Rothwell NJ, Luheshi GN (2000) Detection of the interleukin 18 family in rat brain by RT-PCR. *Mol Brain Res* 77: 290–293

76 Conti B, Park LC, Calingasan NY, Kim Y, Kim H, Bae Y, E Gibson G, Joh TH (1999) Cultures of astrocytes and microglia express interleukin 18. *Mol Brain Res* 67: 46–52

77 Shi FD, Takeda K, Akira S, Sarvetnick N, Ljunggren HG (2000) IL-18 directs autoreactive T cells and promotes autodestruction in the central nervous system *via* induction of IFN-gamma by NK cells. *J Immunol* 165: 2099–3104

78 D'Alessandro JS, Wang EA (1994) Bone morphogenetic proteins inhibit proliferation, induce reversible differentiation and prevent cell death in astrocyte lineage cells. *Growth Factors* 11: 45–52

79 D'Alessandro JS, Yetz-Aldape J, Wang EA (1994) Bone morphogenetic proteins induce differentiation in astrocyte lineage cells. *Growth Factors* 11: 53–62

80 Barres BA, Schmid R, Sendtner M, Raff MC (1993) Multiple extracellular signals are required for long-term oligodendrocyte survival. *Development* 8: 283–295

81 Johe KK, Hazel TG, Muller T, Dugich-Djordjevic M, McKay R (1996) Single factors direct the differentiation of stem cells from the fetal and adult central nervous system. *Genes Dev* 10: 3129–3140

82 Marmur R, Mabie PC, Gokhan S, Song Q, Kessler JA, Mehler MF (1998) Isolation and developmental characterization of cerebral cortical multipotent progenitors. *Dev Biol* 204: 577–591

83 Koblar SA, Turnley AM, Classon BJ, Reid KL, Ware CB, Cheema SS, Murphy M, Bartlett PF (1998) Neural precursor differentiation into astrocytes requires signaling through leukemia inhibitory factor receptor. *Proc Natl Acad Sci USA* 95: 3178–3181

84 Rajan P, McKay RDG (1998) Multiple routes to astrocytic differentiation in the CNS. *J Neurosci* 18: 3620–3629

85 Molne M, Studer L, Tabar V, Ting YT, Eiden MV, McKay RD (2000) Early cortical precursors do not undergo LIF-mediated astrocytic differentiation. *J Neurosci Res* 59: 301–311

86 Satoh M, Sugino H, Yoshida T (2000) Activin promotes astrocytic differentiation of a multipotent neural stem cell line and an astrocyte progenitor cell line from murine central nervous system. *Neurosci Lett* 284: 143–146

87 Kondo T, Raff M (2000) Oligodendrocyte precursor cells reprogrammed to become multipotential CNS stem cells. *Science* 289: 1754–1757

88 Grinspan JB, Reeves MF, Coulaloglou MJ, Nathanson D, Pleasure D (1996) Re-entry into the cell cycle is required for bFGF-induced oligodendroglial dedifferentiation and survival. *J Neurosci Res* 46: 456–464

89 Canoll PD, Kraemer R, Teng KK, Marchionni MA, Salzer JL (1999) GGF/neuregulin induces a phenotypic reversion of oligodendrocytes. *Mol Cell Neurosci* 13: 79–94

90 Marmur R, Mehler, MF, Mabie P, Papavasilou AK, Cohen RI, Chandross KJ, Kessler JA (1995) Characterization of pre-O2A progenitor cultures from mouse embryonic subventricular zone progenitor cells: effects of neurotrophin 3. *Soc Neurosci Abstr* 21: 287

91 Keshet E Lyman SD, Williams DE, Anderson DM, Jenkins NA, Copeland NG, Parada LF (1991) Embryonic RNA expression patterns of the c-kit receptor and its cognate ligand suggest multiple functional roles in mouse development. *EMBO J* 10: 2425–2435

92 Morii E, Hirota S, Kim HM, Mikoshiba K, Nishimune Y, Kitamura Y, Nomura S (1992) Spatial expression of genes encoding c-kit receptors and their ligands in mouse cerebellum as revealed by in situ hybridization. *Dev Brain Res* 65: 123–129

93 De-Fraja C, Conti L, Magrassi L, Govoni S, Cattaneo E (1998) Members of the JAK/STAT proteins are expressed and regulated during development in the mammalian forebrain. *J Neurosci Res* 54: 320–330

94 Lowell CA, Soriano P (1996) Knockouts of Src-family kinases: stiff bones, wimpy T cells and bad memories. *Genes Develop* 10: 1845–1857

95 Grant SG, O'Dell TJ, Karl KA, Stein PL, Soriano P, Kandel ER (1992) Impaired long-term potentiation, spatial learning, and hippocampal development in fyn mutant mice. *Science* 258: 1903–1910.

96 Ignelzi MA Jr, Miller DR, Soriano P, Maness PF (1994) Impaired neurite outgrowth of src-minus cerebellar neurons on the cell adhesion molecule L1. *Neuron* 12: 873–883.

97 Mehler MF, Mabie PC, Zhang D, Kessler JA (1997) Bone morphogenetic proteins in the nervous system. *Trends Neurosci* 20: 309–317

98 Finch CE, Laping NJ, Morgan TE, Nichols NR, Pasinetti GM (1993) TGF-beta 1 is an organizer of responses to neurodegeneration. *J Cell Biochem* 53: 314–322

99 Chalazonitis A, Kalberg J, Twardzik DR, Morrison RS, Kessler JA (1992) Transforming growth factor β has neurotrophic actions on sensory neurons *in vitro* and is synergistic with nerve growth factor. *Develop Biol* 152: 121–132

100 Flanders KC, Ludecke G, Engels S, Cissel DS, Roberts AB, Kondaiah P, Lafyatis R,

Sporn MB, Unsicker K (1991) Localization and actions of transforming growth factor-beta in the embryonic nervous system. *Development* 113: 183–191

101 Soderstrom S, Bengtsson H, Ebendal T (1996) Expression of serine/threonine kinase receptors including the bone morphogenetic factor type II receptor in the developing and adult rat brain. *Cell Tissue Res* 286: 269–279

102 Mehler MF, Marmur R, Gross R, Mabie PC, Zang Z, Papavasiliou A, Kessler JA (1995) Cytokines regulate the cellular phenotype of developing neural lineage species. *Int J Dev Neurosci* 13: 213–240

103 Mabie PC, Mehler MF, Marmur R, Song, Q, Kessler JA (1996) Oligodendroglial and astroglial differentiation during development and remyelination. *Ann Neurol* 40: 546

104 Mabie PC, Mehler MF, Papavasiliou A, Song Q, Kessler JA (1997) Bone morphogenetic proteins induce astroglial differentiation of oligodendroglial-astroglial progenitor cells. *J Neurosci* 17: 4112–4120

105 Schluesener HJ, Meyermann R (1994) Expression of BMP-6, a TGFβ related morphogenetic cytokine, in rat radial glia. *GLIA* 12: 161–164

106 Tomizawa K, Matsui H, Kondo E,Miyamoto K, Tokuda M, Itano T, Nagahata S, Akagi T, Hatase O (1995) Developmental alterations and neuron-specific expression of bone morphogenetic protein-6 mRNA in rodent brain. *Mol Brain Res* 28: 122–128

107 Zhang D, Mehler MF, Song Q, Kessler JA (1998) Development of bone morphogenetic protein receptors in the nervous system and possible roles in regulating TrkC expression. *J Neurosci* 18: 3314–3326

108 Bjorklund A, Lindvall O (2000) *Cell* replacement therapies for central nervous system disorders. *Nat Neurosci* 3: 537–544

109 Hodges H, Sowinski P, Fleming P, Kershaw TR, Sinden JD, Meldrum BS, Gray JA (1996) Contrasting effects of fetal CA1 and CA3 hippocampal grafts on deficits in spatial learning and working memory induced by global cerebral ischaemia in rats. *Neuroscience* 72: 959–988

110 Sinden JD, Rashid-Doubell F, Kershaw TR, Nelson A, Chadwick A, Jat PS, Noble MD, Hodges H, Gray JA (1997) Recovery of spatial learning by grafts of a conditionally immortalized hippocampal neuroepithelial cell line into the ischaemia-lesioned hippocampus. *Neuroscience* 81: 599–608

111 Mattsson B, Sorensen JC, Zimmer J, Johansson BB (1997) Neural grafting to experimental neocortical infarcts improves behavioral outcome and reduces thalamic atrophy in rats housed in enriched but not in standard environments. *Stroke* 28: 1225–1231

112 Young D, Lawlor PA, Leone P, Dragunow M, During MJ (1999) Environmental enrichment inhibits spontaneous apoptosis, prevents seizures and is neuroprotective. *Nat Med* 5: 448–453

113 Van Praag H, Kempermann G, Gage FH (1999) Running increases cell proliferation and neurogenesis in the adult mouse dentate gyrus. *Nat Neurosci* 2: 266–270

114 Sorensen JC, Grabowski M, Zimmer J, Johansson BB (1996) Fetal neocortical tissue blocks implanted in brain infarcts of adult rats interconnect with the host brain. *Exp Neurol* 138: 227–235

115 Borlongan CV, Tajima Y, Trojanowski JQ, Lee VM, Sanberg PR (1998) Transplantation of cryopreserved human embryonal carcinoma-derived neurons (NT2N cells) promotes functional recovery in ischemic rats. *Exp Neurol* 149: 310–321

116 Borlongan CV, Tajima Y, Trojanowski JQ, Lee VM, Sanberg PR (1998) Cerebral ischemia and CNS transplantation: differential effects of grafted fetal rat striatal cells and human neurons derived from a clonal cell line. *Neuroreport* 16: 3703–3709

117 Fukunaga A, Uchida K, Hara K, Kuroshima Y, Kawase T (1999) Differentiation and angiogenesis of central nervous system stem cells implanted with mesenchyme into ischemic rat brain. *Cell Transplant* 8: 435–441

118 Rosenbaum DM, Gupta G, Gokhan S, Singh M, Cohen B, Rosenbaum PS, Kessler JA, Mehler MF (2000) Transplanted embryonic multipotent progenitor cells promote neuronal and glial cell regeneration following cerebral and retinal ischemia. *Soc Neurosci Abstr* 26: 2291

119 Ren J, Tate BA, Sietsma D, Marciniak A, Snyder EY, Finklestein SP (2000) Co-administration of neural stem cells and bFGF enhances functional recovery following focal cerebral infarction in rat. *Soc Neurosci Abstr* 26: 2291

120 Zhao L-R, Duan W-M, Reyes M, Kenne CD, Nussbaum ES, Verfaille CM, Low WC (2000) Human bone marrow stem cells exhibit neural phenotypes after transplantation and ameliorate neurological deficits with ischemic brain injury in rats. *Soc Neurosci Abstr* 26: 2291

121 Takagi Y, Nozaki K, Takahashi J, Yodoi J, Ishikawa M, Hashimoto N (1999) Proliferation of neuronal precursor cells in the dentate gyrus is accelerated after transient forebrain ischemia in mice. *Brain Res* 831: 283–287

122 Johansson BB (2000) Brain plasticity and stroke rehabilitation. The Willis lecture. *Stroke* 31: 223–230

123 Kondziolka D, Wechsler L, Goldstein S, Meltzer C, Thulborn KR, Gebel J, Jannetta P, DeCesare S, Elder EM, McGrogan M et al (2000) Transplantation of cultured human neuronal cells for patients with stroke. *Neurology* 55: 565–569

124 Justicia C, Planas AM (1999) Transforming growth factor-alpha acting at the epidermal growth factor receptor reduces infarct volume after permanent middle cerebral artery occlusion in rats. *J Cereb Blood Flow Metab* 19: 128–132

125 Huang Z, Chen K, Huang PL, Finklestein SP, Moskowitz MA (1997) bFGF ameliorates focal ischemic injury by blood flow-independent mechanisms in eNOS mutant mice. *Am J Physiol* 272: H1401–405

126 Tretter YP, Hertel M, Munz B, ten Bruggencate G, Werner S, Alzheimer C (2000) Induction of activin A is essential for the neuroprotective action of basic fibroblast growth factor *in vivo*. *Nat Med* 6: 812–815

127 Ruocco A, Nicole O, Docagne F, Ali C, Chazalviel L, Komesli S, Yablonsky F, Roussel S, MacKenzie ET, Vivien D et al (1999) A transforming growth factor-beta antagonist unmasks the neuroprotective role of this endogenous cytokine in excitotoxic and ischemic brain injury. *J Cereb Blood Flow Metab* 19: 1345–1353

128 Ren J, Kaplan PL, Charette MF, Speller H, Finklestein SP (2000) Time window of

intracisternal osteogenic protein-1 in enhancing functional recovery after stroke. *Neuropharmacology* 39: 860–865

129 Lin SZ, Hoffer BJ, Kaplan P, Wang Y (1999) Osteogenic protein-1 protects against cerebral infarction induced by MCA ligation in adult rats. *Stroke* 30: 126–133

130 Baetta R, Soma M, De-Fraja C, Comparato C, Teruzzi C, Magrassi L, Cattaneo E (2000) Upregulation and activation of Stat6 precede vascular smooth muscle cell proliferation in carotid artery injury model. *Arterioscler Thromb Vasc Biol* 20: 931–939

131 Lin TN, Wang PY, Chi SI, Kuo JS (1998) Differential regulation of ciliary neurotrophic factor (CNTF) and CNTF receptor alpha (CNTFR alpha) expression following focal cerebral ischemia. *Mol Brain Res* 55: 71–80

132 Sadamoto Y, Igase K, Sakanaka M, Sata K, Otsuka H, Sakaki S, Masuda S, Sasaki R (1998) Erythropoietin prevents place navigation disability and cortical infarction in rats with permanent occlusion of the middle cerebral artery. *Biochem Biophys Res Commun* 253: 26–32

133 Nawashiro H, Martin D, Hallenbeck JM (1997) Neuroprotective effects of TNF binding protein in focal cerebral ischemia. *Brain Res* 778: 265–271

134 Slevin M, Krupinski J, Slowik A, Kumar P, Szczudlik A, Gaffney J (2000) Serial measurement of vascular endothelial growth factor and transforming growth factor-beta1 in serum of patients with acute ischemic stroke. *Stroke* 31: 1863–1870

135 Marti HJ, Bernaudin M, Bellail A, Schoch H, Euler M, Petit E, Risau W (2000) Hypoxia-induced vascular endothelial growth factor expression precedes neovascularization after cerebral ischemia. *Am J Pathol* 156: 965–976

136 Spera PA, Ellison JA, Feuerstein GZ, Barone FC (1998) IL-10 reduces rat brain injury following focal stroke. *Neurosci Lett* 251: 189–192

137 Grilli M, Barbieri I, Basudev H, Brusa R, Casati C, Lozza G, Ongini E (2000) Interleukin-10 modulates neuronal threshold of vulnerability to ischaemic damage. *Eur J Neurosci* 12: 2265–2272

138 Van Wagoner NJ, Benveniste EN (1999) Interleukin-6 expression and regulation in astrocytes. *J Neuroimmunol* 100: 124–139

139 Vila N, Castillo J, Davalos A, Chamorro A (2000) Proinflammatory cytokines and early neurological worsening in ischemic stroke. *Stroke* 31: 2325–2329

140 Sallmann S, Jüttler E, Prinz S, Petersen N, Knopf U, Weiser T, Schwaninger M (2000) Induction of interleukin-6 by depolarization of neurons. *J Neurosci* 20: 8637–8642

141 Marz P, Heese K, Dimitriades-Schmutz B, Rose-John S, Otten U (1999) Role of interleukin-6 and soluble IL-6 receptor in region-specific induction of astrocytic differentiation and neurotrophin expression. *GLIA* 26: 191–200

142 Carlson NG, Wieggel WA, Chen J, Bacchi A, Rogers SW, Gahring LC (1999) Inflammatory cytokines IL-1 alpha, IL-1 beta, IL-6, and TNF-alpha impart neuroprotection to an excitotoxin through distinct pathways. *J Immunol* 163: 3963–3968

143 Feuerstein GZ, Wang X, Barone FC (1998) The role of cytokines in the neuropathology of stroke and neurotrauma. *Neuroimmunomodulation* 5: 143–159

144 Mattson MP, Culmsee C, Yu ZF (2000) Apoptotic and antiapoptotic mechanisms in stroke. *Cell Tissue Res* 301: 173–187

145 Xian CJ, Zhou XF (2000) Roles of transforming growth factor-alpha and related molecules in the nervous system. *Mol Neurobiol* 20: 157–183

146 Ye W, Shimamura K, Rubenstein JL, Hynes, MA, Rosenthal A (1998) FGF and Shh signals control dopaminergic and serotonergic cell fate in the anterior neural plate. *Cell* 93: 755–766

147 Le Roux P, Behar S, Higgins D, Charette M (1999) OP-1 enhances dendritic growth from cerebral cortical neurons *in vitro*. *Exp Neurol* 160: 151–163

148 Bengtsson H, Soderstrom S, Kylberg A, Charette MF, Ebendal T (1998) Potentiating interactions between morphogenetic proteins and neurotrophic factors in developing neurons. *J Neurosci Res* 53: 559–568

149 Zhu G, Mehler MF, Mabie PC, Kessler JA (1999) Developmental changes in progenitor cells responsiveness to cytokines. *J Neurosci Res* 56: 131–145

150 Mehler MF, Gokhan S (1999) Postnatal cerebral cortical multipotent progenitors: regulatory mechanisms and potential role in the development of novel neural regenerative strategies. *Brain Pathol* 9: 515–526

151 Nakashima K, Yanagisawa M, Arakawa,H, Kimura N, Hisatsune T, Kawabata M, Miyazono K , Taga T (1999) Synergistic signaling in fetal brain by STAT3-Smad1 complex bridged by p300. *Science* 284: 479–482

152 Wrana JL (2000) Regulation of smad activity. *Cell* 100: 189–192

153 Liu F, Massague J, Ruiz i Altaba A (1998) Carboxy-terminally truncated Gli3 proteins associate with Smads. *Nat Genet* 20: 325–326

154 De Luca A, Weller M, Frei K, Fontana A (1996) Maturation-dependent modulation of apoptosis in cultured cerebellar granule neurons by cytokines and neurotrophins. *Eur J Neurosci* 8: 1994–2005

155 Ezzeddine ZD, Yang X, DeChiara T, Yancopoulos G, Cepko CL (1997) Postmitotic cells fated to become rod photoreceptors can be respecified by CNTF treatment of the retina. *Development* 124: 1055–1067

156 Bernaudin M, Bellail A, Marti HH, Yvon A, Vivien D, Duchatelle I, Mackenzie ET, Petit E (2000) Neurons and astrocytes express EPO mRNA: oxygen-sensing mechanisms that involve the redox-state of the brain. *GLIA* 30: 271–278

157 Mehler MF, Kessler JA (1997) Hematolymphopoietic and inflammatory cytokines in neural development. *Trends Neurosci* 20: 357–365

Interleukin-10 in cerebral ischemia and stroke

John R. Bethea[1,2], Ricardo Prado[3] and W. Dalton Dietrich[1,2,3]

[1]The Miami Project to Cure Paralysis, Departments of [2]Neurological Surgery and [3]Neurology, University of Miami School of Medicine, P.O. Box 016960 (R-48), Miami, FL 33101, USA

Introduction

Ischemic neuronal cell death induced by transient ischemic attacks, cardiopulmonary arrest followed by resuscitation and acute stroke are leading causes of death and disability in industrialized countries. Early (< 3 h) treatment with tissue plasminogin activator (t-PA) was approved in 1996 for the treatment of acute stroke [1]. Nevertheless, the therapeutic challenge remains to determine what specific pharmacologic or nonpharmagologic interventions can be developed to reduce neuronal cell death and functional abnormalities from strokes or ischemic injury. In this regard, inflammatory processes are thought to participate in neuronal cell death following cerebral ischemia.

Inflammation is a very complex biological process. Inflammatory processes are essential for host defense and wound healing. However, if inflammation becomes dis-regulated it can induce and enhance neuronal injury following ischemia or diseases of the CNS. Important effectors of inflammatory responses are a family of proteins called cytokines. Cytokines play a central role in the initiation, perpetuation, regulation and attenuation of immune and inflammatory responses. Because cytokines have such diverse biological functions their expression is tightly regulated and not constitutive, as is the case for many growth factors. Pro-inflammatory cytokines such as tumor necrosis factor-α (TNFα), interleukin-1 (IL-1) and interleukin-6 (IL-6) are generally produced during the effector phase of an immune response. Anti-inflammatory cytokines such as interleukin-4 (IL-4), interleukin-10 (IL-10) and interleukin-13 (IL-13) that are essential for turning off an immune response are synthesized during the attenuation phase.

Several recent studies have documented the role pro-inflammatory cytokines have in ischemia [2–7]. In one study, Spera and colleagues [7] reported that IL-10 treatment given centrally and systemically reduced overall infarct volume after permanent middle cerebral artery occlusion (MCA). Therefore, the purpose of this

Inflammation and Stroke, edited by Giora Z. Feuerstein
© 2001 Birkhäuser Verlag Basel/Switzerland

chapter is to review recent data regarding the neuroprotective effects of the anti-inflammatory cytokine IL-10 in treating experimental models of focal and global ischemia.

Interleukin-10

IL-10 is a potent anti-inflammatory cytokine that has been used to successfully reduce *in vivo* inflammation and improve functional outcome in humans and experimental models of human inflammatory diseases such as traumatic brain injury, spinal cord injury, multiple sclerosis and meningitis [8–19]. IL-10 is synthesized by numerous cell types including T-helper lymphocytes (Th$_2$), monocytes/macrophages, astrocytes, and microglia [20, 21]. In the peripheral immune system, IL-10 suppresses the majority of monocyte/macrophage inflammatory responses. IL-10 blocks the production of numerous cytokines, matrix degrading metalloproteins (MMPs) and chemokines [13, 18, 20, 22–24]. One of the ways in which IL-10 reduces peripheral inflammation is by reducing the phosphorylation, translocation and subsequent DNA binding of NF-κB family members, while having little or no effect on other transcription factors [25, 26]. Additionally, IL-10 can abrogate the activation of monocytes by blocking tyrosine kinase activity and the Ras signaling pathway [20]. With respect to the CNS, IL-10 reduces TNFα production by astrocytes and antigen presentation by both astrocytes and microglia, and prevents experimental allergic encephalomyelitis in Lewis rats [11, 13, 16]. In an *in vivo* model of cerebral malaria, a single systemic dose (but not intrathecal) of IL-10 was sufficient to block cytokine production and infiltration of inflammatory cells [14].

IL-10 exerts its biological responses by binding to its receptor, a member of the class II cytokine receptor family [27–31]. It was recently demonstrated that, like other members of this family, the IL-10 receptor has two chains, designated alpha and beta [30]. Furthermore, through the use of chimeric receptor constructs it was determined that the beta chain is essential for IL-10 signal transduction to occur [30]. Upon interacting with its receptor IL-10 induces phosphorylation and the subsequent activation of Jak1 and Tyk2 and STAT 1, STAT 3 and in certain cells, STAT5 [30-33]. Jak1 and the STATs interact with the alpha chain and Tyk 2 binds to the beta chain [30-33]. One hypothesis is that the beta chain is required for positioning Tyk 2 along side the alpha chain so signal transduction can be activated [30]. Site directed mutagenesis of the membrane-distal tyrosine residues in the alpha chain along with STAT 3 dominant negative mutations demonstrated that these tyrosines are essential for the anti-inflammatory properties of IL-10 and that STAT 3 is not required [33]. While the anti-inflammatory effects and neuroprotective potential of IL-10 is clear, the mechanism(s) through which it exerts these effects have not been totally elucidated and appear to be cell-type and target-gene dependent.

It is therefore important to determine under what specific experimental conditions is IL-10 treatment neuroprotective. For this aim we summarize three recent ischemic studies that determined the effects of IL-10 treatment on histopathological outcome.

Thrombotic stroke

Thromboembolic mechanisms are believed to play a major role in the pathogenesis of transient ischemic attacks and acute stroke [51]. In an attempt to more accurately mimic the early pathological events associated with vascular thrombosis, rodent models of photochemically-induced vascular thrombosis have been developed and tested [34]. One such photochemical model allows a well demarcated infarct of consistent size and location to be produced non-invasively [35]. Photochemical reactions lead to endothelial damage, blood-brain barrier permeability, and platelet accumulation resulting in severe hemodynamic perturbations and focal ischemia. In this study, we determined whether IL-10 treatment would influence infarct size following photochemically induced thrombotic infarction.

Male Wistar rats weighing 260–360 g were anesthetized with 4% halothane in a mixture of 70 : 30 nitrous oxide and oxygen. Femoral arterial and venous catheters were inserted for arterial blood gas determination, mean arterial blood pressure monitoring, and fluid administration. All animals were mechanically ventilated *via* endotracheal tube followed by muscle paralysis with pancourounium bromide (0.35 mg/kg/h). Brain and body temperature were maintained at 37° C by utilizing both heating pads and lamps.

The methods involved with photochemical induction of cerebral cortical infarction have been described previously [35]. Briefly, rats were mounted in a sterotaxic frame and the exposed skulls were irradiated for 3 min with a 4 mm/diameter 26 mW beam from a 562 nm argon-pumped dye laser *via* 400 μm diameter Mitsubishi optical fiber. The exit beam was collimated with a 30 mm focal length plano spherical lens. The center of the beam was positioned 3 mm lateral to bregma. The photosensitive dye, Rose bengal (10 mg/kg), was injected intravenously over a 1-min period beginning 30 s before the initiation of irradiation. 15 min post-irradiation, IL-10 (5.0 μg) was administered IP. At 24 h after irradiation, a second similar dose of IL-10 was given. Nontreated animals received a similar volume of saline.

Seven days following infarct induction, animals were anesthetized with halothane and the animals were perfused and fixed with 40% formaldehyde, acetic acid, and absolute methanol at 1 : 1 : 8 by volume. Brains were removed and embedded in paraffin and semiserially sectioned at 10 μm intervals. Coronal sections (9 levels/animal) were scanned into a MCID Image Analysis System and areas of infarction were determined. Infarct volume was derived by integration of infarct areas using the trapezoidal rule. Differences in infarct size and volume among the treated groups were determined by one-way analysis of variance.

As previously described, a well-demarcated infarct was visible underlying the irradiated site. No significant effect on infarct area (Fig. 1a) or infarct volume (Fig. 1b) was demonstrated. These data indicate that IL-10 treatment at this specific dose and treatment regimen does not provide significant neuroprotection following experimentally induced thrombotic stroke.

Transient global ischemia

Animal models of transient global ischemia were developed to simulate the type of brain injury produced by human cardiac arrest. This leads to selective neuronal vulnerability of the CA1 hippocampus. Thus, many studies have used this cerebral ischemia model to test novel therapies to protect against neuronal cell death. In this study, we attempted to determine whether IL-10 treatment following 12.5 min of transient global ischemia would lead to significant protection of the CA1 hippocampus.

A model of transient global ischemia that has been previously described was used in these studies [36]. Experiments were conducted on 21 male Wistar rats weighing between 250 and 300 g. Rats were initially anesthetized with 3% halothane, 30% oxygen, and the balance nitrous oxide. The femoral arteries and veins were cannulated and common carotid arteries exposed bilaterally. Close-fitting PV tubing contained within another dual bore silastic tubing was looped around each carotid artery. Rats then underwent intubation and were immobilized with pancuronium bromide, and maintained with repeated doses. Animals were connected to a rodent respirator and ventilated using 70% nitrous oxide, 2% halothane, and the balance oxygen. Brain temperature was indirectly monitored with a thermocoupled probe placed in the temporalis muscle. Temperature was controlled between 36.5 and 37° C because of the known benefits of mild hypothermia on histopathological outcome after cerebral ischemia.

Animals were prepared for bilateral common carotid artery occlusion combined with systemic hypotension (50 mm Hg). Mean arterial blood pressure was first lowered to approximately 60 mm Hg and the ischemic insult initiated by tightening the carotid ligatures bilaterally. Blood was withdrawn until arterial blood pressure declined to 50 mm Hg. The onset of 12.5 min of ischemic insult was timed from that point. The ischemic insult was terminated by loosening the carotid ligatures and slowly reinfusing the shed blood (maintained at 36–37° C) to restore normotension. At 30 min post-ischemia, treated animals received 5 μg of IL-10 IP ($n = 7$). Non-treated animals received a similar volume of saline ($n = 7$). A third group of rats ($n = 7$), in addition to receiving IL-10, 30 min after ischemia, received a second dose of IL-10, 24 h later. Animals were allowed to survive for 3 days prior to perfusion

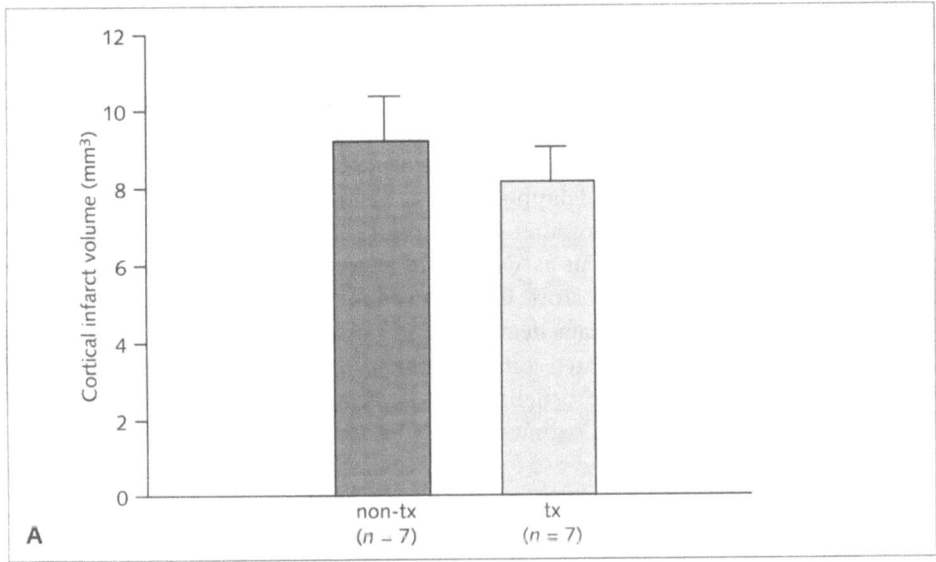

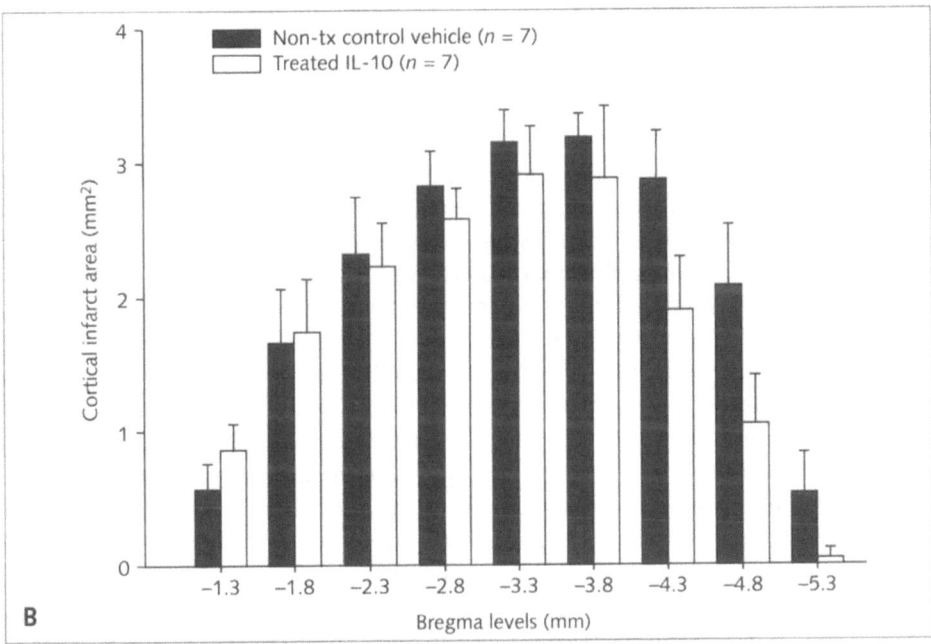

Figure 1
Bar graphs of cortical infarct volumes (A) and areas (B) following photochemically induced cortical infarction. No significant difference in infarct volumes or areas was demonstrated between nontreated and IL-10 treated rats.

fixation and tissue embedding. Semi-quantitative analysis of the CA1 hippocampus was undertaken using a four-point scale where 0 = normal appearing neurons; 1 = few necrotic neurons; 2 = many necrotic neurons; and 3 = few normal appearing neurons.

As previously reported, 12.5 min of transient global ischemia led to severe neuronal cell death within the CA1 hippocampus. A single injection of IL-10, 30 min after the ischemic period did not alter this response. Likewise, in the treated group that received the acute treatment as well as the second IL-10 treatment 24 h after ischemia, a high frequency of necrotic CA1 neurons was again observed. Semi-quantitative assessment of CA1 damage demonstrated no significant effect of IL-10 treatment as compared to nontreated rats $(p > 0.05)$. Thus, in this transient global ischemia model, no significant benefit of IL-10 treatment was observed on CA1 pathology using two treatment regimes.

IL-10 and hypothermia treatment following transient global ischemia

Mild to moderate brain hypothermia has been shown in models of transient global ischemia to be neuroprotective [37]. While intraischemic hypothermia has been shown to provide long-lasting neuroprotection, periods of post-ischemic hypothermia, to a large degree, delay rather than provide long lasting neuroprotection of the CA1 hippocampus [38]. For example, 3 h of moderate hypothermia (30° C) following transient global ischemia provides marked protection to the CA1 hippocampus at 3 days survival. However, in animals allowed to live for 2 months, no significant protection of the CA1 hippocampus has been reported [38]. Recently, it has been reported that hypothermia plus pharmacotherapy can provide some degree of long lasting protection. Hypothermia plus treatment with the noncompetitive NMDA antagonist, MK-801, the free radical scavenger PBN, and treatment with an anti-inflammatory/antipyretic drug (dipyrone) have all been shown to provide a greater degree of long-term protection than hypothermia alone [39–41]. Thus, we questioned whether mild hypothermia plus IL-10 treatment would provide long-lasting neuroprotection in this model of transient global ischemia [36].

Animals underwent 12.5 min of transient global ischemia, as previously described. Animals were randomized into five groups, each containing five animals. Sham-operated control animals underwent brain temperature measurements and all surgical procedures except for the induction of brain ischemia. In the normothermic-ischemic series, intraischemic and post-ischemic brain temperatures were maintained at 36.7–37.0° C during the 4-h post-ischemia observation period. In the post-ischemic hypothermic series, animals underwent normothermic ischemia followed by a 4-h hypothermic period (33–34° C). In the IL-10 treated groups, 5 µg in 100 µl were injected IP in the immediate post-ischemic period, as well as 3 days after ischemia. At 2 months following the ischemic period, rats were perfusion fixed and brain sections analyzed by an observer blinded to the experimental protocol. In this study, normal-appearing pyramidal neurons were counted in the lateral, middle, and medial subsectors of the hippocampus CA1 region.

Figure 2 shows representative light microscopic changes within the CA1 hippocampus for sham-operated and ischemic groups 2 months after surgery. Following normothermic ischemia, post-ischemic hypothermia, or IL-10 treatment alone, few viable neurons were observed in the CA1 hippocampus (Fig. 2a). In contrast, in animals receiving both mild hypothermia and IL-10 treatment, large numbers of viable neurons were seen throughout the CA1 subsector (Fig. 2b). In addition, quantitative cell counts for viable neurons demonstrated that combined treatment with hypothermia and IL-10 produced a significant increase in normal neuronal counts compared with the normothermic ischemic group groups (Fig. 3). Taken together, these data indicate that mild hypothermia combined with IL-10 treatment leads to long-term survival of a neuronal population selectively vulnerable to this ischemic insult.

Discussion

IL-10 and neuroprotection

Recent studies have demonstrated that IL-10 is effective in treating some progressive inflammatory disorders and models of cerebral ischemia or traumatic brain injury [7, 42]. In addition, IL-10 has recently been demonstrated to reduce inflammation and improve functional recovery in *in vivo* models of spinal cord injury [19, 43, 44]. The inability of IL-10 to reduce infarct volume in a thromboembolic stroke model, or protect CA1 neurons from transient global ischemia in the absence of hypothermia remains an enigma. One explanation for this observation is that early cell death in these models is not primarily the result of inflammatory processes but is comprised of excitotoxic, free radical and inflammatory events that prohibit the use of a single therapeutic agent. We are currently studying the effectiveness of combining IL-10 with hypothermia in the photothrombotic model and assessing more chronic survival times.

In addition to being a potent anti-inflammatory cytokine and potentially exerting its neuroprotective effects by attenuating inflammation, recent studies suggest that IL-10 promotes some of its neuroprotecive effects by acting directly on neurons [45]. Using neurons isolated from the brains of mice deficient in IL-10 it was determined that these cells were more susceptible to NMDA toxicity and to deprivation of oxygen and glucose induced cell death [45]. Furthermore, using cerebellar granule cells isolated from wild type mice, IL-10, in a dose dependent manner, protected these cells from excitotoxic cell death [45]. Similarly, IL-10 was shown to prevent apoptosis, in cultures of cerebellar granule cells as determined by TUNEL stain-

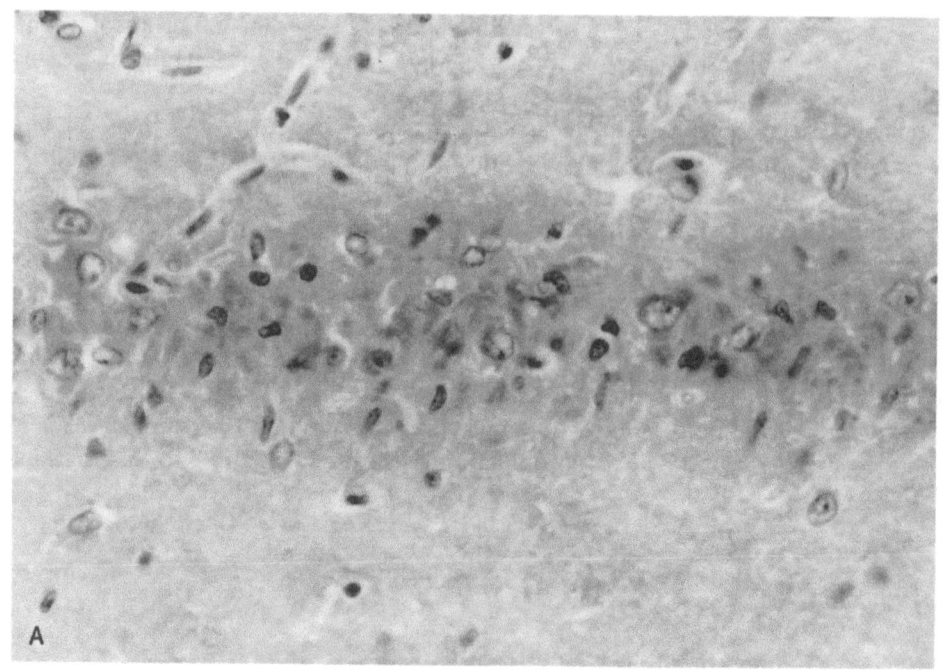

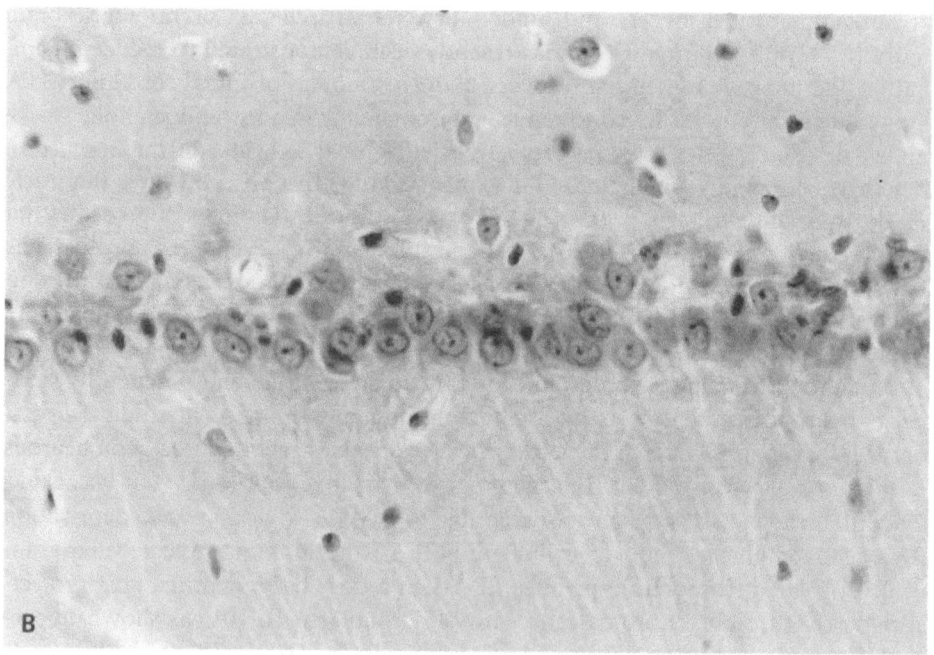

ing [46]. In fact, IL-10 elicited greater neuroprotection than when high concentrations (300 mM) of glutamate were used [46] brain-derived neurotrophic factor or fibroblast growth factor 2. In each of these studies the neuroprotective effects of IL-10 were observed only when the cells were pre-treated with IL-10 for 12–24 h. This suggests that IL-10 may be "altering" the cellular environment and making neurons more resistant to glutamate mediated neuronal toxicity. Two possible ways in which IL-10 could be improving neuronal survival would be by the downregulation of glutamate receptors and or the upregulation of Bcl-2, Bcl-xl or other anti-apoptotic proteins. In this regard, we have recently demonstrated that IL-10 reduces the activation of caspases 8 and 3 and ICAD cleavage following CNS injury [48]. Furthermore, IL-10 has been shown to prevent apoptosis by upregulating Bcl-2 expression in other systems [48, 49]. Thus, IL-10 treatment may be most effective in injury models where apoptotic cell death is a dominant injury mechanism.

The precise mechanisms by which hypothermia and IL-10 following transit global ischemia are protecting neurons from injury have not been elucidated. There are, however, several explanations that could account for the additive neuroprotective effects of IL-10. IL-10 could increase the local synthesis of nerve growth factors, reduce astrogliosis and attenuate specific secondary injury mechanisms following injury. For example, it has recently been demonstrated that IL-10 induced nerve growth factor production in astrocytes and reduced reactive astrogliosis following brain injury in rats [8, 50]. The failure of a restricted period of post ischemic hypothermia to protect chronically has been the subject of recent publications [36, 38]. One hypothesis is that because post-ischemia hypothermia only protects partially, inflammatory processes are activated that may represent a secondary injury mechanism once the hypothermia period has been terminated [38]. Thus, it will be important in future studies to determine the effects of IL-10 treatment on CA1 microglial activation with and without hypothermia.

In conclusion, further studies need to be performed to demonstrate whether the combination of IL-10 and hypothermia are effective strategies for treating other cerebrovascular disorders. However, the effectiveness of combining hypothermia with IL-10 in treating transient global ischemia appears very promising. Once we better understand the mechanisms responsible for the observed chronic neuroprotection then more effective treatment strategies may be developed and tested.

Figure 2
Paraffin-embedded sections of rat brain stained with hematoxylin and eosin (H&E) 2 months after 12.5 min of transient global ischemic showing CA1 hippocampus. (A) Normothermia ischemia. (B) Immediate postishemic hypothermia plus IL-10 treatment. Increased numbers of normal appearing neurons are present in CA1 subsector following hypothermia plus IL-10 treatments.

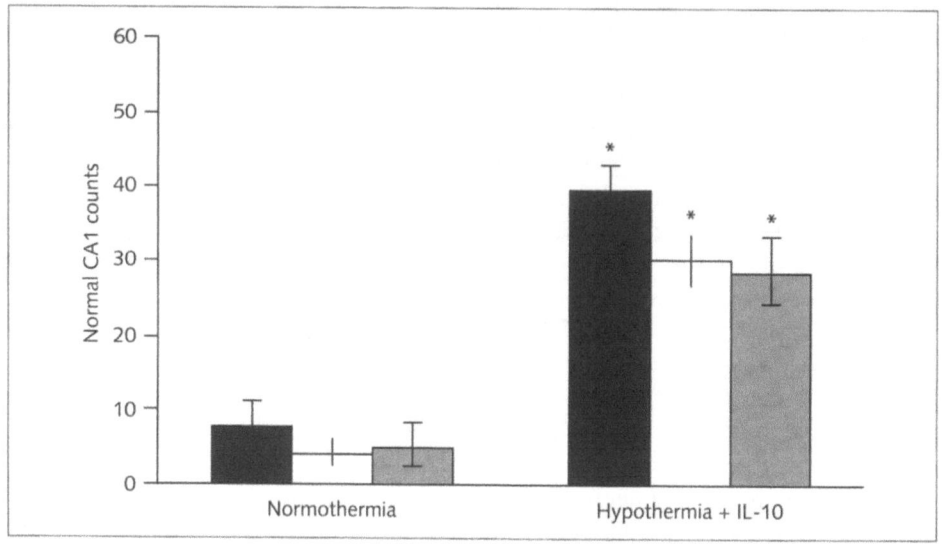

Figure 3
Bar graph of the number of normal-appearing CA1 hippocapal neurons in lateral (black), middle (white) and medial (shaded) CA1 subsectors in the normothermia and hypothermia plus IL-10 treated groups.
*Significantly different from normothermia values.

Acknowledgements

This study was supported by US PHS grants NS27127 and NS37130. The authors thank Olfelia Alonso and Susan Kraydieh for technical support, Judith Cox for word processing, and Charlaine Rowlette for editorial assistance.

References

1   Grotta T (1997) t-PA – The best current option for most patients. *N Engl J Med* 337: 1310–1312

2   Feuerstein GZ, Liu T, Barone FC (1994) Cytokines, inflammation, and brain injury: role of tumor necrosis factor-α. *Cerebrovasc Brain Metabol Rev* 6: 341–360

3   Barone FC, Arvin B, White RF, Miller A, Webb CL, Willete RN, Lysko PG, Feuerstein GZ (1997) Tumor necrosis factor α: a mediator of focal ischemic brain injury. *Stroke* 28: 1233–1244

4   Dawson DA, Martin D, Hallenbeck JM (1996) Inhibition of tumor necrosis factor-alpha reduces focal cerebral ischemic injury in the spontaneously hypertensive rat. *Neurosci Lett* 218: 41–44

5   Liu T, Clark RK, McDonnell PC, Young PR, White RF, Barone FC, Feuerstein GZ (1994) Tumor mecrosis factor α expression in ischemic neurons. *Stroke* 25: 1481–1488

6   Rothwell NJ, Relton JK (1993) Involvement of interleukin-1 and lipocortin-1 in ischaemic brain damage. *Cerebrovasc Brain Metabol Rev* 5: 178–198

7   Spera PA, Ellison, JA, Feuerstein GZ, Barone FC (1998) IL-10 reduces rat brain injury following focal stroke. *Neurosci Lett* 251: 189–192

8   Balasingam V, Wong VW (1996) Attenuation of astroglial reactivity by interleukin-10. *J Neurosci* 16: 2945–2955

9   Berg DJ, Kuhn R, Rajewsky K et al (1995) Interleukin-10 is a central regulator of the response to LPS in murine models of endotoxic shock and the Schwartzman reaction but not endotoxin tolerance. *J Clin Invest* 96: 2339–2347

10 Berman RM, Suzuki T, Tahara H, Robbins PD, Narula SK, Lotze MT (1996) Systemic administration of cellular IL-10 induces an effective specific, and long-lived immune response against established tumors in mice. *J Immunol* 157: 231–238

11 Crisi GM, Santambrogio L, Hochwald GM, Smith SR, Carlino JA Thorbecke GJ (1995) Staphylococcal enterotoxin B and turmor-necrosis factor-α-induced relapses of experimental allergic encephalomyelitis: protection by transforming growth factor-β and interleukin-10. *Eur J Immunol* 25: 3035–3040

12 Cua DJ, Coffman RL Stohlman SA (1996) Exposure to T helper 2 cytokines *in vivo* before encounter with antigen selects for T helper subsets *via* alterations in antigen-presenting cell function. *J Immunol* 157: 2830–2836

13 Issazaseh S, Lorentzen JC, Mustafa MI, HÖjeberg B, Müssener Å Olsson T (1996) Cytokines in relapsing experimental autoimmune encephalomyelitis in DA rats: persistent mRNA expression of proinflammatory cytokines and absent expression of interleukin-10 and transforming growth factor-β. *J Neuroimmunol* 103–115

14 Koedel U, Bernatowicz A, Frei K, Fontana A Pfister H-W (1996) Systemically (but not intrathecally) administered IL-10 attenuates pathophysiologic alterations in experimental pneumococcal meningitis. *J Immunology* 157: 5185–5191

15 Rogy MA, Auffenberg T, Espat NJ, Philip R, Remick D Wollenberg GK (1995) Human tumor necrosis factor receptor (p55) and interleukin 10 gene transfer in the mouse reduces mortality to lethal endotoxemia and also attenuates local inflammatory responses. *J Exp Med* 181: 2289–2293

16 Rott O, Fleisher B Cash E (1994) Interleukin-10 prevents experimental allergic encephalomyelitis in rats. *Eur J Immunol* 24: 1434–1440

17 Rudick RA, Ransohoff RM, Peppler R, Medendorp SV, Lehmann P Alam J (1996) Interferon beta induces interleukin-10 expression: Relevance to multiple sclerosis. *Ann Neurol* 40: 618–627

18 Bethea JR, Castro M, Keane RW, Lee TT, Dietrich DW, Yezierski RP (1998) Traumatic spinal cord injury induces nuclear factor Kapa-B activation. *J Neurosci* 18: 3251–3260

19 Bethea JR, Nagashima H, Acosta MC, Briceno C, Gomez F, Marcillo AE, Loor K, Green J, Dietrich WD (1999) Systemically administered interleukin-10 reduces tumor necrosis

factor-alpha production and significantly improves functional recovery following traumatic spinal cord injury in rats. *J Neurotrauma* 16: 851–863

20   Geng Y, Gulbins E, Altman A Lotz M (1994) Monocyte deactivation by interleukin 10 *via* inhibition of tyrosine kinase activity and the Ras signaling pathway. *Proc Natl Acad Sci USA* 91: 8602–8606

21   Liang FY, Moret V, Wiesendanger M, Roiveller EM (1991) Corticomotoneuronal connections in the rat: evidence from double-labeling of motor neurons and corticospinal axon arborizations. *J Comp Neurol* 311 (3) 356–366

22   Frei K, Lins H, Schwerdel C Fontana A (1994) Antigen presentation in the central nervous system: The inhibitory effect of IL-10 on MHC class II expression and production of cytokines depends on the inducing signals and the type of cell analyzed. *J Immunol* 152: 2720–2728

23   Mertz PM, DeWitt DL, Stetler-Stevenson WG Wah LM (1994) Interleukin 10 suppression of monocyte prostaglandin H synthase-2. *J Biol Chem* 269: 21322–21329

24   Berkman N, John M, Roesems G, Jose PJ, Barnes PJ Chung KF (1995) Inhibition of macrophage inflammatory protein-1α expression by IL-10. *J Immunol* 155: 4412–4418

25   Romano MF, Lamberti A, Petrella A et al (1996) IL-10 inhibits nuclear factor-κB/Rel nuclear activity in CD2-Stimulated human peripheral T Lymphocytes. *J Immunol* 156: 2119–2123

26   Wang P, Wu P, Siegel MI, Egan RW Billah MM (1995) Interleukin (IL)-10 inhibits nuclear factor κB (NF-κB) activation in human monocytes. *J Biol Chem* 270: 9558–9563

27   Bazan JF (1990) Structural design and molecular evolution of a cytokine receptor super family. *Proc Natl Acad Sci USA* 87: 6934–6938

28   Bazan JF (1990) Shared architecture of hormone binding domains in type I and II interferon receptors. *Cell* 61: 753–754

29   Thoreau E, Petridou B, Kelly PA, Mornon JP (1991) Structural symmetry of the extracellular domain of the cytokine/growth hormone/prolactin receptor family and interferon receptors revealed by hydrophobic cluster analysis. *FEBS Lett* 282: 26–31

30   Kotenko KV, Krause CD, Izotova LS, Pollack BP, Wu W, Pestka S (1997) Identification and functional characterization of a second chain of the interleukin-10 receptor complex. *EMBO J* 16: 5894–5903

31   Findbloom DS, Winestock KD (1995) IL-10 induces the tyrosine phosphorylation of Tyk 2 and Jak 1 and the differential assembly of STAT1a and STST 3complexes in human T cells and monocytes. *J Immunol* 155: 1079–1090

32   Ho ASY, Moore KW (1994) Interleukin-10 and its receptor. *Ther Immunol* 1: 173–185

33   O'Farrel AM, Liu Y, Moore KW, Mui ALF (1998) IL-10 inhibits macrophage activation and proliferation by distinct signaling mechanisms: evidence for Stat3-dependent and independent pathways. *EMBO J* 17: 1006–1018

34   Watson BD, Dietrich WD, Prado R, Nakayama H, Kamemitsu H, Futrell NN, Yao H, Markgraf CG, Wester P (1995) Concepts and techniques of experimental stroke induced

by cerebrovascular photothrombosis. In: ST Ohnishi, T Ohnishi T (eds): *Central nervous system trauma: research techniques*. Boca Raton, FL, CRC Press, 169–194

35   Watson BD, Dietrich WD, Busto R, Wachtel M, Ginsberg MD (1985) Induction of reproducible brain infarction by photochemically initiated thrombosis. *Ann Neurol* 17: 497–504

36   Dietrich WD, Busto R, Bethea JR (1999) Postischemic hypothermia and IL-10 treatment provide long-lasting neuroprotection of CA1 hippocampus following transient global ischemia in rats. *Exp Neurol* 158: 444–450

37   Busto R, Dietrich WD, Globus MY-T, Martinez E, Valdes I, Scheinberg P, Ginsberg MD (1987) Small differences in intraischemic brain temperature critically determine the extent of ischemic neuronal injury. *J Cereb Blood Flow Metab* 7: 729–738

38   Dietrich WD, Busto R, Alonso O, Globus M Y-T, Ginsberg MD (1993) Intraischemic but not postischemic brain bypothermia protects chronically following global forebrain ischemia in rats. *J Cereb Blood Flow Metab* 13: 541–549

39   Dietrich WD, Lin B, Globus M Y-T, Green EJ, Ginsberg MD, Busto R (1995) Effect of delayed MK-801 (dizocilpine) treatment with or without immediate postischemic hypothermia on chronic neuronal survival after global forebrain ischemia in rats. *J Cereb Blood Flow Metab* 15: 960–968

40   Coimbra C, Drake M, Boris-Moeller F, Wieloch T (1996) Long-lasting neuroprotective effect of postischemic hypothermia and treatment with an anti-inflammatory/antipyretic drug: Evidence for chronic encephalopathic processes following ischemia. *Stroke* 27: 1578–1585

41   Pazos AJ, Green EJ, Busto R, McCabe PM, Baena RC, Ginsberg MD, Globus MY-T, Schneiderman N, Dietrich WD (1999) Effects of combined postischemic hypothermia and delayed N-tert-butyl-a-phylnitrone (PBN) administration on histopathological and behavioral deficits associated with transient global ischemia in rats. *Brain Res* 846: 186–195

42   Knoblach SM, Faden AI, (1998) Interleukin-10 improves outcome and alters proinflammatory cytokine expression after experimental traumatic brain injury. *Exp Neurol* 153: 143–151

43   Brewer K, Yezierski RP, Bethea JR (1999) Neuroprotective effects of interleukin-10 following excitotoxic spinal cord injury. *Exp Neurol* 159: 484–493

44   Plunkett JA, Yu Cg, Easton JM, Bethea JR, Yezierski RP (2001) Effects of interleukin-10 (IL-10) on pain behavior and gene expression following excitotoxic spinal cord injury in the rat. *Exp Neurol* 168: 144–154

45   Barbieri I, Brusa R, Basudev H, Casati C and Grilli M (1998) Neuroprotective action of interleukin-10 in mouse primary neuronal cultures. *J Neuroscience Abstr* 24: 1446

46   Sanna A, Pflug B, Colangelo AM, and Mocchetti I (1998) Interleukin-10 prevents glutamate-induced apoptosis in cerebellar granule cells. *J Neuroscience Abstr* 24: 1781

47   Mosser HC, Chen J, Bethea JR (2000) Effect of IL-10 treatment on ICAD expression following spinal cord injury. *Soc Neurosci Abstr* 26: 2304

48   Levy Y, Brouet JC (1994) Interleukin-10 prevents spontaneous death of germinal center B cells by induction of the BCL-2 protein. *J Clin Invest* 93: 424–428

49   Taga K, Chretien J, Cherney B (1994) Interleukin-10 inhibits apoptotic cell death in infectious mononucleosis T cells. *J Clin Invest* 94: 251–260

50   Brodie C (1996) Differential effects of Th1 and Th2 derived cytokines on NGF synthesis by mouse astrocytes. *FEBS Lett* 394: 117–120

51   Cerebral Embolism Task Force (1986) Carcinogenic brain embolism. *Arch Neurol* 43: 71–87

Chemokines and ischemic stroke

Elaine E. Peters and Giora Z. Feuerstein

Cardiovascular Sciences, DuPont Pharmaceuticals Company, Experimental Station E400/6220E, Route 141 & Henry Clay Road, Wilmington, DE 19880-0400, USA

Introduction

Chemokines (chemoattractant cytokines) play a vital role in the development and function of the immune system. In addition to this well characterized role, recent evidence has suggested chemokines may be produced by both neurons and glial cells in response to various stimuli, thus implicating chemokines in a number of neurological disorders, including ischemic stroke, trauma, Alzheimer's disease, multiple sclerosis and brain tumors.

Chemokines and chemokine receptors

The chemokines are a growing family of more than 50 structurally and functionally related proteins involved in inflammatory cell recruitment. These relatively small (8–10 kDa) proteins are usually subdivided into four subfamilies on the basis of their structural conservation of specific cysteine residues [1–3]. The C–X–C or α family which includes interleukin 8 (IL-8) and interferon-inducible protein-10 (IP-10); the C–C or β family, macrophage inflammatory protein-1α (MIP-1α) and monocyte chemoattractant protein-1 (MCP-1) are examples; the CX_3C or δ family which only has a single member at present, namely fractalkine or neurotactin and; the C or γ family which also only has one member, lymphotactin, and is distinguished by possessing only two conserved cysteine residues rather than the four found in the C–X–C and C–C families. It is possible to further subdivide the C–X–C family into those chemokines which contain the amino acid sequence glutamic acid-leucine-arginine (ELR motif) close to the N terminus (for example IL-8) and those which do not (e.g. IP-10).

The individual members of each chemokine family generally exhibit marked sequence homology with each other and this is reflected in their similar chemoattractant profiles. Generally, but not exclusively, ELR motif C–X–C chemokines attract neutrophils but not monocytes. In comparison, non-ELR C–X–C chemokines are chemoattractant for monocytes and lymphocytes but not neutrophils. C–C chemokines similarly have little effect on neutrophils but will attract lymphocytes, monocytes, basophils and eosinophils.

The diverse biological activities of chemokines are mediated by G-protein coupled receptors with a nomenclature based on ligand preference (Tab. 1) [4–6]. The most notable feature of chemokine receptors is their "promiscuity". Individual chemokines may bind to different receptor subtypes and the receptors may be activated by chemokines from different families. One interesting example is the CXCR3 receptor. In addition to binding the C–X–C chemokine IP-10, it may bind the C–C chemokines eotaxin and MCP-4 although these do not activate the receptor and may instead be viewed as endogenous antagonists [7].

Chemokines and the brain

Chemokines and their receptors are constitutively expressed throughout the brain [3]. Microglia [8], astrocytes [9] and neurons [10] all express chemokines in structures as diverse as the cerebellum, hippocampus and spinal cord. Cerebrovascular endothelial cells are also reported to produce chemokines [11]. With the increasing prevalence of reports of leukocyte infiltration in various neurological disorders, chemokines, with their chemoattractant actions, have become the focus of an increasing number of investigations.

Chemokines and cerebral ischemia

Cytokine-induced neutrophil chemoattractant (CINC)

CINC is a member of the C–X–C family of chemokines originally identified as chemoattractant following interleukin-1 activation of epithelial cells. It is the homologue of human GRO and murine KC gene and is markedly chemoattractant for neutrophils [12]. Increased expression of CINC mRNA may be detected as early as 3 h after transient cerebral ischemia [13]. Peak mRNA expression occurs at 24 h with levels returning to baseline within 2–5 days [12]. The reported time-course of CINC expression precedes that of post-ischemic leukocyte infiltration and, may occur in response to interleukin-1 (IL-1) and tumor necrosis factor-α (TNFα) which are capable of inducing its production [14]. These data suggest a role for CINC in the detrimental post-ischemic neutrophil recruitment. Using an antibody directed against CINC it is possible to reduce both ischemic damage and edema formation [15].

Table 1 - Chemokines and their receptors.

Chemokine	Receptor	Cell types
C–C chemokines		
MIP-1α	CCR1, CCR4, CCR5	monocytes, T lymphocytes, natural killer (NK) cells, basophils, eosinophils, dendritic cells, hematopoetic progenitors
MIP-1β	CCR5, CCR8	monocytes, T lymphocytes, NK cells, dendritic cells, hematopoetic progenitors
MIP-3α	CCR6	lymphocytes, dendritic cells
MCP-1	CCR2, CCR4	monocytes, memory T lymphocytes, basophils, NK cells, hematopoetic progenitors
MCP-2	CCR1, CCR2	monocytes, memory and naïve T lymphocytes, eosinophils, NK cells
MCP-3	CCR1, CCR2, CCR3	monocytes, memory T lymphocytes, eosinophils, basophils, NK cells, dendritic cells
MCP-4	CCR2, CCR3	monocytes, T lymphocytes, eosinophils
MCP-5	CCR2	monocytes, T lymphocytes, eosinophils, dendritic cells
RANTES	CCR1, CCR3, CCR4, CCR5	monocytes, memory T lymphocytes, eosinophils, basophils, NK cells, dendritic cells
Eotaxin	CCR3	eosinophils
C–X–C chemokines		
IL-8	CXCR1, CXCR2	neutrophils
IP-10	CXCR3	T lymphocytes, NK cells
GRO-α, GRO-β, GRO-γ	CXCR2	neutrophils
SDF-1	CXCR4	T lymphocytes, dendritic cells
C chemokines		
Lymphotactin	XCR1	lymphocytes
CX$_3$C chemokines		
neurotactin/fractalkine	CX$_3$CR1	?

Abbreviations: MIP, macrophage inflammatory protein; MCP, monocyte chemoattractant protein; IL-8, interleukin-8; IP-10, interferon-inducible protein-10; GRO, growth-related oncogene; SDF, stromal cell-derived factor.

Interleukin-8 (IL-8)

Elevated levels of IL-8 (a C–X–C chemokine), are evident in plasma from patients with ischemic stroke [16]. In comparison, experimental studies have reported significant increases in brain IL-8 may be detected by 6 h without changes in plasma IL-8 levels [17] implying local production. The exact post-ischemic role of IL-8 is as yet unclear. However, peak cerebrospinal fluid levels after traumatic brain injury appear to correlate with disruption of the blood brain barrier [18] and this would support the experimental data of reductions in edema formation and ischemic damage, with antibodies to IL-8 [17]. Interestingly, a correlation between IL-8 levels and nerve growth factors has been reported [18], a finding reproduced by *in vitro* studies of astrocytes. The localization of post-ischemic IL-8 appears confined to endothelial cells [11] and, to a lesser extent, neutrophils.

Interferon-inducible protein-10 (IP-10)

Monocytes and T lymphocytes are the principal targets for IP-10. This C–X–C chemokine also has potent chemoattractant actions on vascular smooth muscle and astrocytes [19, 20]. The time-course of mRNA expression for this chemokine in response to ischemia is complex; IP-10 mRNA detected by Northern analysis was significantly increased compared to control by 3 h after middle cerebral artery occlusion with a peak level at 6 h. The secondary increase appeared to occur 10–15 days post-ischemia. Immunohistochemical staining revealed the expression of IP-10 was localized in neurons (3–12 h) and astrocytes (6 h onwards). Based on these data it is likely IP-10 mediates extended leukocyte infiltration and astrocytic activation after ischemic stroke.

Monocyte chemoattractant protein-1 (MCP-1)

The C–C chemokine MCP-1 is chemoattractant for monocytes and basophils but not neutrophils. It is constitutively expressed by glia and endothelial cells at low levels, but is rapidly upregulated in response to cytokine stimuli [21]. The temporal expression of MCP-1 is almost identical after permanent and transient focal ischemia. Increased expression occurs by 3 h after transient ischemia and by 6 h after permanent ischemia. Peak levels in both cases occur between 12 and 48 h [21, 22] and do not decline by 5 days post-insult. MCP-1 is initially (6–48 h) expressed by astrocytes surrounding the ischemic lesion [23]. Later expression (after 4 days) is localized to microglia/macrophages. Presently there are no reports where specific antagonists of MCP-1 have been used to further investigate its role in cerebral ischemia.

Monocyte chemoattractant protein-3 (MCP-3)

The post-ischemic expression of MCP-3 has, to date, only been the subject of one report [24]. Marked increases in MCP-3 mRNA were detected by 12 h after either permanent or transient ischemia with permanent ischemia displaying the greatest relative increase, 49-fold compared to 17-fold for transient ischemia. Expression was confined to the ischemic cortex and was sustained up to 5 days with infiltrating leukocytes being the most probable source.

Macrophage inflammatory protein-1 (MIP-1)

MIP-1 is a member of the C–C chemokine family which, in addition to its chemoattractant actions, has potent pyrogenic activity [25]. Identical changes in MIP-1α mRNA and MIP-1β mRNA have been reported after cerebral ischemia. Increased levels may be observed as early as 1 h post-insult with peak levels reached between 8 and 16 h [25]. In contrast with MCP-3, transient ischemia results in the greater magnitude of expression. Immunohistochemical staining and *in situ* hybridization have demonstrated that microglia/macrophages and not astrocytes are responsible for the MIP-1 expression [25, 26].

Fractalkine

Fractalkine is a novel CX_3C which has the distinction of existing in two forms: a membrane bound form with adhesive actions and a chemoattractant soluble form [27]. Permanent middle cerebral artery occlusion does not appear to affect fractalkine mRNA expression [27], so it is presently unclear whether or not this chemokine has a role in post ischemic inflammation. Fractalkine itself is expressed by neurons while its receptor CX_3CR1 is predominately located on resident microglial cells [28]. This distribution pattern has been suggested to represent a role in signaling between microglia and neurons. However, it is possible the microglial expression of the receptor may have a role in the post-ischemic actions of these cells.

Concluding remarks

The normal brain has low levels of chemokines yet they and their receptors are rapidly upregulated in response to cerebral ischemia. There is considerable data for post-ischemic chemokine production but, as yet, little direct evidence for their involvement in the pathophysiology of ischemic stroke. Certainly, the post-ischemic inflammatory response involves leukocyte adhesion and infiltration and chemokines play a vital role in regulating leukocyte traffic. However, until specific chemokine antagonists become available it will not be possible to fully elucidate their pathological role nor to fully exploit their obvious potential to yield new therapeutic opportunities for ischemic stroke.

References

1   Rollins BJ (1997) Chemokines. *Blood* 90: 909–928
2   Luster AD (1998) Chemokines – chemotactic cytokines that mediate inflammation. *N Eng J Med* 338: 436–445
3   Mennicken F, Maki R, De Souza EB, Quirion R (1999) Chemokines and chemokine receptors in the CNS: a possible role in neuroinflammation and patterning. *Trends Pharmacol Sci* 20: 73–78
4   Wells TNC, Power CA, Proudfoot AEI (1998) Definition, function and pathophysiological significance of chemokine receptors. *Trends Pharmacol Sci* 19: 376–380
5   Premack BA, Schall TJ (1996) Chemokine receptors: gateways to inflammation and infection. *Nat Med* 2:1174–1178
6   Murphy PM (1994) The molecular biology of leukocyte chemotactic receptors. *Ann Rev Immunol* 12: 593–633
7   Weng Y, Siciliano SJ, Waldburger KE, Sirotina-Meisher A, Staruch MJ, Duagherty BL, Gould SL, Springer MS, DeMartino JA (1998) Binding and functional properties of recombinant and endogenous CXCR3 chemokine receptors. *J Biol Chem* 273: 18288–18291
8   He J, Chen Y, Farzan M, Choe H, Ohagen A, Gartner S, Busciglio J, Yang X, Hofmann W, Newman W et al (1997) CCR3 and CCR5 are co-receptors for HIV-1 infection of microglia. *Nature* 385: 645–649
9   Tanabe S, Heesen M, Berman MA, Fischer MB, Yoshizawa I, Luo Y, Dorf ME (1997) Murine astrocytes express a functional chemokine receptor. *J Neurosci* 17: 6522–6528
10 Bacon KB, Harrison JK (2000) Chemokines and their receptors in neurobiology: perspectives in physiology and homeostasis. *J Neuroimmunol* 104: 92–97
11 Zhang W, Smith C, Shapiro A, Monette R, Hutchison J, Stanimirovic D (1999) Increased expression of bioactive chemokines in human cerebrovascular endothelial cells and astrocytes subjected to ischemia *in vitro. J Neuroimmunol* 101: 148–160
12 Liu T, Young PR, McDonnell PC, White RF, Barone FC, Feuerstein GZ (1993) Cytokine-induced neutrophil chemoattractant mRNA expressed in cerebral ischemia. *Neurosci Lett* 164: 125–128
13 Yamasaki Y, Matsuo Y, Matsuura N, Onodera H, Itoyama Y, Kogure K (1995) Transient increase of cytokine-induced neutrophil chemoattractant, a member of the interleukin-8 family, in ischemic brain areas after focal ischemia in rats. *Stroke* 26: 318–322
14 Baggiolini M, Dewald B, Moser B (1994) Interleukin-8 and related chemotactic cytokines – CXC and CC chemokines. *Adv Immunol* 55: 97–179

15 Yamasaki Y, Matsuo Y, Zagorski J, Matsuura N, Onodera H, Itoyama Y, Kogure K (1997) New therapeutic possibility of blocking cytokine-induced neutrophil chemoattractant on transient ischemic brain damage in rats. *Brain Res* 759: 103–111

16 Kostulas N, Kivisakk P, Huang Y, Matusevicious D, Kostulas V, Link H (1998) Ischemic stroke is associated with a systemic increase of blood mononuclear cells expressing interleukin-8 mRNA. *Stroke* 29: 462–466

17 Matsumoto T, Ikeda K, Mukaida N, Harada A, Matsumoto Y, Yamashita J, Matsushima K (1997) Prevention of cerebral edema and infarct in cerebral reperfusion injury by an antibody to interleukin-8. *Lab Invest* 77: 119–125

18 Kossmann T, Stahel PF, Lenzlinger PM, Redl H, Dubs RW, Trentz O, Schlag G, Morganti-Kossmann MC (1997) Interleukin-8 released into the cerebrospinal fluid after brain injury is associated with blood-brain barrier dysfunction and nerve growth factor production. *J Cereb Blood Flow Metab* 17: 280–289

19 Wang X, Ellison JA, Siren AL, Lysko PG, Yue TL, Barone FC, Shatzman A, Feuerstein GZ (1998) Prolonged expression of interferon-inducible protein-10 in ischemic cortex after permanent occlusion of the middle cerebral artery in rat. *J Neurochem* 71: 1194–1204

20 Wang X, Li X, Schmidt DB, Foley JJ, Barone FC, Ames RS, Sarau HM (2000) Identification and molecular characterization of rat CXCR3: receptor expression and interferon-inducible protein-10 binding are increased in focal stroke. *Mol Pharmacol* 57: 1190–1198

21 Wang X, Yue TL, Barone FC, Feuerstein GZ (1995) Monocyte chemoattractant protein-1 messenger RNA expression in rat ischemic cortex. *Stroke* 26: 661–665

22 Yamagami S, Tamura M, Hayashi M, Endo N, Tanabe H, Katsuura Y, Komoriya K (1999) Differential production of MCP-1 and cytokine-induced neutrophil chemoattractant in the ischemic brain after transient focal ischemia in rats. *J Leukoc Biol* 65: 744–749

23 Gourmala NG, Buttini M, Limonta S, Sauter A, Boddeke HW (1997) Differential and time dependent expression of monocyte chemoattractant protein-1 mRNA by astrocytes and macrophages in rat brain: effects of ischemia and peripheral lippopolysaccharide administration. *J Neuroimmunol* 74: 35–44

24 Wang X, Li X, Yaish-Ohad S, Sarau HM, Barone FC, Feuerstein, GZ (1999) Molecular cloning and expression of the rat monocyte chemotactic protein-3 gene: a possible role in stroke. *Brain Res Mol Brain Res* 71: 304–312

25 Gourmala NG, Limonta S, Bochelen D, Sauter A, Boddeke HW (1999) Localization of macrophage inflammatory protein: macrophage inflammatory protein-1 expression in rat brain after peripheral administration of lipopolysaccharide and focal cerebral ischemia. *Neuroscience* 88: 1255–1266

26 Takami S, Nishikawa H, Minami M, Nishiyori A, Sato M, Satoh M (1997) Induction of macrophage inflammatory protein MIP-1alpha mRNA on glial cells after focal cerebral ischemia in the rat. *Neurosci Lett* 227: 173–176

27 Chapman GA, Moores K, Harrison D, Campbell CA, Stewart BR, Strijbos PJLM (2000)

Fractalkine cleavage from neuronal membranes represents an acute event in the inflammatory response to excitoxic brain damage. *J Neurosci* 20: RC87 (1–5)

28 Harrison JK, Jiang Y, Chen SZ, Xia YY, Maciejewski D, Botti P, McNamara RK, Streit WJ, Salafranca MN, Adhikari S et al (1998) Role for neuronally derived fractalkine in mediating interactions between neurons and CX3CR1-expressing microglia. *Proc Natl Acad Sci USA* 95: 10896–10901

Biphasic activity of tumor necrosis factor in stroke and brain trauma: interaction with reactive oxygen species

Esther Shohami

Department of Pharmacology, The Hebrew University School of Pharmacy, Jerusalem, 91120, Israel

Introduction

Traumatic brain injury, which is the leading cause of death in young adults and children, is associated with motor, mental and behavioral disabilities in many of its survivors [1]. To date, none of the drugs which had been successfully tested in animal models made a breakthrough in the treatment of head injured patients.

The primary traumatic event triggers a cascade of secondary mechanisms in which mediators such as glutamate, reactive oxygen species (ROS), arachidonic acid and its oxidation products, cytokines and more, are released, each with a specific time-course. When acting simultaneously, some mediators may have either an additive or a synergistic effect to augment the devastating outcome of trauma. Therefore, when elucidating mechanisms of brain damage on the one hand, and while studying the effect of an experimental drug on the other, the interplay between various harmful mediators has to be considered.

In recent years, the concept of an inflammatory response by brain resident cells after injury as a part of both the detrimental and the healing processes has emerged, and the role of inflammatory mediators in both processes is now suggested [2–6]. Accumulating evidence demonstrates that within the acute (hours) post-traumatic period there is local synthesis of tumor necrosis factor, interleukins and chemokines, collectively referred to as cytokines. In the healthy brain, most cytokines are expressed at very low (or even non-detectable) levels; however, they are upregulated in response to injury, as has been shown both in clinical [7, 8] and experimental brain injury [9–15].

Tumor necrosis factor-α (TNFα) is a multifunctional proinflammatory cytokine that is implicated in the pathogenesis of acute ischemic and traumatic brain injury. However, it has also been shown to exert neuroprotective effects, and to play a trophic role in brain development [3] and during repair or regeneration. This proinflammatory cytokine is produced upon stimulation by monocytes, macrophages, T and B lymphocytes, neutrophils and mast cells. Ischemic or traumatic brain injury activates proteolytic enzymes that hydrolyze membrane-bound pro-TNFα, and

Inflammation and Stroke, edited by Giora Z. Feuerstein

release soluble TNFα into the extracellular space. Upon TNFα binding, intracellular signals activate the transcription factor NF-κB, starting with hydrolysis of the inhibitory protein IκB in complex with the heterodimer polypeptides p50 and p65. This allows the p65/p50 complex to be translocated to the nucleus and to bind to κB consensus sequences in enhancers of many genes. The beneficial or detrimental outcome of such activation depends upon its extent and the involvement of other cellular mediators, in particular ROS (reviewed in [16]).

ROS are highly reactive molecules that induce lipid-peroxidation, DNA-damage, activation of NF-κB and transcription of various genes encoding toxic products. The brain is particularly vulnerable to oxidative damage and there is a delicate balance between the production of ROS and their neutralization. Antioxidant enzymes (superoxide dismutase, catalase and peroxidase) and low molecular weight antioxidants (LMWA) are the endogenous protective agents that act against oxidative stress.

This chapter focuses on the pathological role of TNFα in the early post traumatic period, and special emphasis is given to the synergistic effect of TNFα and ROS.

Temporal changes in brain TNFα levels after traumatic injury

Clinical studies have demonstrated elevated levels of TNFα in inflammatory disorders of the CNS, such as HIV encephalitis [17] and meningitis [18]. TNFα is also involved in the pathogenesis of various immune-mediated processes, and is the key mediator in septic shock [19]. It is now accepted that cytokines play a role in the acute pathophysiology of trauma [20] and in ischemic and traumatic brain injury [9–15]. Elevated levels of TNFα (30–40-fold higher than normal) were reported in the serum [21] and cerebrospinal fluid [22] of head-injured patients. Moreover, human cerebral microvascular endothelium recovered from patients that had experienced percussion trauma produced high levels of IL-1, IL-6 and TNFα at 8 and 24 h [8]. High cytokine levels in the CSF correlated with poor outcome and brain damage in patients who suffer subarachnoid hemorrhage [23]. Similarly, high levels of cytokines (mRNA or bioactivity) 3–8 h after fluid percussion [11, 14, 15] or within 1–4 h after closed head injury [12, 13] were found in experimental models of traumatic brain injury.

Acute detrimental effects of TNFα after brain injury

To explore the role of acute TNFα production after ischemic and traumatic brain injury several investigators inhibited the cytokine by pharmacological means. A TNFα mRNA inhibitor such as rolipram (a phosphdiesterase inhibitor) or tyrphostins, which inhibit protein tyrosine kinases, improved the outcome in TNFα-mediated diseases [24, 25]. CNI-1493, a tetravalent guanylhydrazone compound that inhibits phosphorylation of p38 mitogen-activated protein (MAP) kinase and has been shown to selectively inhibit TNFα synthesis [26] exhibited significant cerebroprotection when used in cerebral ischemia and trauma ([27] and unpublished observations from our laboratory). Using a permanent middle cerebral artery occlusion model in mice, Nawashiro et al. showed reduction in the volume of brain damage after treatment with TNF-binding protein (TNFbp) [28]. In a series of studies in a rat model of closed head injury (CHI) in our laboratory, TNFα translation was inhibited by HU-211 (dexanabinol) [12], expression was inhibited by pentoxyphylline and activity was inhibited by TNFα-binding protein [29]. In all these experiments neuroprotection was achieved after the administration of a single dose (given within 1–4 h after trauma) as reflected by less edema, and BBB disruption, faster and greater clinical recovery and smaller hippocampal cell loss. Dexanabinol was also effective when treating rats subjected to permanent middle cerebral artery occlusion. It reduced infarct volume, improved motor and cognitive function and this was associated with inhibition of TNFα [30, 30a]. IL-10, an anti-inflammatory cytokine that inhibits the production of TNFα, was used in a model of traumatic brain injury to improve clinical outcome [31]. When given as a single dose early (within hours) after spinal cord injury, it inhibited TNFα production, and improved the clinical outcome [32], as expected.

Chronic beneficial effects of TNFα after brain trauma

In contrast to reports on the acute toxicity of TNFα after trauma and ischemia, the opposite effect has been documented, mainly in studies using mice lacking the TNF receptors. TNFR$^{-/-}$ mice subjected to MCAO [33] or to traumatic brain injury [34] had a higher infarct area at 24 h after the insult, as compared with that in the wild-type, and they were under greater oxidative stress. Moreover, these mice were unable to upregulate the antioxidant and neuroprotective enzyme manganese superoxide dismutase (Mn-SOD). In line with these findings, Stahel et al. have also shown that TNF/lymphotoxin-α double knockout mice suffered higher mortality than their matched wild type controls during 7 days of recovery after CHI [35]. They analyzed C5aR mRNA and protein expression after CHI, and observed upregulation of both components mainly in neurons [36]. These findings suggest that post-traumatic neuronal expression of the C5aR is, at least in part, regulated by TNFα and lymphotoxin-α during 7 days after trauma, and that C5a-mediated processes are required for brain repair. While the role of the C5aR-mediated response after brain injury has not been fully elucidated, a recent study on C5a-mediated protection from apoptotic neuronal death in a model of intraventricular kainic acid injection in mice, supports the proposed role of C5a in brain recovery [37].

A solution to the apparently conflicting role of TNFα after trauma was proposed by Scherbel et al [38]. Exploring the acute and chronic effects of TNFα deficiency on recovery from traumatic injury, they showed that during the first post-trauma days (up to 4 days) the TNF(−/−) mice recovered faster than their matched controls, as expected from the pharmacological studies. However, their motor function did not improve after day 1, whereas that of the wild-type mice, who failed most of the clinical tests on days 1–4, improved slowly, and by day 7–14, they performed better in motor testing. A similar bi-phasic effect was also demonstrated by histology. Additional support of this dual and time-dependent role of TNFα after trauma came from the study of Bethea et al. [32]. As mentioned above, rats were treated after spinal cord injury with IL-10, an anti-inflammatory cytokine that inhibits the production of TNFα. When the drug was given within hours after injury, as a single dose, facilitated clinical recovery was evident even at 8 weeks. However, when a second dose of IL-10 was given on day 3 post injury, the beneficial effect of day 1 dose was completely abolished [32]. These findings support the notion that TNFα detrimental and beneficial effect depends upon the time point after injury.

The effect of TNFα is not only time-dependent but also varies with the specific brain region. Thus, TNFbp, when administered into the striatum with NMDA was protective, but aggravated NMDA-induced hippocampal damage in neonates [39]. This finding agrees with other evidence showing that responses to TNFα (and to other inflammatory mediators) are not uniform throughout the brain [40].

Cumulatively, the dual effect of TNFα after brain injury includes a toxic phase, which may persist between 1 and 24 h post injury and can be blocked by inhibitors, and a protective phase that begins within 2–3 days and lasts for the rest of the recovery period.

Neuroprotective effects of TNFα: in vitro studies

The discrepancy between observations of TNFα pathogenic and protective function in animal models of brain injury is also reflected in a series of *in vitro* studies on brain cells. Barger et al. showed that TNFα protects against iron and amyloid-β peptide in a model system of cultured hippocampal and neocortical astrocytes [41], and Mattson et al. [42] demonstrated the protective effect of TNFα under glucose deprivation and glutamate toxicity. The lack of a direct cytotoxic effect by TNFα suggests that in the setting of brain injury, other pathogenic stimuli contribute to TNFα cytotoxicity. We hypothesized that in addition to the time factor, the local neurochemical milieu determines whether a cytokine is protective or detrimental in the injured brain.

In the search for a neurochemical mediator that could switch TNFα function after brain injury from protective to toxic, we proposed that reactive oxygen species

(ROS) may contribute to TNFα-induced toxicity, and that these two mediators might even synergize in the early post-traumatic period.

Reactive oxygen species in the pathophysiology of brain injury

ROS have been implicated as toxic mediators in traumatic brain injury (for review see [43]). In our CHI model we inferred the role of ROS as toxic mediators by showing that nitroxides, a group of molecules displaying SOD-like activity that are able to penetrate the cell and to neutralize intracellular radicals, exerted significant neuroprotection [44]. Additionally, we demonstrated consumption of the endogenous antioxidants, due to the overproduction of ROS [45].

Synergistic effect of TNFα and ROS after brain trauma

Transcription of many pro-inflammatory, immune and apoptotic genes, which are induced by TNFα is dependent on the activation of nuclear factor κB (NF-κB). Each step of NF-κB activation and DNA binding is redox-sensitive, as reviewed by Kaldt-shmidt et al. [16]. Thus, it is conceivable that the point of intersection of TNFα and ROS, both of which are elevated in brain insults, could be NF-κB.

An interaction between TNFα-induced toxicity and ROS was demonstrated recently, using an *in vivo* model of blood-brain barrier (BBB) disruption. Injected intracerebrally, TNFα induced BBB permeability within 3–4 h, which was significantly abolished when the mice were treated with the antioxidant Tempol from the nitroxides family (see above) [46]. To further explore the cellular mechanism of this interaction, we exposed rat and human brain endothelial cells, rat astrocytes or PC12 cells to sub-lethal doses of TNFα and H_2O_2 and found that the combination had a synergistic effect on the viability of these cells. When treated with TNFα alone, HBEC, RBEC and astrocytes showed no morphological signs of apoptosis. However, the addition of low doses of H_2O_2 simultaneously with TNFα resulted in early DNA fragmentation, followed by the appearance of TUNEL-positive apoptotic cells [47]. Moreover, TNF induced the activation of transcription factor κB as evidenced by translocation of the p65 subunit into the nucleus. Sublethal doses of H_2O_2 inhibited the translocation of the p65 subunit of NF-κB, although it had no effect on the degradation of the NF-κB inhibitor in the cytoplasm [47]. Similarly, when PC12 cells were exposed to a combination of sub-toxic doses of TNFα and H_2O_2, there was significant release of PGE_2 and LDH, indicating cell activation and death, respectively [48].

Taken together, our findings suggest that when the neurochemical milieu of the early post-traumatic or ischemic brain is simulated, at least in part, the cellular response differs from that observed when cells are exposed to normal conditions

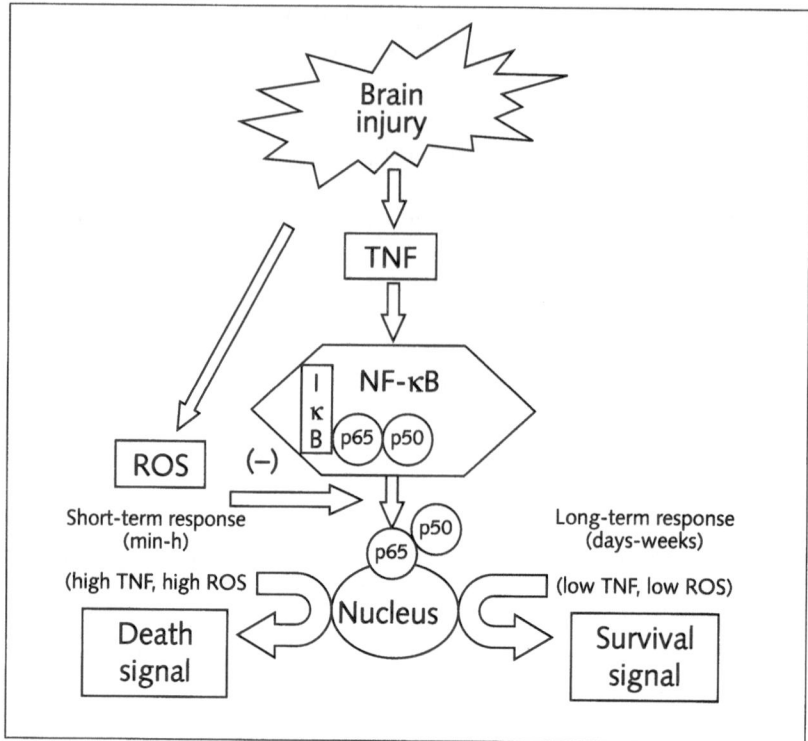

Figure 1

Upon TNFα binding, the cytosolic portions of its receptors recruit multiple intracellular adapter proteins. Following a series of steps, the transcription factor NF-κB is activated, starting with hydrolysis of the inhibitory protein IκB that is complexed with the heterodimer polypeptides p50 and p65. The p65/p50 complex is translocated to the nucleus and binds to κB consensus sequences in enhancers of many genes. The outcome of such activation depends upon its extent and the involvement of other cellular mediators. Under low levels of TNFα and ROS the major products may be protective (e.g. MnSOD, calbindin etc.), whereas under acute post-injury conditions (high levels of TNFα and ROS), the major product may be toxic (e.g. inflammatory cytokines). A possible mechanism by which ROS switches the NF-κB response is inhibition of the p65 nuclear translocation.

(e.g. TNFα alone). Figure 1 summarizes the proposed interaction between TNFα and ROS after brain injury, as discussed in this chapter.

A broader understanding of the effect of ROS on TNFα-induced activation of NF-κB in the injured brain by both mediators and the modulation of this factor by the cellular redox state is required to reconcile the apparently conflicting reports on the role of TNFα after brain injury.

References

1   Waxweiler RJ, Thurman D, Sniezek J, Sosin D, O'Neil J (1995) Monitoring the impact of traumatic brain injury: a review and update. *J Neurotrauma* 12: 509–516

2   Rothwell NJ, Hopkins SJ (1995) Cytokines and the nervous system II: action and mechanisms of action. *Trends Neurosci* 18: 130–136

3   Merril JE, Benveniste EN (1996) Cytokines in inflammatory brain lesions: helpful and harmful. *Trends Neurosci* 19: 331–338

4   Barger S (1998) Tumor necrosis factor, the good, the bad and the umbra. In: MP Mattson (ed): *Neuroprotective signal transduction.* Humana Press, Totowa, NJ, 163–183

5   Munoz-Fernandez M, Fresno M (1998) The role of tumor necrosis factor, interleukin-6, Interferon-γ and inducible nitric oxide synthase in the development and pathology of the nervous system. *Prog Neurobiol* 56: 307–340

6   Barone FC, Feuerstein, GZ (1999) Inflammatory mediators and stroke: new opportunities for novel therapeutics. *J Cereb Blood Flow Metab* 19: 819–834

7   Morganti-Kossman MC, Lenzlinger PM, Hans V, Stahel P, Csuka E, Ammann E, Stocker R, Trentz O, Kossmann T (1997) Production of cytokines following brain injury: beneficial and deleterious for the damaged tissue. *Mol Psych* 2: 133–136

8   Gourin CG, Shackford SR (1997) Production of tumor necrosis factor-alpha and interleukin-1 beta by human cerebral microvascular endothelium after percussive trauma. *J Trauma* 42: 1101–1107

9   Feuerstein GZ, Wang X, Barone FC (1997) Inflammatory gene expression in cerebral ischemia and trauma. Potential new therapeutic targets. *Ann NY Acad Sci* 825: 179–193 (review)

10 Liu T, Clark RK, McDonnel PC, Toung PR, White RF, Barone FC, Feuerstein FZ (1994) Tumor necrosis factor-alpha expression in ischemic neurons. *Stroke* 25: 1481–1488

11 Taupin V, Toulmond S, Serrano A, Benavides J, Zavala F (1993) Increase in IL-6, IL-1 and TNF levels in rat brain following traumatic lesion. Influence of pre- and post-traumatic treatment with Ro5 4864, a peripheral-type (p site) benzodiazepine ligand. *J Neuroimmunol* 42: 177–185

12 Shohami E, Gallily R, Mechoulam R, Bass, Ben-Hur T (1997) Cytokine production in the brain following closed head injury: Dexanabinol (HU-211) is a novel TNFα inhibitor and an effective neuroprotectant. *J Neuroimmunol* 72: 169–177

13 Shohami E, Novikov M, Bass R, Yamin A, Gallily R (1994) Closed head injury triggers early production of TNF and IL-6 by brain tissue. *J Cereb Blood Flow Metab* 14: 615–619

14 Fan L, Young PR, Barone FC, Feuerstein GZ, Smith DH, McIntosh TK (1996) Experimental brain injury induces differential expression of tumor necrosis factor-α mRNA in the CNS. *Mol Br Res* 36: 287–291

15 Kita T, Liu L, Tanaka N, Kinoshita Y (1997) The expression of tumor necrosis factor-alpha in the rat brain after fluid percussive injury. *Int J Legal Med* 110: 305–311

16 Kaltschmidt B, Sparna T, Kaltschmidt C (1999) Activation of NF-κB by reactive oxygen intermediates in nervous system. *Antiox Redox Signal* 1: 129–144

17 Grimaldi LM, Martino GV, Franciotta DM, Brustia R, Castagna A, Pristera R, Prizzarin A (1991) Elevated tumor necrosis factor-alpha levels in spinal fluid from HIV-1 infected patients with central nervous system involvement. *Ann Neurol* 29: 21–25

18 Leist TP, Frei K, Kam-Hansen S, Zinkernagel RM, Fontana A (1988) Tumor necrosis factor α in cerebrospinal fluid during bacterial, but not viral, meningitis: evaluation in murine model infections and in patients. *J Exp Med* 167: 1743–1758

19 Tracey KJ (1991) Tumor necrosis factor (cachectin) in the biology of septic shock syndrome. *Circ Shock* 35: 123–128

20 Jiang J, Tian K, Chen H, Zhu P, Wang Z (1997) Kinetics of plasma cytokines and its clinical significance in patients with severe trauma. *Chin Med J* 110: 923–926

21 Goodman JC, Robertson CS, Grossman RG, Narayan RK (1990) Elevation of tumor necrosis factor in head injury. *J Neuroimmunol* 30: 213–217

22 Ross SA, Halliday MI, Campbell GC, Byrnes DP,. Rowlands BJ (1994) The presence of tumor necrosis factor in CSF and plasma after severe head injury. *Br J Neurosurg* 8: 419–425

23 Mathiesen T, Edner G, Ulfarsson E, Andersson B (1997) Cerebrospinal fluid interleukin-1 receptor antagonist and tumor necrosis factor-alpha following subarachnoid hemorrhage. *J Neurosurg* 87: 215–220

24 Buttini M, Mir A, Appel K, Wiederhold KH, Limonta S, Gebicke-Haerter PJ, Boddeke HW (1997) Lipopolysaccharide induces expression of tumor necrosis factor alpha in rat brain: inhibition by methylprednisolone and by rolipram. *Br J Pharmacol* 122: 1483–1489

25 Novogrodsky A, Vanichkin A, Patya M, Gazit A, Osherov N, Levitzki A (1994) Prevention of lipopolysaccharide-induced lethal toxicity by tyrosine kinase inhibitors. *Science* 264: 1319–1322

26 Bianchi M, Bloom O, Raabe T, Cohen PS, Chesney J, Sherry B, Schmidtmayerova H, Calandra T, Zhang X, Bukrinsky M et al (1996) Suppression of proinflammatory cytokines in monocytes by a tetravalent guanylhydrazone. *J Exp Med* 183: 927–936

27 Meistrell ME 3rd, Botchkina GI, Wang H, Di Santo E, Cockroft KM, Bloom O, Vishnubhakat JM, Ghezzi P, Tracey K (1997) Tumor necrosis factor is a brain damaging cytokine in cerebral ischemia. *Shock* 8: 341–348

28 Nawashiro H, Martin D, Hallenbeck JM (1997) Inhibition of tumor necrosis factor ameliorated brain infarction in mice. *J Cereb Blood Flow Metab* 17: 229–232

29 Shohami E, Bass R, Wallach D, Yamin A, Gallily R (1996) Inhibition of tumor necrosis factor (TNFa) activity in rat brain is associated with cerebroprotection after closed head injury. *J Cerebr Blood Flow Metab* 16: 378–384

30 Leker R, Shohami E, Abramsky O, Ovadia H. (1999) Dexanabinol; a novel neuroprotective drug in experimental focal cerebral ischemia. *J Neurol Sci* 162: 114–119

30a Lavie G, Teichner A, Shohami E, Ovadia H, Leker RR (2001) Long term cerebroprotective effects of dexanabinol in a model of focal cerebral ischemia. *Brain Res* 901: 195–201

31 Knoblach SM, Faden AI (1998) Interleukin-10 improves outcome and alters proinflammatory cytokine expression after experimental traumatic brain injury. *Exp Neurol* 153: 143–151

32 Bethea JR, Nagashima H, Acosta MC, Briceno C, Gomez F, Marcillo AE, Loor K, Green J, Dietrich WD (1999) Systemically administered Interleukin-10 rescues tumor necrosis factor-alpha production and significantly improves functional recovery following traumatic spinal cord injury in rats. *J Neurotrauma* 16: 851–863

33 Bruce AJ, Boling W, Kindy MS, Peschon J, Kraemer PJ, Carpenter MK, Holtsberg FW, Mattson MP (1996) Altered neuronal and microglial responses to excitotoxic and ischemic brain injury in mice lacking TNF receptors. *Nature Med* 2: 788–794

34 Sullivan PG, Bruce-Keller AJ, Rabchevsky AG, Christakos S, Clair DK, Mattson MP, Scheff SW (1999) Exacerbation of damage and altered NF-kappaB activation in mice lacking tumor necrosis factor receptors after traumatic brain injury. *J Neurosci* 19: 6248–6256

35 Stahel PF, Shohami E, Younis FM, Kariya K, Otto VI, Lenzlinger PM, Grosjean MB, Eugster HP, Trentz O, Kossmann T et al (2000) Experimental closed head injury: Analysis of neurological outcome, blood brain barrier dysfunction, intracranial neutrophil infiltration and neuronal cell death in mice deficient in genes for pro-inflammatory cytokines. *J Cereb Blood Flood Metabol* 20: 369–380

36 Stahel PF, Kariya K, Shohami E, Barnum SR, Eugster H, Trentz O, Kossmann T, Morganti-Kossmann MC (2000) Intracerebral complement C5a receptor (CD88) expression is regulated by TNF and lymphtoxin-α following closed head injury in mice. *J Neuroimmunol* 109:164–172

37 Osaka H, Mukherjee P, Aisen P, Pasinetti GM, (1999) Complement-derived anaphylatoxin C5a protects against glutamate-mediated neurotoxicity. *J Cell Biochem* 73: 303–311

38 Scherbel U, Raghupathi R, Nakamura M, Saatman KE, Trojanowski JQ, Neugebauer E, Marino MW, McIntosh TK (1999) Differential acute and chronic responses of tumor necrosis factor-deficient mice to experimental brain injury. *Proc Natl Acad Sci USA* 96: 8721–8726

39 Galasso JM, Wang P, Martin D, Silverstein FS (2000) Inhibition of TNFα can attenuate or exacerbate excitotoxic injury in neonatal rat barin. *NeuroReport* 11: 231–235

40 Phillips LM, Simon PJ, Lampson LA (1999) Site-specific immune regulation in the brain: differential modulation of major histocompatibility complex (MHC) proteins in brainstem vs. hippocampus. *J Comp Neurol* 405: 322–333

41 Barger SW, Horster D, Furukawa K, Goodman Y, Krieglstein J, Mattson MP (1995) Tumor necrosis factors alpha and beta protect neurons against amyloid beta-peptide toxicity: evidence for involvement of a kappa B-binding factor and attenuation of peroxide and Ca^{2+} accumulation. *Proc Nat Acad Sci USA* 92: 9328–9332

42 Mattson MP, Cheng B, Baldwin SA, Smith-Swintosky VL, Keller J, Geddes JW, Scheff

SW, Christakos S. (1995) Brain injury and tumor necrosis factors induce calbindin D-28k in astrocytes: evidence for a cytoprotective response. *J Neur Res* 42: 357–370

43 Chan PH, (1996) Role of oxidants in ischemic brain damage. *Stroke* 27: 1124–1129

44 Beit-Yannai E, Zhang R, Trembovler V, Samuni A, Shohami E. (1996) Cerebroprotective effect of stable nitroxide radicals in closed head injury in the rat. *Brain Res* 717: 22–28

45 Beit-Yannai E, Kohen R, Horowitz M, Trembovler V, Shohami E (1997) Changes in biological reducing activity in rat brain following closed head injury: a cyclic voltammetry study in normal and acclimated rats. *J Cereb Blood Flow Metabol* 17: 273–279

46 Trembovler V, Beit-Yannai E, Younis F, Gallily R, Horowitz M, Shohami E (1999) Antioxidants attenuate acute toxicity of tumor necrosis factor α induced by brain injury in Rat. *J Interferon Cytokine Res* 19: 791–795

47 Ginis I, Hallenbeck JM, Liu J, Spatz M, Jaiswal R, Shohami E (2000) Tumor necrosis factor and reactive oxygen species cooperative cytotoxicity is mediated *via* inhibition of NF-κB. *Mol Med* 6: 1028–1041

48 Trembovler V, Abu-Raya S, Lazarovic P, Shohami E (2000) Toxic effects of tumor necrosis factor alpha are enhanced by reactive oxygen species. 5th Intl. Neurotrauma symposium, Garmisch, Germany (abstract)

Interleukin-1 and IL-1 receptor antagonist in stroke: mechanisms and potential therapeutics

Nancy J. Rothwell and and Sarah A. Loddick

Biological Sciences, 1.124, Stopford Building, University of Manchester, Manchester M13 9PT, UK

The interleukin-1 family

The IL-1 family comprises two agonists, IL-1α and IL-1β, the products of separate genes, which exert virtually identical actions. Both ligands are produced as precursors; pro-IL-1α is biologically active, but pro-IL-1β is inactive and must be cleaved by the enzyme caspase-1. The mechanisms through which IL-1α and β are released from the cell are unknown. IL-1α appears to remain largely intracellular, whereas IL-1β is released more readily, but has no classical leader sequence. It now seems likely that release of IL-1β is linked directly to cleavage by caspase-1 (see [1]). Recent evidence suggests that these events are regulated by extracellular ATP acting on purinergic P2x7receptors; pharmacological activation of these receptors leads to IL-1β cleavage and release from macrophages and microglia [2, 3].

The third member of the IL-1 family, IL-1 receptor antagonist (IL-1ra) appears to act solely as a competitive receptor antagonist which blocks all actions of IL-1α and β [1]. Recent genome analysis has revealed a number of putative, new IL-1 ligands. IL-18, originally identified as interferon γ inducing factor (IGIF) and also termed IL-1γ, shares homology with IL-1, is cleaved by caspase-1 and acts on similar receptors to the IL-1 family, but does not have identical actions (see [4]). More recently, six further genes with homology to the IL-1 family have been identified by several groups and assigned various names including FIL-1 delta; epsilon; zeta; eta; theta and H1 (IL-1raβ) [5–8], but the functions of these proteins are at present unknown.

IL-1α and β are believed to signal exclusively through an 80 kDa cell surface receptor (IL-1RI) [9], which must interact with an accessory protein (AcP) to elicit signal transduction through phosphorylation of MAP kinases and activation of NF-κB [9, 10]. A second IL-1 receptor (IL-1RII) binds IL-1 (particularly IL-1β), but fails to initiate signal transduction and probably acts as a shed receptor which inhibits the biological activity of extracellular IL-1 [11]. The IL-1 receptor family is also

Inflammation and Stroke, edited by Giora Z. Feuerstein

expanding rapidly, particularly since the realisation that they share homology with the Toll family of receptors in *Drosophila*. The relationship between the new IL-1 ligands and receptors has not yet been identified and their functional role on the brain is not known. All established members of the IL-1 family (IL-1α, IL-1ra, caspase-1, IL-1RI, AcP and IL-1RII) have been identified in the brain on several cell types, and IL-1 has now been established as a mediator of ischaemic brain damage in experimental animals (see [12]).

Evidence for the involvement of IL-1 in ischaemic brain damage

Expression of IL-1 in normal brain is very low, but is increased rapidly in response to cerebral ischaemia or similar stimuli. IL-1 (particularly IL-1β) mRNA is increased within 30 min of experimental ischaemia in rodents [13, 14], and protein is upregulated within 1 h, normally in microglia and perivascular cells, with later expression by astrocytes and invading immune cells (see [12]). IL-1ra seems to be produced slightly later, largely by neurons [15].

IL-1 itself is not toxic to normal rodent brain or neuronal cultures, but can induce responses which are associated with ischaemic brain damage such as induction of oedema, blood brain barrier (BBB) injury, activation of glia, upregulation of prostanoids, nitric oxide, complement, β-amyloid precursor protein and release of free radicals (see [16–17]). Intracerebral injection of IL-1 into rodents exposed to cerebral ischaemia (or excitotoxic or traumatic brain injury) markedly exacerbates injury and can induce damage at distant sites [18–21].

Numerous studies have reported that blocking IL-1 action, mainly by administration of IL-1ra (see below) markedly inhibits ischaemic brain damage, as determined from histological analysis (infarct volume), neuronal survival, edema, glial activation, neutrophil invasion and behavioural outcome (see [12]). Few studies have addressed the specific roles of IL-1α and β, though an antibody against IL-1β reduces ischaemic brain damage in rats [22]. Mice lacking functional caspase-1 show similarly reduced injury [23], though these studies are not conclusive since caspase-1 also cleaves pro-IL-18 and may contribute to activation of apoptosis [4]. Our recent data suggest that mice lacking IL-1α or IL-1β show normal or only slightly reduced damage in response to middle cerebral artery occlusion (MCAo), whereas animals lacking both IL-1 genes exhibit dramatically reduced injury [24]. IL-1ra appears to act as an endogenous inhibitor of IL-1 since blocking its activity in brain enhances ischaemic injury [25].

The mechanisms of action of IL-1 are not fully understood and probably involve multiple sites and effector mechanisms. IL-1 (and IL-1ra) appear to act at specific sites in the brain, most notably the striatum and hypothalamus, and influence neuronal death at distant sites in the cortex, probably by activation of complex neuronal pathways leading to release of glutamate within the cortex [18, 19, 26].

Therapeutic targets

A number of sites for therapeutic intervention exist within the IL-1 family. Little is known about the regulation of expression of IL-1α and β in the brain, but several molecules which inhibit expression, e.g. glucocorticoids, lipocortin, cannabinoids and the cytokine IL-10, some of which are neuroprotective [27–29]. Thus reported protective effects of IL-10, lipocortin and cannabinoids may depend on inhibition of IL-1 expression, while glucocorticoids have complex actions (see [30–32]). There is now considerable interest in the P2x7 receptor and caspase-1 as targets to block IL-1 cleavage and cellular release in peripheral and CNS disease. As yet, few if any data have been published on the effects of selective inhibitors of either processes, though gene knockout animals indicate the validity of these approaches. It is not yet known if modulation of P2x7 receptors or caspase-1 will target IL-1β exclusively, and compensatory upregulation of IL-1α (or other components of the IL-1 system) may limit the effectiveness of these approaches in the long term.

The most effective approach to inhibit IL-1 in experimental ischaemia is IL-1ra (see the following). Efforts to identify small (ideally non-peptide) IL-1 receptor antagonists, have not yet been fruitful. Identification of the signalling pathways and secondary mediators of IL-1 action has provided new targets. These include the MAP kinases, p38, p42/44 and ERK, and also NF-κB. A p38 kinase inhibitor (SB 239063) significantly reduces ischaemic brain damage in the rat [33], but it remains to be determined if the protective effects of this inhibitor are due solely to its effects on IL-1 signalling.

As with many biological systems, maximal specificity is achieved by blocking the receptor which is normally (and almost certainly in the case of IL-1) specific to the ligand. Modification of the expression or release of IL-1, or of post-receptor signalling pathways may have less selectivity for IL-1. Thus the most selective approach currently available is to inhibit IL-1 actions with IL-1ra.

Neuroprotective effects of IL-1ra

Studies on recombinant (r)IL-1ra have provided extensive evidence that *endogenous* IL-1 contributes to neuronal death following a variety of brain insults. Relton and Rothwell were the first to describe neuroprotective effects of IL-1ra, demonstrating that icv injection of rIL-1ra caused a significant reduction of damage induced by permanent occlusion of the middle cerebral artery (pMCAO) in rats [34]. Since this study, IL-1ra has been shown to reduce injury caused by ischaemic, hypoxic, traumatic and excitotoxic insults as well as seizure related brain damage and EAE [see 35]. These data implicate IL-1 in the progression of diverse neurodegenerative conditions, and suggest that IL-1ra may prove useful for the treatment of such conditions. rIL-1ra is effective when administered (icv) up to 30 min after pMCAO [20],

3 h after hypoxic ischaemic injury [36], and 4 h after traumatic brain injury [37] indicating that delayed treatment can be successful. Furthermore, *peripheral* administration of rIL-1ra prevents neuronal loss caused by ischaemic (pMCAO) and heat stroke induced brain injury in adult rats [38–40]. The protective effects of rIL-1ra treatment are sustained, since IL-1ra treated animals still have a reduced lesion volume 7 days after pMCAO [20, 38]. The reduction in lesion volume caused by IL-1ra is associated with increased neuronal survival and improved function; peripheral administration of rIL-1ra reduced infarct volume, brain water content, infiltration of inflammatory cells and the number of necrotic neurones and improved neurological outcome after pMCAO [38].

IL-1ra reduces neuronal death in all forms of experimentally induced ischaemic injury studied (permanent and transient focal; global; hypoxic), in a variety of species (rat, mouse, gerbil) (see [12]), and although it has yet to be tested in higher species, this evidence has led to consideration of rIL-1ra for the treatment of stroke.

Clinical aspects of IL-1 in stroke

Increased IL-1 expression has been reported in the brain or CSF of patients with a diverse range of insults including head injury, Parkinson's disease and Alzheimer's disease [41–44]. Several clinical considerations relate to IL-1 in ischaemic brain damage in patients, for example, whether increased production of endogenous IL-1 (or sensitisation to IL-1) may initiate an ischaemic event or worsen outcome after a stroke. Atherosclerosis, a primary risk factor for stroke, is now recognised as an inflammatory condition associated with cytokine production (see [45]). IL-1 produced within the systemic circulation or cerebrovasculature could gain access to the brain parenchyma or act outside the brain to influence ischaemic brain damage. Systemic infection or inflammation result in production of IL-1 both locally at the site of disease, and within the brain, mainly within the hypothalamus [46, 47]. Recent data suggest that IL-1 expression in the hypothalamus can cause or contribute to cortical neuronal loss [18], which could explain the reported association between infection and stroke [48–50].

Polymorphisms in the IL-1 family have now been associated with a variety of neurodegenerative conditions including Alzheimer's disease, epilepsy and multiple sclerosis [51–55], but have not yet been reported in stroke. Genetic variation in expression of IL-1 or its receptor or indeed the production of inhibitors such as IL-1ra, could lead to altered susceptibility to an ischaemic event. The major area of consideration is now whether inhibitors of IL-1 synthesis, release or action may be of clinical benefit in stroke. Acute blockade of IL-1 is unlikely to have any such detrimental effects because current knowledge suggests that IL-1 has little or no role in normal physiology, and chronic deletion of IL-1 has no apparent adverse effects in animals [12, 47]. Blocking IL-1 may have primary benefits in stroke due to neuroprotection but could also limit the effects of systemic or CNS infection and induction of fever which are associated with poor outcome [56]. No studies on blocking IL-1 in acute clinical stroke have yet been undertaken. A preliminary (safety) study has just begun in Manchester to compare IL-1ra with placebo in a double-blind trial. However, while this is progressing it will be important to test IL-1ra in all types of experimental stroke in lower species, to carefully establish its pharmacological profile and ideally to test IL-1ra in a higher species. Ultimately the question of IL-1's role in cerebral ischaemia in humans will rest on well-designed clinical studies using inhibitors of IL-1 at doses and treatment regimes which are of proven efficacy in a wide range of preclinical models.

References

1   Dinarello CA (1998) Interleukin-1, interleukin-1 receptors and interleukin-1 receptor antagonist. *Int Rev Immunol* 16: 457–499
2   Sanz JM, Di Virgilio F (2000) Kinetics and mechanism of ATP-dependent IL-1 beta release from microglial cells. *J Immunol* 164: 4893–4898
3   Ralevic V, Burnstock G (1998) Receptors for purines and pyrimidines. *Pharmacol Rev* 50: 413–492
4   Fantuzzi G, Dinarello CA (1999) Interleukin-18 and interleukin-1 beta: two cytokine substrates for ICE (caspase-1). *J Clin Immunol* 19: 1–11
5   Busfield SJ, Comrack CA, Yu G, Chickering TW, Smutko JS, Zhou H, Leiby KR, Holmgren LM, Gearing DP, Pan Y (2000) Identification and gene organization of three novel members of the IL-1 family on human chromosome 2. *Genomics* 66: 213–216
6   Kumar S, McDonnell PC, Lehr R, Tierney L, Tzimas MN, Griswold DE, Capper EA, Tal-Singer R, Wells GI, Doyle ML et al (2000) Identification and initial characterization of four novel members of the interleukin-1 family. *J Biol Chem* 275: 10308–10314
7   Mulero JJ, Pace AM, Nelken ST, Loeb DB, Correa TR, Drmanac R, Ford JE (1999) IL1HY1: A novel interleukin-1 receptor antagonist gene. *Biochem Biophys Res Commun* 263: 702–706
8   Smith DE, Renshaw BR, Ketchem RR, Kubin M, Garka KE, Sims JE (2000) Four new members expand the interleukin-1 superfamily. *J Biol Chem* 275: 1169–1175
9   Sims J, Gayle MA, Slack JL, Alderson MR, Bird TA, Giri JG, Colotta F, Re F, Mantovani A, Shanebeck K et al (1993) Interleukin-1 signalling occurs exclusively via the type I receptor. *Proc Natl Acad Sci USA* 90: 6155–6159
10 O'Neill LA, Dinarello CA (2000) The IL-1 receptor/toll-like receptor superfamily: crucial receptors for inflammation and host defense. *Immunol Today* 21: 206–209
11 Colotta F, Re F, Muzio M, Bertini B, Polentarutti N, Sironi M, Giri JG, Dower SK, Sims JE, Mantovani A (1993) Interleukin-1 type II receptor: a decoy target for IL-1 that is regulated by IL-4. *Science* 261: 472–475

12 Touzani O, Boutin H, Chuquet J, Rothwell N (1999) Potential mechanisms of inter-
    leukin-1 involvement in cerebral ischaemia. *J Neuroimmunol* 100: 203–215

13 Buttini M, Sauter A, Boddeke HW (1994) Induction of interleukin-1 beta mRNA after
    focal cerebral ischaemia in the rat. *Brain Res Mol Brain Res* 23: 126–134

14 Minami M, Kuraishi Y, Yabuuchi K, Yamazaki A, Satoh M (1992) Induction of inter-
    leukin-1 beta mRNA in rat brain after transient forebrain ischemia. *J Neurochem* 58:
    390–392

15 Toulmond S, Rothwell NJ (1995) Time-course of IL-1 receptor antagonist (IL-1ra)
    expression after brain trauma in the rat. *Soc Neurosci Abstr* 21: 200

16 Rothwell N, Allan S, Toulmond S (1997) The role of interleukin 1 in acute neurode-
    generation and stroke: pathophysiological and therapeutic implications. *J Clin Invest*
    100: 2648–2652

17 Rothwell NJ, Luheshi GN (2000) Interleukin-1 in the brain: biology, pathology and
    therapeutic target. *Trends Neurosci* 23: 618–625

18 Allan SM, Parker LC, Collins B, Davies R, Luheshi GN, Rothwell NJ (2000) Cortical
    cell death induced by IL-1 is mediated via actions in the hypothalamus of the rat. *Proc
    Natl Acad Sci USA* 97: 5580–5585

19 Lawrence CB, Allan SM, Rothwell NJ (1998) Interleukin-1beta and the interleukin-1
    receptor antagonist act in the striatum to modify excitotoxic brain damage in the rat.
    Eur J Neurosci 10: 1188–1195

20 Loddick SA, Rothwell NJ (1996) Neuroprotective effects of human recombinant inter-
    leukin-1 receptor antagonist in focal cerebral ischaemia in the rat. *J Cereb Blood Flow
    Metab* 16: 932–940

21 Toulmond S, Relton JK, Lawrence CB, Loddick S, Benavides J, Rothwell NJ (1993)
    Neurotoxic effects of interleukin-1 (IL-1) *in vivo*. *Soc Neurosci Abstr* 19: 771

22 Yamasaki Y, Matsuura N, Shozuhara H, Onodera H, Itoyama Y, Kogure K (1995) Inter-
    leukin-1 as a pathogenetic mediator of ischemic brain damage in rats. *Stroke* 26: 676–
    680

23 Schielke GP, Yang GY, Shivers BD, Betz AL (1998) Reduced ischemic brain injury in
    interleukin-1 beta converting enzyme-deficient mice. *J Cereb Blood Flow Metab* 18:
    180–185

24 Boutin H, Luheshi G, Rothwell N (2000) Effect of IL-1α and IL-1β deletion on cerebral
    ischaemia. *Soc Neurosci Abstr* 670.15

25 Loddick SA, Wong ML, Bongiorno PB, Gold PW, Licinio J, Rothwell NJ (1997) Endoge-
    nous interleukin-1 receptor antagonist is neuroprotective. *Biochem Biophys Res Com-
    mun* 234: 211–215

26 Stroemer RP, Rothwell NJ (1998) Exacerbation of ischemic brain damage by localized
    striatal injection of interleukin-1beta in the rat. *J Cereb Blood Flow Metab* 18: 833–839

27 Knoblach SM, Faden AI (1998) Interleukin-10 improves outcome and alters proinflam-
    matory cytokine expression after experimental traumatic brain injury. *Exp Neurol* 153:
    143–151

28 Louw DF, Yang FW, Sutherland GR (2000) The effect of delta-9-tetrahydrocannabinol on forebrain ischemia in rat. *Brain Res* 857: 183–187

29 Relton JK, Strijbos PM, O'Shaugnessy CT, Carey F, Forder RA, Tilders FH, Rothwell NJ (1991) Lipocortin-1 is an endogenous inhibitor of ischaemic damage in the rat brain. *J Exp Med* 174: 305–310

30 Distelhorst CW (1997) Glucocorticoid-induced apoptosis. Advances Pharmacol 41: 247–270

31 McEwen BS, Gould EA, Sakai RR (1992) The vulnerability of the hippocampus to protective and destructive effects of glucocorticoids in relation to stress. *Br J Psychiatry* (Suppl): 18–23

32 Reagan LP, McEwen BS (1997) Controversies surrounding glucocorticoid-mediated cell in the hippocampus. *J Chem Neuroanat* 13: 149–167

33 Barone FC, Feuerstein GZ, White RF, Irving EA, Parsons AA, Hadingham SJ, Roberts J, Hunter AJ, Archer G, Kumar S et al (1999) Selective inhibition of p38 mitogen activated kinase reduces brain injury and neurological deficits in rat focal stroke models. *J Cereb Blood Flow Metab* 19: S613

34 Relton JK, Rothwell NJ (1992) Interleukin-1 receptor antagonist inhibits ischaemic and excitotoxic neuronal damage in the rat. *Brain Res Bull* 29: 243–246

35 Martin D, Miller G, Neuberger T, Relton J, Fischer N (1998) Role of IL-1 in neurodegeneration. Pre-clinical findings with IL-1ra and ICE inhibitors. In: PL Wood (ed): *Neuroinflammation: mechanisms and management.* Humana Press, Totowa, 197–219

36 Martin D, Chinookoswong N, Miller G (1994) The interleukin-1 receptor antagonist (rhIL-1ra) protects against cerebral infarction in a rat model of hypoxia-ischemia. *Exp Neurol* 130: 362–367

37 Toulmond S, Rothwell N (1995) Interleukin-1 receptor antagonist inhibits neuronal damage caused by fluid percussion injury in the rat. *Brain Res* 671: 261–266

38 Garcia JH, Liu KF, Relton JK (1995) Interleukin-1 receptor antagonist decreases the number of necrotic neurons in rats with middle cerebral artery occlusion. *Am J Pathol* 147: 1477–1486

39 Lin MT, Kao TY, Jin YT, Chen CF (1995) Interleukin-1 receptor antagonist attenuates the heat stroke-induced neuronal damage by reducing the cerebral ischemia in rats. *Brain Res Bull* 37: 595–598

40 Relton JK, Martin D, Thompson RC, Russell DA (1996) Peripheral administration of Interleukin-1 Receptor antagonist inhibits brain damage after focal cerebral ischemia in the rat. *Exp Neurol* 138: 206–213

41 Blum-Degen D, Muller T, Kuhn W, Gerlach M, Przuntek H, Riederer P (1995) Interleukin-1 beta and interleukin-6 are elevated in the cerebrospinal fluid of Alzheimer's and *de novo* Parkinson's disease patients. *Neurosci Lett* 202: 17–20

42 McClain CJ, Cohen D, Ott L, Dinarello CA, Young B (1987) Ventricular fluid interleukin-1 activity in patients with head injury. *J Lab Clin Med* 110: 48–54

43 Mogi M, Harada M, Kondo T, Riederer P, Inagaki H, Minami M, Nagatsu T (1994)

Interleukin-1β, interleukin-6, epidermal growth factor and transforming growth factor-α are elevated in the brain from parkinsonian patients. *Neurosci Lett* 180: 147–150

44 Mogi M, Harada M, Narabayashi H, Inagaki H, Minami M, Nagatsu T (1996) Interleukin (IL)-1b, IL-2, IL-4, IL-6 and transforming growth factor-α levels are elevated in ventricular cerebrospinal fluid in juvenile parkinsonism and Parkinson's disease. *Neurosci Lett* 211: 13–16

45 Ross R (1999) Atherosclerosis – an inflammatory disease. *N Engl J Med* 340: 115–126

46 Hopkins SJ, Rothwell NJ (1995) Cytokines and the nervous system I: expression and recognition. *Trends Neurosci* 18: 83–88

47 Rothwell NJ, Hopkins SJ (1995) Interactions between cytokines and the nervous system II: Actions and mechanisms. *Trends Neurosci* 18: 130–136

48 Bornstein NM, Bova IY, Korczyn AD (1997) Infections as triggering factors for ischemic stroke. *Neurology* 49: S45–S46

49 Bova IY, Bornstein NM, Korczyn AD (1996) Acute infection as a risk factor for ischemic stroke. *Stroke* 27: 2204–2206

50 Grau AJ, Buggle F, Becher H, Zimmermann E, Spiel M, Fent T, Maiwald M, Werle E, Zorn M, Hengel H et al (1998) Recent bacterial and viral infection is a risk factor for cerebrovascular ischemia: clinical and biochemical studies. *Neurology* 50: 196–203

51 Du Y, Dodel RC, Eastwood BJ, Bales KR, Gao F, Lohmuller F, Muller U, Kurz A, Zimmer R, Evans RM et al (2000) Association of an interleukin 1 alpha polymorphism with Alzheimer's disease. *Neurology* 55: 480–483

52 Rogers J (2000) An IL-1 alpha susceptibility polymorphism in Alzheimer's disease: new fuel for the inflammation hypothesis. *Neurology* 55: 464–465

53 Mrak RE, Griffin WS (2000) Interleukin-1 and the immunogenetics of Alzheimer disease. *J Neuropathol Exp Neurol* 59: 471–476

54 Kanemoto K, Kawasaki J, Miyamoto T, Obayashi H, Nishimura M (2000) Interleukin (IL)1beta, IL-1alpha, and IL-1 receptor antagonist gene polymorphisms in patients with temporal lobe epilepsy. *Ann Neurol* 47: 571–574

55 Schrijver HM, Crusius JB, Uitdehaag BM, Garcia Gonzalez MA, Kostense PJ, Polman CH, Pena AS (1999) Association of interleukin-1beta and interleukin-1 receptor antagonist genes with disease severity in MS. *Neurology* 52: 595–599

56 Grau AJ, Buggle F, Steichen-Wiehn C, Heindl S, Banerjee T, Seitz R, Winter R, Forsting M, Werle E, Bode C (1995) Clinical and biochemical analysis in infection-associated stroke. *Stroke* 26: 1520–1526

Inflammatory cytokines in CNS trauma

V. Wee Yong[1] and Richard M. Ransohoff[2]

[1]Departments of Oncology and Clinical Neurosciences, University of Calgary, 3330 Hospital Drive, Calgary, Alberta T2N 4N1, Canada; [2]The Lerner Research Institute, Cleveland Clinic Foundation, 9500 Euclid Avenue, Cleveland, OH 44195-5244, USA

Inflammatory cytokines are elevated in CNS trauma

In this section, issues to be considered include whether the normal brain expresses inflammatory cytokines, in what cellular compartment, and which inflammatory cytokines are upregulated as a result of CNS trauma. As to the latter, the cellular sources and time-course of expression are also issues to be discussed.

Multiple reports have indicated that inflammatory cytokines, including interleukin (IL)-1 (α and β), tumor necrosis factor-α (TNFα), IL-2, IL-6 and transforming growth factors β (TGFβ) are expressed at basal levels in the normal brain (reviewed in [1]). In this regard, IL-1 has been found to be expressed by neurons [2], microglia [3], endothelial cells, oligodendrocytes and their progenitors [4], and astrocytes, suggesting that all cellular components of the CNS have the capacity to express cytokines. Nonetheless, caution should be exercised in interpreting the results since several of these reports have utilised immunohistochemistry to locate cytokines; the specificity of the various antibodies for their targets was not often demonstrated in these studies. Other reports, using different methods including polymerase chain reaction (PCR), have found minimal, if at all, expression of IL-1 in the normal brain [5].

In contrast to basal expression, it is clear that many cytokines are present in the brains of rodents following a mechanical injury to this tissue. Notably, IL-1, TNFα and TGFβs are found to be commonly elevated [6, 7]. Human brains from a variety of pathologies have also been found to express IL-1 [8]. Apart from infiltrating leukocytes, the cells that upregulate cytokines within the CNS parenchyma after experimental trauma have been determined to include microglia/macrophages [7, 9], endothelial cells, astrocytes and even neurons [10].

There is discrepancy as to the source of cytokines in CNS trauma. Tchelingerian et al. [9] noted that 24 h after a penetrating injury to the hippocampus, intense IL-1 and TNFα immunoreactivity was confined to neurons, while positive signals appeared in microglia and astrocyte process only at day 6. In contrast, after spinal cord contusion in rats, semi-quantitative PCR showed IL-1β and TNFα to be increased by 1 h of injury, and the cellular source was proposed to be microglia [11]. Bartholdi et al. [12] had also suggested that the early increase of inflammatory cytokines after spinal cord injury was microglial in origin. In recent analyses of a corticectomy (aspiration of a piece of cerebral cortex) injury to the adult mouse brain, we detected an early elevation of IL-1β transcript (using *in situ* hybridization) in immunohistochemically-identified microglia [5]. It was clear that while not all microglia expressed IL-1β transcript at the 3 h time point that was analysed, all IL-1β expressing cells were microglia [5]. Furthermore, the elevation of IL-1β peaked at 3 h, and declined thereafter, as was also observed by others [13]. Since neurophils and monocytes traffic into the CNS parenchyma from 6–12 h after trauma, these findings suggest that the CNS-intrinsic increase of IL-1β far outweighs the amounts that are produced by leukocytes upon their subsequent transit into the CNS.

The nature and location of the injury may also dictate the time-course and cellular source of the cytokine in question. For instance, while Streit et al. [11] showed elevation of IL-1β and TNFα by 1 h of spinal cord contusion, studies of facial nerve axotomy by the same group indicated that the induction of IL-1 did not occur until about 3 days after the insult. Interestingly, the acute inflammatory responses to mechanical lesions in the CNS differ between the brain and spinal cord [14].

Interactions of inflammatory cytokines with other molecules in CNS trauma

While the focus of this chapter is inflammatory cytokines, other molecules are also elevated in CNS trauma and these have the capacity to impact on cytokine activity. In particular, the chemokines and matrix metalloproteinases (MMPs) that are also increased in CNS trauma can interact with inflammatory cytokines in several ways.

Chemokines are small molecules that were traditionally described in the context of providing a migrational gradient for the transit of leukocytes [15]. In early studies involving brain stab wound injury in neonatal rats, we discovered that the chemokine macrophage chemoattractant protein (MCP)-1 was promptly elevated by astrocytes, before any prominent infiltrates could be found [16]. Subsequently, others have reported that MCP-1 and other chemokines, including RANTES, MIP-1β, GRO-α and IP-10, were upregulated in the CNS parenchyma by 1–2 h of experimental brain trauma in animals [17–21]. Chemokines are also increased following traumatic brain injuries in humans [22]. Cellular sources at early timepoints include cells intrinsic to the CNS, and, indeed, all neural cell types can produce chemokines in various situations [23–25].

What are the stimuli for the CNS expression of chemokines in trauma? Because several tissue culture based studies demonstrate that chemokines expressed by astrocytes and microglia are upregulated by inflammatory cytokines, particularly IL-1

[26–29], the latter are viable candidates as regulators of chemokine expression in CNS insults. As IL-1β is increased by 15 min of a corticectomy insult to the CNS [5], this time frame is consistent with the hypothesis that this cytokine is a transcriptional regulator of chemokine expression in the brain following trauma. The consequences of cytokine-induced chemokine expression will be elaborated in the next section.

Notably, cytokines may also downregulate chemokine expression by glial cells. In this regard, the anti-inflammatory cytokines, IL-10 and TGFβ were found to inhibit the production of RANTES by microglia in culture [28].

The family of matrix metalloproteinases (MMPs) consists of proteolytic enzymes that can degrade all components of the ECM. MMPs are implicated in a variety of physiological and pathological processes that involve some degree of ECM turnover (reviewed in [30]). It has become evident that MMPs are elevated in CNS trauma [31]. In this regard, a rise in several MMP members was observed 6–12h after corticectomy [31]. The functions of MMPs in trauma remain elusive but will be discussed in the next section. Of relevance to this section, IL-1β was found to be a potent transcriptional regulator of the production of MMP-9 by cultured neurons and astrocytes [31]. Furthermore, IL-1β likely regulates the production of MMP-9 *in vivo* since the application of IL-1 receptor antagonist to the corticectomy injury site in CNS trauma prevents the subsequent elevation of MMP-9 [31].

Besides regulating chemokine and MMP transcription, cytokines can interact with these molecules in complex ways. MMPs can process several pro-cytokines, including pro-TNFα [32] and pro-IL-1β [33], into their active forms. Conversely, MMPs may degrade mature IL-1β into inactive fragments [33]. Ito et al. [34] also demonstrated that prolonged incubation with MMP-1, -2, -3 and –9 resulted in IL-1β (but not IL-1α) degradation and loss of its biological activity. Interestingly, the primary site of cleavage of IL-1β by MMP-2 was identified as the Glu^{25}–Leu^{26} bond, not unlike the glutamate-leucine bond of chemokines with the ELR (glutamate-leucine-arginine) motif. Further, MMP-2 was shown to cleave MCP-3, yielding a truncated peptide that acted as an antagonist at chemokine receptors CCR1, CCR2 and CCR3 [35]. MCP-1 was recently found to induce MMP-1 in primary skin fibroblasts, but this required the intermediary of IL-1 [36]. Thus, there is a complex interaction between cytokines, chemokines and MMPs in the CNS to achieve multiple endpoints.

Possible functions of inflammatory cytokines in CNS trauma

Several studies implicate cytokines in producing pathology to the CNS. For example, TNFα has been found to be toxic to oligodendrocytes [37], to cause demyelination *in vivo* [38] and to inflict neuronal death (reviewed in [39]) or glial apoptosis [40] in CNS trauma. The intracerebral infusion of a selective TNFα antagonist, sTNFR fusion protein, 15 min before and 1 h after a fluid percussion injury to the brain, improved behavioral recovery [41]. A large literature links IL-1 to acute neurodegeneration in ischemia (reviewed in [42]). In correspondence with the detrimental effects of pro-inflammatory cytokines, the use of IL-10, an anti-inflammatory cytokine which downregulates the levels of IL-1β, TNFα and inducible nitric oxide synthase among others, decreased traumatic [43] or quisqualate-induced [44, 45] damage in the injured rat spinal cord.

Nonetheless, the evidence also supports a beneficial role for inflammatory cytokines in CNS trauma. Several cytokines induce the production of neurotrophic factors, particularly nerve growth factor (NGF), from astrocytes in culture (reviewed in [1]). The infusion of IL-1β into the brain increased the content of NGF [46], fibroblast growth factors and glial derived neurotrophic factor [47]. When fibroblasts overexpressing leukemia inhibitory factor were implanted into the injured adult rat spinal cord, expression of neurotrophin-3 and corticospinal axon regrowth were increased compared to controls [48]. Moreover, using enriched cultures, many inflammatory cytokines can directly provide for neuronal survival or neurite extension [1].

Recently, we described that the neurotrophic factor, ciliary neurotrophic factor (CNTF), was upregulated in the CNS parenchyma following a corticectomy insult [5]. This upregulation was prevented by the exogenous adminstration of an IL-1 receptor antagonist. Strikingly, CNTF induction was not observed after corticectomy in mice genetically null for IL-1β, but expression could be "rescued" by the application of IL-1β to the lesion site [5]. These observations strengthen the concept that the expression of cytokines post-trauma may serve to enhance CNS repair, by virtue of regulating the activity or levels of neurotrophic factors. Genetic models of CNS inflammation, in mice that transgenically express particular cytokines [49], may help to decipher the roles of cytokines in CNS injuries.

A provocative recent revelation is that autoreactive T cells that migrate into a crush lesion site might attenuate the degree of neuronal loss that arises as a result of secondary degeneration to that area [50]. This concept is referred to as "protective autoimmunity" [51], where the presence of T cells confers neuroprotection to the damaged area. A mechanism to explain the neurotrophic potential of autoreactive T cells is that these cells elaborate neurotrophic factors at the area of injury [52, 53]. Thus, while extensive tissue damage can occur in response to T cell infiltration as evident from the multiple sclerosis literature, T cells in other circumstances exert beneficial properties.

There are other roles of inflammation in CNS trauma, by virtue of the indirect effect of cytokines on non-neuronal cells. For instance, the phenomenon of reactive astrogliosis, where astrocytes undergo characteristic changes in response to CNS insults, may serve to enhance CNS repair [1, 54], although detrimental properties of astrogliosis have also been reported. Inflammatory cytokines are thought to regulate the phenomenon of astrogliosis [54–58], and, in this regard, would limit CNS damage or enhance CNS repair.

The interactions of cytokines with MMPs and chemokines, noted above, will likely impact on CNS recovery. By virtue of transcriptionally regulating the production of MMPs and chemokines, cytokines unleash within the CNS this battery of effectors. While a principal role for chemokines in CNS trauma may be to influence the composition of inflammatory cells in the lesioned area, chemokines likely have functions that alter CNS toxicity or repair. All CNS cells, including neurons, have receptors for chemokines [24] and these may have a role in remodeling following injury. Mice genetically deficient for the chemokine receptor, CXCR4, or its ligand, stromal derived factor (SDF)-1, have derailed migration of granule cells in the cerebellum [59]. MCP-1 regulates the migration of astrocytes while SDF-1β alters microglia chemotaxis [60]. Chemokines may also regulate the proliferation and migration of neural progenitor cells to sites of CNS trauma in an attempt to replenish lost cells. In this regard, GRO-α has been shown to be a potent mitogen for spinal cord oligodendrocyte precursors [61]. In addition to promoting CNS remodeling following trauma, chemokines may also confer trophic activity on neurons that survive the initial insult. *In vitro*, the chemokine IL-8 was noted to mediate a pronounced survival of hippocampal neurons [62]. Finally, yet another potential activity of chemokines following CNS trauma is that of angiogenesis. CXC chemokines with an ELR motif at their N-terminus (e.g. GRO-α and IL-8) have a positive role in angiogenesis [63], and may help to recruit new blood vessels to areas of repair.

As noted above, MMPs are transcriptionally regulated by cytokines, particularly IL-1. The functions of MMPs that are elevated in CNS trauma remain elusive. Since MMPs can kill neurons [64], and mice deficient for MMP-9 have less behavioral deficits and smaller lesion volumes following spinal cord injury when compared to wild-type controls [65], the presence of MMPs in CNS trauma appears detrimental. Nonetheless, there could be possible beneficial roles of MMPs in CNS trauma given their rapid and consistent upregulation following the injury [31]. These favorable roles may include the remodeling of the post-injury ECM to modulate cell migration, signaling and survival. Also, MMPs regulate growth factor availability, by virtue of releasing ECM- or cell surface-bound growth factors [66–68]. MMPs may also act as an intermediary in growth factor signaling [69]. When active MMP-9 is focussed on the cell membrane by its interaction with CD44 (hyaluronan receptor), angiogenesis is promoted through the conversion of pro-TGFβ to TGFβ [70]. MMPs are involved in growth cone activity since MMP inhibitors attenuate this process [30]. Furthermore, MMP-2 produced by dorsal root ganglion neurons inactivates inhibitory chondroitin sulfate proteoglycans and expose the permissive laminin substrate to facilitate the elongation of neurites [71]. In this context, the roles of cytokines in inducing MMPs following CNS trauma would have favorable outcomes.

Conclusions

It is clear that much remains to be investigated with respect to the roles of inflammatory cytokines that are present in the CNS following an insult. It is apparent that both beneficial and detrimental functions of cytokines exist. The pendulum that swings the balance of a cytokine towards favorable or detrimental outcomes likely depends on a variety of competing factors. These include the magnitude of induction of the cytokine following the injury, and the persistence of the elevation of cytokines. Also, since each cytokine is multi-functional, both good and bad properties of the cytokine are unleashed simultaneously. The presence of other factors will also modulate the activity of the cytokine of interest; Liu et al. [72] demonstrated that IL-1β and TNFα signaling in astrocytes is modulated by the P2 purinergic receptors, and purine nucleotides are found in the extracellular space following trauma. A particular cytokine may also be time-dependent in its functions. Results from TNF null mice subjected to a cortical impact injury suggest that although the presence of TNF in the acute post-trauma period may be deleterious, this cytokine may facilitate long-term behavioral recovery and histological repair [73].

Overall, the challenge is for us to swing the pendulum towards beneficial roles for cytokines, so that the multiple favorable functions of the ubiquitously expressed inflammatory cytokines can be tipped in favor of repair and recovery of the CNS following insults.

References

1   Yong VW (1996) Cytokines, astrogliosis and neurotrophism following CNS trauma. In: E Benveniste, R Ransohoff (eds): *Cytokines and the CNS: development, defense and disease*. CRC Press, Boca Raton, 309–327

2   Breder CD, Dinarello CA, Saper CB (1988) Interleukin-1 immunoreactive innervation of the human hypothalamus. *Science* 240: 321–324

3   Giulian D, Woodward J, Young DG, Krebs JF, Lachman LB (1988) Interleukin-1 injected into the mammalian brain stimulates astrogliosis and neovascularization. *J Neurosci* 8: 2485–2490

4   Blasi F, Riccio M, Brogi A, Strazza M, Taddei ML, Romagnoli S, Luddi A, D'Angelo R, Santi S, Costantino-Ceccarini E et al (1999) Constitutive expression of interleukin-1 beta (IL-1beta) in rat oligodendrocytes. *Biol Chem* 380: 259–264

5   Herx LM, Rivest S, Yong VW (2000) Central nervous system-initiated inflammation and neurotrophism in trauma: IL-1β is required for the production of ciliary neurotrophic factor. *J Immunol* 165: 2232–2239

6   Nieto-Sampedro M, Berman MA (1987) Interleukin-1 like activity in rat brain: sources, targets, and effect of injury. *J Neurosci* Res 17: 214–219

7   Woodroofe MN, Sarna GS, Wadha M et al (1991) Detection of interleukin-1 and inter-

leukin-6 in adult rat brain, following mechanical injury, *in vivo* microdialysis: evidence of a role for microglia in cytokine production. *J Neuroimmunol* 33: 227–236

8   Da Cunha A, Jefferson JJ, Tyor WR, Glass JD, Jannotta FS, Vitkovic L (1993) Control of astrocytosis by interleukin-1 and transforming growth factor-β1 in human brain. *Brain Res* 631: 39–45

9   Tchelingerian J, Quinonero J, Booss J, Jacque C (1993) Localization of TNFα and IL-1α immunoreactivities in striatal neurons after surgical injury to the hippocampus. *Neuron* 10: 213–224

10   Tchelingerian JL, Le Saux F, Jacque C (1996) Identification and topography of neuronal cell populations expressing TNFα and IL-1α in response to hippocampal lesion. *J Neurosci Res* 43: 99–106

11   Streit WJ, Semple-Rowland SL, Hurley SD, Miller RC, Popovich PG, Stokes BT (1998) Cytokine mRNA profiles in contused spinal cord and axotomized facial nucleus suggest a beneficial role for inflammation and gliosis. *Exp Neurol* 152: 74–87

12   Schnell L, Fearn S, Klassen H, Schwab ME, Perry VH (1999) Acute inflammatory responses to mechanical lesions in the CNS: differences between brain and spinal cord. *Eur J Neurosci* 11: 3648–3658

13   Bartholdi D, Schwab ME (1997) Expression of pro-inflammatory cytokine and chemokine mRNA upon experimental spinal cord injury in mouse: an *in situ* hybridization study. *Eur J Neurosci* 9: 1422–1438

14   Tonai T, Taketani Y, Ueda N, Nishisho T, Ohmoto Y, Sakata Y, Muraguchi M, Wada K, Yamamoto S (1999) Possible involvement of interleukin-1 in cyclooxygenase-2 induction after spinal cord injury in rats. *J Neurochem* 72: 302–309

15   Gerard C, Rollins BJ (2001) Chemokines and disease. *Nat Immunol* 2: 108–110

16   Glabinski AR, Balasingam V, Tani M, Kunkel SL, Strieter RM, Yong VW, Ransohoff RM (1996) Chemokine monocyte chemoattractant protein 1 is expressed by astrocytes after mechanical injury to the brain. *J Immunol* 156: 4363–4368

17   Berman JW, Guida MP, Warren J, Amat J, Brosnan CF (1996) Localization of monocyte chemoattractant peptide-1 expression in the central nervous system in experimental autoimmune encephalomyelitis and trauma in the rat. *J Immunol* 156: 3017–3023

18   Ghirnikar RS, Lee YL, He TR, Eng LF (1996) Chemokine expression in rat stab wound brain injury. *J Neurosci Res* 46: 727–733

19   McTigue DM, Tani M, Krivacic K, Chernosky A, Kelner GS, Maciejewski D, Maki R, Ransohoff RM, Stokes BT (1998) Selective chemokine mRNA accumulation in the rat spinal cord after contusion injury. *J Neurosci Res* 53: 368–376

20   Muessel MJ, Berman NE, Klein RM (2000) Early and specific expression of monocyte chemoattractant protein-1 in the thalamus induced by cortical injury. *Brain Res* 870: 211–221

21   Le YL, Shih K, Bao P, Ghirnikar RS, Eng LF (2000) Cytokine chemokine expression in contused rat spinal cord. *Neurochem Int* 36: 417–425

22   Whalen MJ, Carlos TM, Kochanek PM, Wisnewski SR, Bell MJ, Clark RS, DeKosky ST,

Marion DW, Adelson PD (2000) Interleukin-8 is increased in cerebrospinal fluid of children with severe head injury. *Crit Care Med* 28: 929–934

23 Arsenio VC, Campbell IL (1999) Chemokines in the CNS: plurifunctional mediators in diverse states. *Trends Neurosci* 22: 504–512

24 Hesselgesser J, Horuk R (1999) Chemokine and chemokine receptor expression in the central nervous system. *J Neurovirol* 5: 13–26

25 Glabinski AR, Ransohoff RM (1999) Chemokines and chemokine receptors in CNS pathology. *J Neurovirol* 5: 3–12

26 Barna BP, Pettay J, Barnett GH, Zhou P, Iwasaki K, Estes M (1994) Regulation of monocyte chemoattractant protein-1 expression in adult human non-neoplastic astrocytes is sensitive to tumor necrosis factor (TNF) or antibody to 55-kDa TNF receptor. *J Neuroimmunol* 50: 101–107

27 McManus CM, Brosnan CF, Berman JW (1998) Cytokine-induced MIP-1α and MIP-1β expression in human fetal microglia. *J Immunol* 160: 1449–1455

28 Hu S, Chao CC, Ehrlich LC, Sheng WS, Sutton RL, Rockswold GL, Peterson PK (1999) Inhibition of microglial cell RANTES production by IL-10 and TGF-β. *J Leuk Biol* 65: 815–821

29 Miyamoto Y, Kim SU (1999) Cytokine-induced production of macrophage inflammatory protein-1α (MIP-1α) in cultured human astrocytes. *J Neurosci Res* 55: 245–251

30 Yong VW, Krekoski CA, Forsyth PA, Bell R, Edwards DR (1998) Matrix metalloproteinases and diseases of the central nervous system. *Trends Neurosci* 21: 75–80

31 Vecil GG, Larsen PH, Herx LM, Besson A, Goodyer CG, Yong VW (2000) Interleukin-1 is a key regulator of matrix metalloproteinase-9 in human neurons in culture and following mouse brain trauma *in vivo*. *J Neurosci Res* 61: 212–224

32 English WR, Puente XS, Freije JM, Knauper V, Amour A, Merryweather A, Lopez-Otin C, Murphy G (2000) Membrane type 4 matrix metalloproteinase (MMP17) has tumor necrosis factor-alpha convertase activity but does not activate pro-MMP2. *J Biol Chem* 275: 14046–14055

33 Schonbeck U, Mach F, Libby P (1998) Generation of biologically active IL-1 beta by matrix metalloproteinases: A novel caspase-1-independent pathway of IL-1β processing. *J Immunol* 161: 3340–3346

34 Ito A, Mukaiyama A, Itoh Y, Nagase H, Thogersen IB, Enghild JJ, Sasaguri Y, Mori Y (1996) Degradation of interleukin 1β by matrix metalloproteinases. *J Biol Chem* 271: 14557–14660

35 McQuibban GA, Gong JH, Tam EM, McCulloch CA, Clark-Lewis I, Overall CM (2000) Inflammation dampened by gelatinase A cleavage of monocyte chemoattractant protein-3. *Science* 289: 1202–1206

36 Yamamoto T, Eckes B, Mauch C, Hartmann K, Krieg T (2000) Monocyte chemoattractant protein-1 enhances gene expression and synthesis of matrix metalloproteinase-1 in human fibroblasts by an autocrine IL-α loop. *J Immunol* 164: 6174–6179

37 Louis J-C, Magal E, Takayama S (1993) CNTF protection of oligodendrocytes against natural and tumor necrosis factor α-induced death. *Science* 259: 689

38   Jenkins HG, Ikeda H (1992) Tumor necrosis factor causes an increase in axonal transport of protein and demyelination in the mouse optic nerve. *J Neurol Sci* 108: 99–104

39   Shohami E, Ginis I, Hallenbeck JM (1999) Dual role of tumor necrosis factor alpha in brain injury. *Cytokine Growth Factor Rev* 10: 119–130

40   Lee YB, Yune TY, Baik SY et al. (2000) Role of tumor necrosis factor-α in neuronal and glial apoptosis after spinal cord injury. *Exp Neurol* 166: 190–195

41   Knoblach SM, Fan L, Faden AI (1999) Early neuronal expression of tumor necrosis factor-alpha after experimental brain injury contributes to neurological impairment. *J Neuroimmunol* 95 (1–2): 115–125

42   Rothwell NJ, Luheshi GN (2000) Interleukin 1 in the brain: biology, pathology and therapeutic target. *Trends Neurosci* 23: 618–625

43   Bethea JR, Nagashima H, Acosta M, Briceno C, Gomez F, Marcillo AE, Loor K, Green J, Dietrich WD (1999) Systemically administered interleukin-10 reduced tumor necrosis factor alpha production and significantly improves functional recovery following traumatic spinal cord injury in rats. *J Neurotrauma* 16: 851–863

44   Brewer KL, Bethea JR, Yezierski RP (1999) Neuroprotective effects of interleukin-10 following excitotoxic spinal cord injury. *Exp Neurol* 159: 484–493

45   Plunkett JA, Yu CG, Easton JM, Bethea JR, Yezierski RP (2001) Effects of interleukin-10 (IL-10) on pain behavior and gene expression following excitotoxic spinal cord injury in the rat. *Exp Neurol* 168: 144–154

46   Dekosky ST, Goss JR, Miller PD, Styren SD, Kochanek PM, Marion D (1994) Upregulation of nerve growth factor following cortical trauma. *Exp Neurol* 130: 173–177

47   Ho A, Blum M (1997) Regulation of astroglial-derived dopaminergic neurotrophic factors by interleukin-1β in the striatum of young and middle-aged mice. *Exp Neurol* 148: 348–359

48   Blesch A, Uy HS, Grill RJ, Cheng JG, Patterson PH, Tuszynski MH (1999) Leukemia inhibitory factor augments neurotrophin expression and corticospinal axon growth after adult CNS injury. *J Neurosci* 19: 3556–3566

49   Owens T, Wekerle H, Antel J (2001) Genetic models of CNS inflammation. *Nature Med* 7: 161–166

50   Moalem G, Leibowitz-Amit R, Yoles E, Mor F, Cohen IR, Schwartz M (1999) Autoimmune T cells protect neurons from secondary degeneration after central nervous system axotomy. *Nat Med* 5: 49–55

51   Schwartz M, Cohen IR (2000) Autoimmunity can benefit self-maintenance. *Immunol Today* 21: 265–268

52   Kerschensteiner M, Gallmeier E, Behrens L, Leal VV, Misgeld T, Klinkert WE, Kolbeck R, Hoppe E, Oropeza-Wekerle RL, Bartke I et al (1999) Activated human T cells, B cells, and monocytes produce brain-derived neurotrophic factor *in vitro* and in inflammatory brain lesions: a neuroprotective role of inflammation? *J Exp Med* 189: 865–870

53   Hammarberg H, Lidman O, Lundberg C, Eltayeb SY, Gielen AW, Muhallab S, Svenningsson A, Linda H, van der Meide PH, Cullheim S et al (2000) Neuroprotection by

encephalomyelitis and neurotrophin production by CNS-infiltrating T and natural killer cells. *J Neurosci* 20: 5283–5291

54   Streit WJ, Hurley SD, McGraw TS, Semple-Rowland SL (2000) Comparative evaluation of cytokine profiles and reactive gliosis supports a critical role for interleukin-6 in neuron-glia signaling during regeneration. *J Neurosci Res* 61: 10–20

55   Balasingam V, Yong VW (1996) Attenuation of astroglial reactivity by interleukin-10. *J Neurosci* 16: 2945–2955

56   Chiang CS, Powell HC, Gold LH, Samimi A, Campbell IL (1996) Macrophage/microglial-mediated primary demyelination and motor disease induced by the central nervous system production of interleukin-3 in transgenic mice. *J Clin Invest* 97: 1512–1524

57   Logan A, Green J, Hunter A, Jackson R, Berry M (1999) Inhibition of glial scarring in the injured rat brain by a recombinant human monoclonal antibody to transforming growth factor-β2. *Eur J Neurosci* 11: 2367–2374

58   Brunello AG, Weissenberger J, Kappeler A, Vallan C, Peters M, Rose-John S, Weis J (2000) Astrocytic alterations in interleukin-6/soluble interleukin-6 receptor α double-transgenic mice. *Am J Pathol* 157: 1485–1493

59   Ma Q, Jones D, Borghesani PR, Segal RA, Nagasawa T, Kishimoto T, Bronson RT, Springer TA (1998) Impaired B-lymphopoiesis, myelopoiesis, and derailed cerebellar neuronal migration in CXCR4- and SDF-1-deficient mice. *Proc Natl Acad Sci USA* 95: 9448–9453

60   Tanabe S, Heesen M, Yoshizawa I, Berman MA, Luo Y, Bleul CC, Springer TA, Okuda K, Gerard N, Dorf ME (1997) Functional expression of the CXC-chemokine receptor-4/fusin on mouse microglial cells and astrocytes. *J Immunol* 159: 905–911

61   Robinson S, Tani M, Streiter RM, Ransohoff RM, Miller RH (1998) The chemokine growth-regulated oncogene-α promotes spinal cord oligodendrocyte precursor proliferation. *J Neurosci* 18: 10457–10463

62   Araujo DM, Cotman CW (1993) Trophic effects of interleukin-4, -7 and -8 on hippocampal neuronal cultures: potential involvement of glial-derived factors. *Brain Res* 600: 49–55

63   Belperio JA, Keane MP, Arenberg DA, Addison CL, Ehlert JE, Burdick MD, Strieter RM (2000) CXC chemokines in angiogenesis. *J Leukoc Biol* 68: 1–8

64   Johnston JB, Zhang K, Silva C, Shalinsky DR, Conant K, Ni W, Corbett D, Yong VW, Power C, (2001) HIV-1 Tat neurotoxicity is prevented by matrix metalloproteinase inhibitors. *Ann Neurol* 49: 230–241

65   Wang X, Jung J, Asahi M, Chwang W, Russo L, Moskowitz MA, Dixon CE, Fini ME, Lo EH (2000) Effects of matrix metalloproteinase-9 gene knock-out on morphological and motor outcomes after traumatic brain injury. *J Neurosci* 20: 7037–7042

66   Levi E, Fridman R, Miao HQ, Ma YS, Yayon A, Vlodavsky I (1996) Matrix metalloproteinase-2 releases active soluble ectodomain of fibroblast growth factor receptor 1. *Proc Natl Acad Sci USA* 93: 7069–7074

67   Whitelock JM, Murdoch AD, Iozzo RV, Underwood PA (1996) The degradation of

human endothelial cell-derived perlecan and release of bound basic fibroblast growth factor by stromelysin, collagenase, plasmin, and heparanases. *J Biol Chem* 271: 10079–10086

68 Suzuki M, Raab G, Moses MA, Fernandez CA, Klagsbrun M (1997) Matrix metallo-proteinase-3 releases active heparin-binding EGF-like growth factor by cleavage of a specific juxtamembrane site. *J Biol Chem* 272: 31730–31737

69 Prenzel N, Zwick E, Daub H, Leserer M, Abraham R, Wallasch C, Ullrich A (1999) EGF receptor transactivation by G-protein-coupled receptors requires metalloproteinase cleavage of proHB-EGF. *Nature* 402: 884–888

70 Yu Q, Stamenkovic I (2000) Cell surface-localized matrix metalloproteinase-9 prote-olytically activates TGF-beta and promotes tumor invasion and angiogenesis. *Genes Dev* 14: 163–176

71 Zuo J, Ferguson TA, Hernandez YJ, Stetler-Stevenson WG, Muir D (1998) Neuronal matrix metalloproteinase-2 degrades and inactivates a neurite-inhibiting chondroitin sulfate proteoglycan. *J Neurosci* 18: 5203–5211

72 Liu JSH, John GR, Sikora A, Lee SC, Brosnan CF (2000) Modulation of interleukin-1β and tumor necrosis factor α signaling by P2 purinergic receptors in human fetal astro-cytes. *J Neurosci* 20: 5292–5299

73 Scherbel U, Raghupathi R, Nakamura M, Saatman KE, Trojanowski JQ, Neugebauer E, Marino MW, McIntosh TK (1999) Differential acute and chronic responses of tumor necrosis factor-deficient mice to experimental brain injury. *Proc Natl Acad Sci USA* 96: 8721–8726

Inflammation in cerebral thrombosis, angiogenesis
and matrix regulation:
a new perspective in stroke research and therapeutics

Microvessel integrin expression during focal cerebral ischemia

Gregory J. del Zoppo

Department of Molecular and Experimental Medicine, The Scripps Research Institute, 10550 North Torrey Pines Road, MEM 132, La Jolla, CA 92037, USA

Introduction

Occlusion of the middle cerebral artery (MCA:O) initiates reactive changes in the downstream microvasculature, which represent responses to ischemia and a preparation for tissue repair. Changes in microvessel integrity and permeability [1, 2], presentation of adhesion receptors for leukocytes [3, 4], activation of platelets and expression of their fibrin(ogen) receptor [3, 5], loss of basal lamina integrity [6, 7], simultaneous alteration in cell-matrix adhesion receptors [8, 9], and changes in astrocyte ultrastructure [10, 11] occur rapidly following MCA:O. These processes all involve alterations in integrin receptor expression. Integrins are $\alpha\beta$ heterodimeric transmembrane glycoproteins which participate in vascular development, tissue and vascular structural integrity, and intercellular communication [12–14]. Integrin receptors mediate cell-matrix interactions which appear essential for brain tissue structure and function. In resting brain tissue integrin expression is constitutive or inducible under conditions of focal ischemia and inflammation.

Cell receptor responses occur swiftly to an ischemic challenge. Endothelial cell leukocyte adhesion receptors respond to ischemia in a rapid and orderly way, to initiate the cellular inflammatory response. P-selectin appears on the endothelium by 2 h MCA:O, followed by ICAM-1 by 4 h, and E-selectin between 7 and 24 h following MCA:O (during reperfusion) [3, 4]. An intact vascular matrix appears to be required for the expression of the adhesion receptors [4]. The adhesion of polymorphonuclear (PMN) leukocytes to the activated microvascular endothelium is required for their transit into the tissue, and contributes to microvascular perfusion defects [15–17] and the focal "no-reflow" phenomenon [5, 18, 19] following MCA:O and reperfusion. These multiple and simultaneous events underscore the

Inflammation and Stroke, edited by Giora Z. Feuerstein

role of the cerebral microvessel as the interface for the transition from ischemic injury to cellular inflammation [20]. They emphasize the viability of cerebral microvascular cells in the face of ischemia. The importance of the upregulation of the microvascular endothelial cell-leukocyte adhesion receptors P-selectin, E-selectin, and ICAM-1 in active inflammatory (e.g., demyelinating) lesions of the CNS have been explored by Benveniste [21] and Hartung [22]. These fundamental observations of endothelial cell receptor expression in both acute ischemia and chronic inflammation presage the involvement of integrin receptors in both conditions.

Cerebral microvessel structure and matrix integrity

Cerebral capillaries consist of endothelial cells, basal lamina (an extension of the extracellular matrix [ECM]), and astrocyte end-feet. Anatomic and functional relationships support their consideration as a unique ternary complex [20, 23]. In the adult brain, the ECM is found as the basal lamina in microvessels, basement membrane within the meninges, and at other intercellular sites [24]. In non-capillary microvessels, individual smooth muscle cells are encased in the vascular ECM, which is continuous with the basal lamina [23]. The basal lamina serves also as one important vascular barrier to the transmigration or extravasation of circulating blood cells [6, 7]. In addition, proteoglycans contribute to the matrix which separates neurons and glia from neighboring cells within the neuropil [24]. The matrix forms the framework for cellular and microvascular development within the central nervous system (CNS) and, therefore, together with their integrin receptors is required for the construction and proper function of the brain.

Integrins and intravascular responses

Integrin receptor expressions mediate intercellular interactions between circulating cells within blood vessels of the CNS. Firm adhesion of activated PMN leukocytes to endothelial cell ICAM-1 entails an interaction of the β_2-integrins $\alpha_M\beta_2$ (MAC-1) and $\alpha_L\beta_2$ (LFA-1) with ICAM-1 on microvascular endothelium [25, 26], while lymphocytes interact with VCAM-1 *via* the integrin $\alpha_4\beta_1$ [27]. The β_2-integrin-ICAM-1 interaction is a prerequisite for transmigration of PMN leukocytes in a number of inflammatory conditions [25]. The platelet integrin $\alpha_{IIb}\beta_3$-fibrin(ogen) interaction is the terminal step in platelet activation [28, 29]. Integrin $\alpha_{IIb}\beta_3$, in addition to binding activated platelets to the growing fibrin matrix, signals the environment to the platelet [30]. Well-described in circulating cells, β_2-integrins of leukocytes and the integrin $\alpha_{IIb}\beta_3$ of platelets can signal the environment through the condition of specific ligands ("outside-in" signaling) and the response of cell

196

activation ("inside-out" signaling) [30]. These dynamic intravascular cell integrin-ligand interactions can serve as targets for intervention.

Endothelial cell-astrocyte-neuron interrelationships

The proximity of the endothelium to the neighboring astrocyte end-feet in cerebral capillaries and postcapillary venules suggests a close functional relationship for communication and nutrient supply. Adhesion receptors on endothelial cells and on astrocyte end-feet are presumed to maintain this close cell-cell apposition [1, 8, 9]. The endothelium and astrocyte end-feet attach to matrix laminins and collagen IV by integrin receptors. It is postulated that β_1-integrins (e.g., α_1, α_3, and α_6) mediate adherence of endothelial cells to the basal lamina [1], while the integrin $\alpha_6\beta_4$ is expressed at the interface of the astrocyte end-feet and the basal lamina in select microvessels [9]. In addition, it is attractive to consider that signaling of environmental status or intercellular communication are mediated by integrin receptors on endothelial cells and astrocytes in the CNS; however, evidence for this is as yet sketchy.

Extracellular matrix and the microvessel basal lamina

The ECM is a fabric woven of laminins, type IV collagen, fibronectin, proteoglycans, and heparin sulfates studded with entactin, thrombospondin, nidogen, and other proteins [31]. Generated by endothelial cells and astrocytes in concert during development, the basal lamina forms a biologically active connection between these two cell compartments. Organotypic tissue cultures have shown that intact basal lamina requires the juxtaposition of microvascular endothelial cells and astrocytes [32, 33]. Microvascular endothelial cells and astrocytes play reciprocal roles in the generation of matrix proteins. In culture, astrocytes secrete laminin, fibronectin, and chondroitin sulfate proteoglycan, while collagens stimulate astrocyte-induced endothelial cell maturation [34–36]. Conversely, endothelial cell-derived ECM components stimulate astrocyte growth and function (e.g., glutamine synthetase activity) [37, 38]. The blood-brain barrier also relies upon the interdependence of endothelial cells and astrocytes. This has been elegantly shown in chick-quail adrenal vascular tissue/brain tissue xenograft [39] and fetal-adult hippocampal/neocortex allograft preparations [40]. Soluble factor(s) generated by astrocytes are necessary to maintain endothelial blood-brain barrier characteristics including the induction of tight-junctions, transendothelial resistance, and glucose/amino acid transport polarity [40–42]. The basal lamina and blood-brain barriers, then, depend exquisitely upon cooperation between these two unrelated cell types. Disruption of both barriers, as during focal cerebral ischemia, contributes to edema formation and hemorrhagic transformation.

Integrin expression

Integrin α and β subunits are expressed in the resting and activated CNS. A growing body of histological and immunocytochemical evidence suggests potential roles of integrin receptors in cell-cell interactions and chronic inflammation in the CNS. Pinkstaff et al. have suggested a diverse distribution of specific integrin subunit transcripts with neuronal cells within cerebral subfields in the adult rat [43]. Correlation with receptor presentation has not been reported, however. While the cellular transcript distributions appear to follow identifiable topographical landmarks, the cell localization, function, and specificity of the signals remain open for further study.

Neurons in culture have been shown to express the α_8 subunit among others, however β_1 integrins appear to play roles in proliferation and chain migration of neural precursor cells in the absence of glia [44, 45]. While astrocytes can express integrin $\alpha_V\beta_5$ in the presence of vitronectin [46], integrin $\alpha_V\beta_8$ appears to play a role in astrocyte migration *in vitro* [46]. Oligodendrocytes can express $\alpha_6\beta_1$ and α_V integrins *in vitro*; however, migration appears to be mediated exclusively by integrin $\alpha_V\beta_1$, and not $\alpha_6\beta_1$ or $\alpha_V\beta_3$ [47, 48]. In rodent (murine/rat) brain, the β_8 subunit has been localized to cells of the hippocampus and the molecular layer of the cerebellum [49]. Human microglia express both β_1 and β_2 integrins, and can be distinguished from peripheral monocytes by relatively increased expression of the β_1-integrins α_2, α_4, α_5, and α_6 [50]. These varied reports suggest that expression of integrin receptors on several cell types can be detected most readily in conditions of culture, but do not explain the lack of apparent expression on non-vascular cells in whole brain. They imply potential distinct roles of specific integrins in the proliferation, migration, and organizational integrity of cells in the CNS.

A number of investigators have now identified integrin subunits on vascular structures in the CNS. Subunit β_1 has been found on all microvessel diameter categories of human, baboon, and rat cerebral tissues (Tab. 1) [1, 51–54]. Antigens of subunits α_2, α_3, α_5, α_6, β_1, β_3, and β_4, but not α_V and α_4 were identified by Paulus et al. on *post-mortem* human brain vessels [53]. Subunits α_1 and β_5 were not investigated. Abelda reported differential integrin subunit expression on capillaries and larger vessels; however, specific vessel categories were not identified [52]. Subunits α_1, α_3, and α_6 were found in both vessel groups while α_2, α_5, α_V, and β_3 appeared only on larger vessels. Subunit α_4 was not expressed, and data for subunits β_1, β_4, and β_5 were not reported. McGeer et al. described the capillary distribution of the β_1 integrins α_1, α_2, α_3, α_5, and α_6 in post-mortem human brain specimens [51], and described the presence of α_1 and α_6 together with subunit β_1 on human brain capillaries. The absence of subunit α_2 is discordant with its expression in the non-human primate [1].

Haring et al. surveyed integrin antigen expression in cerebral tissues of the non-human primate. Subunits α_1, α_2, α_3, α_4, α_5, α_V, β_1, β_2, β_3, and β_4 are expressed

Table 1 - Integrin expression on cerebral microvessels (non-ischemic)

Author	Refs.	Species	Integrin subunits												
			α_1	α_2	α_3	α_4	α_5	α_6	α_V	β_1	β_2	β_3	β_4	β_5	β_6
Paulus	[53]	human*	–	m	m		m	m		m		m	m	–	
McGeer	[51]	human*	c	c	c		c	c		c			c		
Abelda	[52]	human*	m	–	m		–	m	–			–			
Haring	[1]	baboon	m	–	m	–	–	m	–	m		m	m	–	
Rooms	[54]	rat								m					

c, capillary; l, large microvessel; m, both capillary and large microvessel (designations per individual citations); –, none detected; blank, not tested; *, post-mortem variously in the cerebral microvasculature (Fig. 1) [1]. No apparent association with non-vascular cells was noted on frozen sections. The β_1 integrins α_1, α_2, and α_3 colocalize with CD31 (PECAM-1) in endothelial cells in all microvessels, and to vascular smooth muscle cells in precapillary arterioles [1, 8]. Integrin $\alpha_1\beta_1$ is associated with fibers of select resting astrocytes around larger microvessels in the non-human primate brain. Confocal microscopic studies indicate that the integrin $\alpha_6\beta_4$ is expressed on the abluminal surface of cerebral microvessels at the interface of astrocyte end-feet with the basal lamina (ECM) ligand laminin-5 [9]. The known association of integrin $\alpha_6\beta_4$ with hemidesmosomes in epithelial cells [55], and the appearance of hemidesmosomes on astrocyte end-feet [56], support the close proximity of astrocytes to endothelial cells through integrin adherent mechanisms.

Murine knockout preparations, homozygous deficient for select integrin receptors demonstrate the requirement of the intact integrin-matrix interactions for CNS development. Complete deficiency of integrin subunits α_5, α_8, or β_1 produces perinatal or peri-implantation lethality [57], but can also produce specific alterations of CNS integrity [58–60]. An integrin β_1 knock-in displays defective neuroepithelial cell migration, and is lethal in the embryonic stages [60, 61]. Defects in the survival of neural crest cells and of neurons are associated with the deficiency of subunits α_5 and α_8, respectively [58, 59]. Mice deficient in integrin subunit α_{6A} are viable, but display defective lamination of the cortical layers [62]. Of interest to cerebral vascular integrity is the phenotype of subunit $\alpha_V^{(-/-)}$ preparations. While lethal in the perinatal period, deficient expression of subunit α_V can also cause intracerebral hemorrhage in mice [63]. These integrin subunits are evidently critical for CNS development, cerebrovascular integrity, and the architecture of the neuropil. It seems likely that subunits β_1 and α_V play roles in many aspects of cerebral tissue viability.

Modulation of integrin expression in the CNS

Regulation of integrin expression within the adult CNS is poorly understood. However, modulation of microvascular and intravascular cell expression occurs in the setting of focal cerebral ischemia and chronic inflammation.

Figure 1

Relative distribution of integrin subunits expressed on microvessels of normal non-human primate (Papio anubis/cynocephalus) brain. Upper panel: α-subunits. Lower panel: β-subunits. Microvessel diameters as given in upper legend are valid for both figures [1].

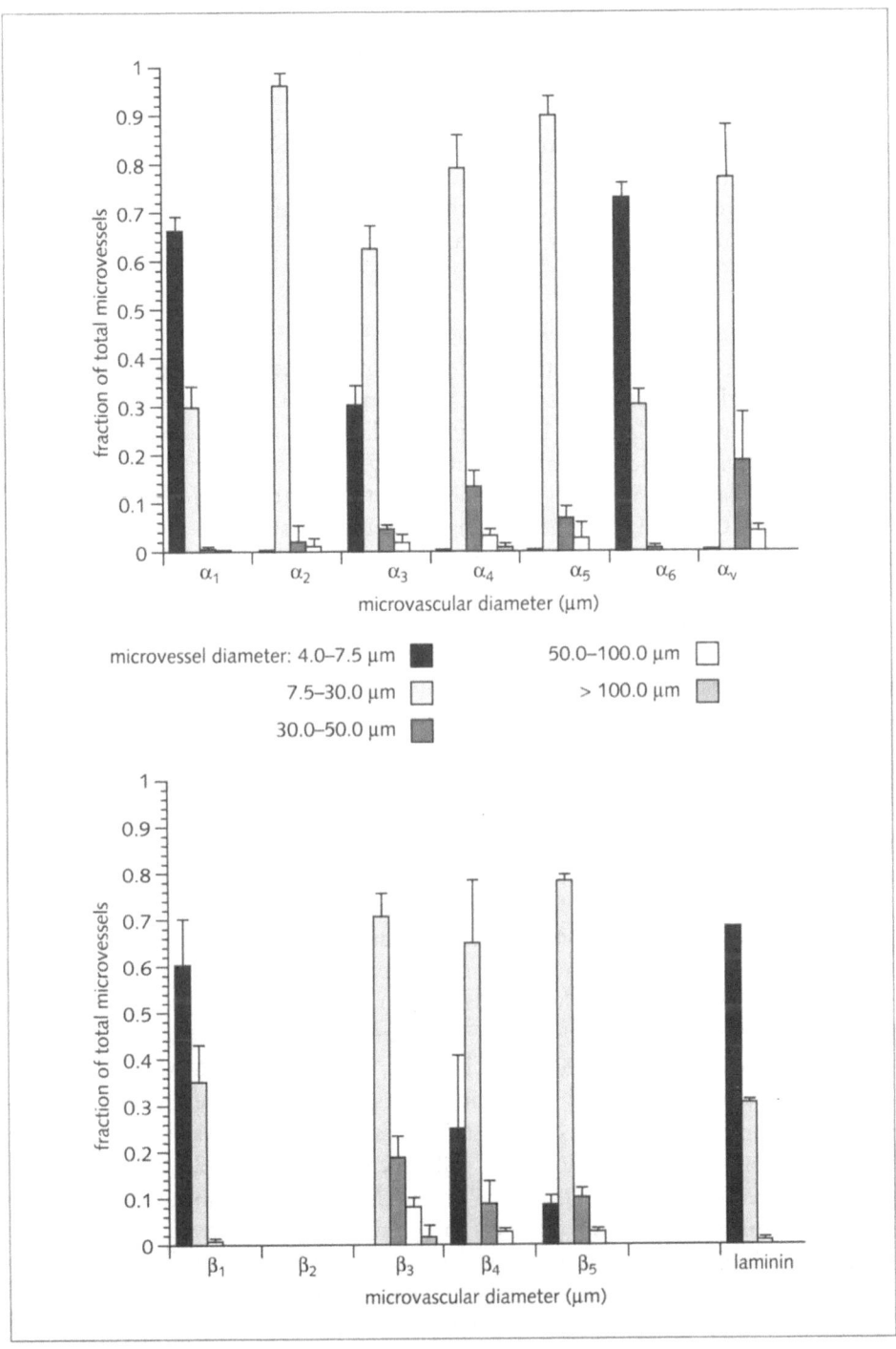

Focal cerebral ischemia

Neuron injury with loss of neurological function accompanies obstruction of a brain-supplying artery. Equally rapid responses are evident in the downstream microvasculature which affect both matrix and structural integrin expression [9, 64, 65]. These events are only partially elucidated, but indicate a temporally and topographically coordinated set of processes that involve integrin receptor biology. Their responses indicate the sensitivity of select microvessels to an ischemic challenge.

Microvessel basal lamina

During focal cerebral ischemia, the antigenicity of selected matrix ligands to vascular integrins within the microvascular basal lamina is lost. ECM components of the basal lamina, including laminin-1, laminin-5, collagen IV, and fibronectin, disappear together following experimental MCA:O [6, 7, 9]. The intermediate filaments laminin-1 and laminin-5, which codistribute in the basal lamina, display identical responses to MCA:O [6, 9]. These changes are most associated with hemorrhagic transformation within the regions of the most severe neuron injury, and are detectable as early as 2 h after MCA:O in experimental preparations [9].

The disappearance of matrix proteins may be due to proteolysis, blockade of transcription, inhibition of translation, or a combination of these. Remodelling of the microvessel basal lamina occurs when secreted proteases including metalloproteinases (MMPs) and plasminogen activators (PAs), which are associated with the cerebral microvasculature, degrade laminin, collagen, or fibronectin [66, 67]. Metalloproteinases are Zn^{2+} endopeptidases which are secreted in a proenzyme form. More than 20 distinct members of the matrixin family have been identified [68]. All members of this family share common structural domains which include a (NH_2-terminal) signal peptide, a pro-domain, a Zn^{2+} containing catalytic site, and one or more (COOH-terminal) hemapexin-like domains. Secreted in latent form as proenzymes, pro-MMP-2 and pro-MMP-9 are activated to their respective 72 kDa and 92 kDa enzymes by separate mechanisms. Latent MMP-2 is activated on cellular membrane surfaces by MT1-MMP (MMP-14) or MT3-MMP (MMP-16), while latent MMP-9 is activated by plasmin (generated by PAs), select serine proteases, and specific MMPs including MMP-1, MMP-2, MMP-3, AND MMP-8 [68].

Latent MMP-2 is expressed in constitutive fashion by a number of cell types, and its active form participates in cellular responses including adhesion, proliferation, and migration. Vascular endothelial cells secrete pro-MMP-2, contributing to detectable levels in plasma. Pro-MMP-2 and MMP-9 are associated with PMN leukocytes, macrophages, and platelets in the circulation. Non-vascular parenchymal cells of the CNS also have the capacity to generate MMPs [69–74]. Activities of MMP-2 and MMP-9 are modulated by the specific inhibitors TIMP-2 and TIMP-1, respectively, which are themselves under regulation [75]. Latent MMP-2 and MMP-

2 have homologous binding sites for TIMP-2. MMP-2, in addition, exposes the Zn^{2+}-containing active site which offers a second binding site for inhibition by TIMP. How the latent MMPs, their activators, and their active products participate in the CNS, is not understood. But activated serine proteases generated during ischemia may augment the effects of active MMPs. In one example, thrombin stimulates MMP-2 and MMP-9 secretion by vascular smooth muscle cells [76, 77]. Also, PMN leukocyte granule enzymes, including collagenase (MMP-8), gelatinase A (MMP-2), gelatinase B (MMP-9), elastase, and cathepsin G are released during the cellular inflammatory phase following ischemia, and degrade laminins and collagens [66, 78–83]. Endothelial cells and astrocytes, microglia, and oligodendrocytes appear to express MMPs under specific conditions of culture [69–74]. Synthesis of plasminogen activators (e.g., urokinase (u-PA)) has also been attributed to a number of cell-types within the CNS, including endothelial cells, neurons, astrocytes, and microglia *in vivo* or *in vitro* [84–87]. The reactions of these cell-types to ischemia within the CNS, their ability to generate MMPs or PAs, potential effects on microvascular matrix, and their impact on neuron integrity are under study.

Pro-MMP-2 activity is constitutively generated in uninjured basal ganglia and cortical tissues in non-human primates and rodents [88, 89] (Tab. 2). Anthony et al. reported the marked expression of latent MMP-9 by PMN leukocytes in human brain within 1 week of stroke, and MMP-2 from macrophages thereafter [82]. In anesthetized Wistar-Kyoto and spontaneously hypertensive (SHR) rats, Rosenberg et al. showed that pro-MMP-9 increases by 12–24 h and MMP-2 by 5 days after MCA:O [90]. Similar findings also have been noted by others [91–93]. In general, they suggest that in rodents subject to MCA:O, increased pro-MMP-9 expression precedes that of pro-MMP-2. By contrast, in the ischemic basal ganglia of the nonhuman primate, a significant rapid increase in the expression of the latent form of MMP-2 occurs 1–2 h after MCA:O, which correlates significantly with the size of the ischemic core (Ic) region [94]. Those findings suggest that MMP-2 secretion may be directly related to early neuron injury. Furthermore, evidence of coexpression of the activators of latent MMP-2 has been obtained. Hence, MMP-2 can be synthesized *de novo* by microvascular cells in direct association with neuron injury, in the same time and location as the loss of microvascular matrix and integrin receptor expression.

Pro-MMP-9 activity is significantly increased in the ischemic regions of those primate subjects displaying hemorrhagic transformation, but is not related to neuron injury. Whether the latent MMP-9 activity is causal or is a product of blood cellular activation within the hemorrhage is unknown. Hence, a clear dichotomy between the expressions of pro-MMP-2 and pro-MMP-9 is seen following MCA:O in the primate, which is differentially related to neuron injury.

Resident nonvascular cells of the CNS appear to express t-PA, u-PA, or PAI-1. t-PA and u-PA have been reported to be secreted by endothelial cells, neurons, astrocytes, and microglia *in vivo* or *in vitro* [67, 84, 85, 87, 95–99]. Expression of PA activity has been reported in nonischemic cerebral tissues of the mouse, sponta-

Table 2 - Responses of matrix metalloproteinases and plasminogen activators to focal cerebral ischema

Authors	Refs.	Species	Ischemia	Assay	MMP-2	MMP-9	TIMP-1
Rosenberg	[89]	SHR	MCA:O	Z	↑ 120 h	↑ 12–120 h	
Anthony	[82]	human	stroke	IH	↑ > 7 days	↑ < 7 days	
Clark	[92]	human	stroke	Z	↑ 4–84 months	↑ 48–96 h	
Romanic	[134]	SHR	MCA:O	Z, IH	↑ >120 h	↑ 6–120 h	?
Heo	[94]	primate	MCA:O/R	Z	↑ 1–2 h	hemorrhage	
Fujimura	[93]	m	MCA:O/R	Z, Z(r)	↑ 23 h	↑ 1–23 h	?
Gasche	[91]	m	MCA:O	Z, Z(r)	↑ 4–24 h	↑ 2–24 h	?

Authors	Refs.	Species	Ischemia	Assay	u-PA	t-PA	PAI-1
Rosenberg	[90]	SHR	MCA:O	Z	↑ 12–240 h	↓ 12–24 h	
Wang	[104]	m	MCA:O/R	ZIS		↑ 24 h	
Ahn	[115]	m	MCA:O	Z	↑ 4–24 h	~	
Zhang	[117]	Wistar	MCA:O	IH, ISH			↑ 4 h
Docagne	[135]	m	MCA:O	RT PCR		~	↑ 24–72 h
Hosomi	[118]	primate	MCA:O	Z, ELISA	↑ 1–2 h	no change	↑ 1–2 h

IH, immunohistochemistry; ISH, in situ hybridization; RT-PCR, reverse transcriptase-PCR; Z, zymography; ZIS, in situ zymography; Z(r), reverse zymography; ELISA, enzyme-linked immunosorbent assay neously hypertensive rat (SHR), and non-human primate [67, 100, 101]. u-PA mRNA is expressed in neurons and oligodendrocytes during process outgrowth in rodent brain [102]. t-PA is expressed by neurons in many brain regions, but extracellular proteolysis seems confined to specific discrete brain regions [103]. Recent studies suggesting that t-PA can mediate hippocampal neurodegeneration during excitotoxicity or following focal cerebral ischemia have opened a discussion that PAs may play roles in cellular viability outside the endogenous (vascular) fibrinolytic system [104]. However, conflicting evidence of increasing injury by t-PA has been balanced against credible reports of no effect or reduction in infarct volume in rodent focal cerebral ischemia models. The potential roles of PAs in the CNS have not yet been clarified by murine knockout preparations. For instance, plasminogen$^{(-/-)}$ constructs subject to MCA:O display larger regions of injury than (strain-specific) wild-type, while t-PA$^{(-/-)}$ constructs have smaller injury regions [105].

Plasmin is capable of degrading selected matrix proteins of the basal lamina, elastin, and myelin basic protein (MBP) either directly or through the activation of latent MMPs [106–110]. In normal cerebral tissue, t-PA is associated with medium sized microvessels of the size of the *vasa vasorum* [67]. The roles of PAs in altering matrix integrity in response to focal cerebral ischemia also have not yet been clearly defined [99, 103, 111], but they may facilitate degradation of basal lamina *via* several paths. Plasmin and u-PA, but not t-PA, can activate latent MMP-1, MMP-3, and MMP-9, or in the case of pro-MMP-2 through the proteolytic activation of MT1-MMP [106, 110, 112–114]. Similarly, other serine proteases can also activate latent MMP-9.

Recently reported studies have focused on the responses of PAs within the CNS to focal ischemia in rodents (Tab. 2). Rosenberg et al. first described increased u-PA-like proteinase activity and decreased t-PA-like proteinase activity by 12–24 h after permanent MCA:O in anesthetized Wistar-Kyoto rats and SHRs [90]. Ahn et al. reported an increase in u-PA-like proteinase activity, but no change in t-PA-like proteinase activity in unperfused cerebral tissues following MCA:O in C57BL/6J mice [115]. Pfefferkorn et al. also observed an increase in PA activity within the caudate putamen by 9 h following MCA:O in Wistar rats, although the exact PA was not defined [116]. In contrast, Wang et al. suggested that increases in t-PA-like proteinase activity following MCA:O contribute to neurodegeneration within the ischemic zone [104], while in separate experiments neuron injury in the hippocampus was thought to be laminin-dependent [99, 111]. t-PA, but not u-PA, has been assigned a role in neuron injury within the murine hippocampus [99, 104]. In short, no consensus about the response of t-PA in brain tissue among these species to MCA:O has appeared. PAI-1 antigen was reported to be increased after 4 h following MCA:O in Wistar rats [117]. However, no relation of PAI-1 with u-PA and t-PA activity in cerebral ischemia has been reported.

By contrast, in the primate ischemic basal ganglia a rapid persistent increase in gelatin-proteolytic activity was due mainly to significantly increased u-PA in the Ic regions followed MCA:O [118]. A transient decrease in t-PA activity 2 h after MCA:O coincided with a significant persistent increase in PAI-1 antigen, producing an increase in t-PA·PAI-1 complex, although total t-PA antigen was unchanged. PAI-1 content within the plasma increased in the same time frame. The increase in u-PA within the ischemic basal ganglia coincided with pro-MMP-2 generation, but was not directly related to neuron injury.

Microvessel integrin expression

The responses of endothelial cell and astrocyte integrin expression to ischemia also have a highly significant temporal and topographical relationship to neuron injury [8, 9]. There is a rapid and significant loss of integrins $\alpha_1\beta_1$ and $\alpha_3\beta_1$ from microvascular endothelium as early as 2 h following MCA:O in the ischemic region (Fig. 2) ([8] and unpublished). This is accompanied by a comparable and highly significant abrupt loss of subunit β_1 from astrocyte fibres in the same time frame [8]. The decreased expression of integrin subunit β_1 antigen parallels blockade of β_1 transcription, which also is evident by 2 h MCA:O [8]. Ischemia also alters the close relationship between the astrocyte end-feet and the basal lamina endothelium [9]. In the Ic region, the number of microvessels expressing integrin $\alpha_6\beta_4$ on astrocyte end-feet falls rapidly by 2 h MCA:O, exceeding the decrease in expression of the ligand laminin-5 (Figs. 2 and 3). Integrins $\alpha_1\beta_1$ and $\alpha_6\beta_4$ are, then, equally sensitive to ischemia. The changes in integrin expression are graded with respect to the degree of neuron injury, being most pronounced in the regions of severe ischemic neuron damage, and much less notable at a distance from the core [119]. These changes in integrin expression affect both capillaries and larger cerebral microvessels.

Integrin expression may be altered in microvessels presenting with evidence of cellular activation. Within 2 h following MCA:O, select microvessels predominantly within the Ic region express the integrin $\alpha_V\beta_3$ [120]. Integrin $\alpha_V\beta_3$ is a receptor for multiple ligands including (fibrin)ogen, fibronectin, vitronection, osteopontin, and von Willebrand factor, and participates in angiogenesis and vascular remodeling. Given identified roles of integrin $\alpha_V\beta_3$ in vascular remodelling, which can occur in preparation for new vessel formation, a putative role for integrin $\alpha_V\beta_3$ expression in vascular responses was expected [120]. Predominantly in the Ic region, VEGF and integrin $\alpha_V\beta_3$ were highly significantly co-expressed in microvessels displaying activation antigen PCNA beginning 1 h following MCA:O [120]. The co-appearance of these antigens was seen predominantly on non-capillary microvessels resembling precapillary arterioles (7.5–30.0 µm diameter), where the primary immunoreactivity was associated with the smooth muscle. These events coincided with evidence of neuron injury and, while spatially codistributed, were independent of time. These findings further support the very rapid activation and integrin responses of microvessels following MCA:O.

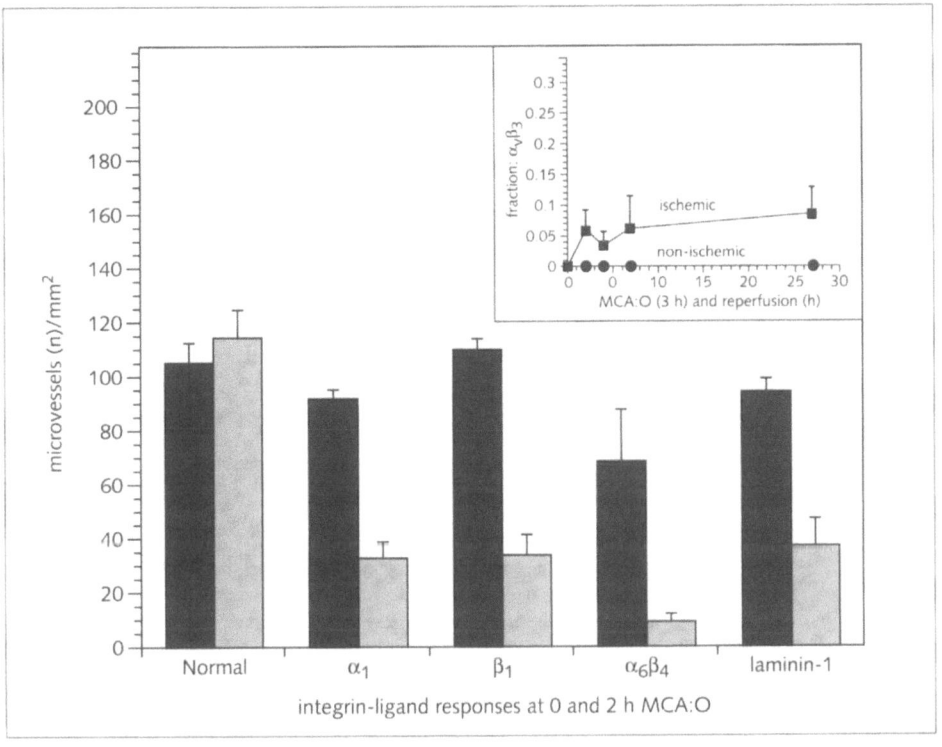

Figure 2
Microvessel integrin and ligand responses to middle cerebral artery occlusion (MCA:O) at 2 h compared to baseline in the basal ganglia.

Expression of integrin $\alpha_V\beta_3$ also occurs in proximity to several of its ligands following MCA:O. Okada et al. reported the highly significant association of arteriolar integrin $\alpha_V\beta_3$ upregulation with intra-luminal fibrin deposition at all timepoints following MCA:O in the non-human primate [65]. Microvascular integrin $\alpha_V\beta_5$ was not altered under the same conditions. Osteopontin was observed in the region of glial activation at some distance from the integrin $\alpha_V\beta_3$ upregulation late following MCA:O in the rat [30]. The relationships of the ligand expression to integrin $\alpha_V\beta_3$ upregulation are unclear; however, the link between VEGF and integrin $\alpha_V\beta_3$ expression and the appearance of intravascular fibrin suggests significant alterations in arteriolar integrity (e.g., permeability) or endothelial cell activation which could promote thrombosis [65, 120, 121].

VEGF transcripts also appeared on cells with the morphology of PMN leukocytes which had penetrated the wall of select microvessels in the Ic region within 2 h following MCA:O [120]. VEGF can be expressed by activated leukocytes, presum-

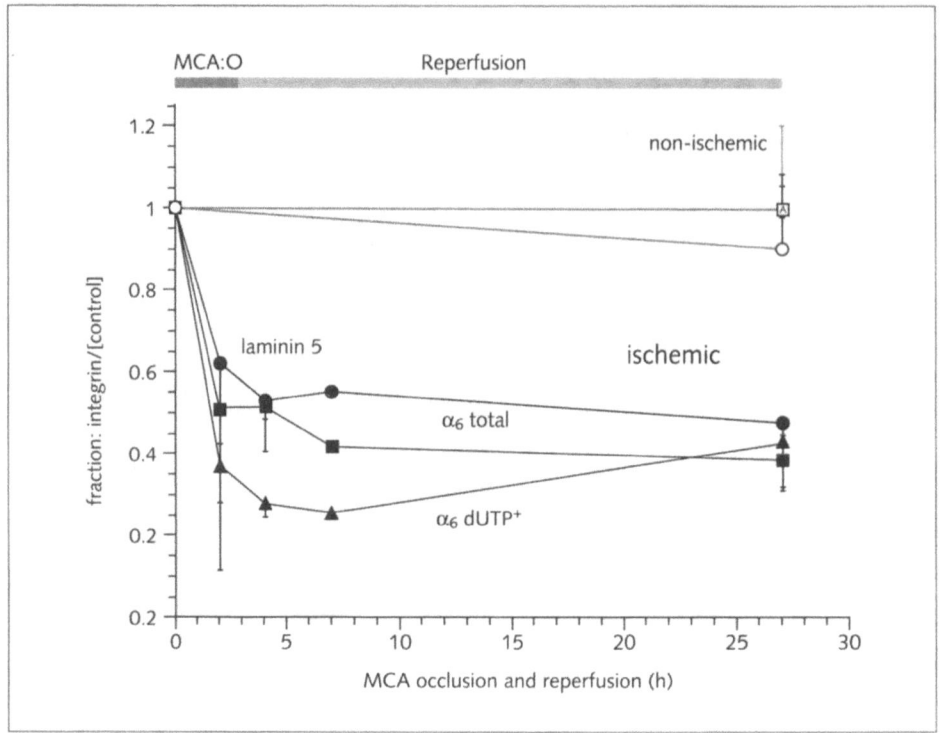

Figure 3
Response of microvessel integrin $\alpha_6\beta_4$ expression following MCA:O in the non-human primate basal ganglia [9].

ably as participants in the inflammatory process [122–124]. To what degree they contribute to the VEGF antigen observed in the microvascular wall during ischemia is unknown. It is certain that, like the expression of integrins, these events coincide with early evidence of neuron injury.

Intravascular integrin-matrix interactions

Early following MCA:O PMN leukocytes, platelets, and fibrin deposit in the microvasculature within [2, 3, 10], or adjacent to [125], the evolving ischemic region(s). These circulating elements contribute to the microvascular "no-reflow" phenomenon associated with focal cerebral ischemia [5, 18, 19]. Strategies which block the leukocyte β_2-integrin can significantly increase cerebral microvessel patency [18], and apparently reduce infarct volume [20] in separate model systems. Recently, direct inhibition of the platelet receptor $\alpha_{IIb}\beta_3$ has been shown to increase microvascular patency, but is associated with a dose-dependent increase in significant hemorrhage in the non-human primate [5]. In separate experiments in a murine MCA:O model, inhibition of platelet $\alpha_{IIb}\beta_3$ was associated with a decrease in apparent infarct volume, but an increase in complicating hemorrhage with dose [126]. While these experimental efforts indicate the potential that specific integrin receptor blockade can alter microvascular patency and perhaps injury volume, unrelated strategies against the leukocyte integrin subunit β_2 and the vascular integrin subunit β_3 so far have been problematic in ischemic stroke [127]. The limited clinical experience with integrin inhibitors supports the broader view that circulating cells participate in the ischemic lesion, and, further, that discrete experimental work is required for well-conceived clinical tests.

Demyelinating disorders

Expression of integrin receptors is also modulated under conditions of chronic inflammation, including experimental autoimmune encephalitis (EAE). The development of the EAE lesions probably involves vascular reactivities similar to acute inflammation, and is likely to cause alterations in receptor expressions similar to other forms of chronic inflammation of the CNS (e.g., neoplasia). In immune-mediated inflammatory/demyelinating disease of the CNS, expression of subunits α_V and β_4 is increased on astrocytes [128]. Subunit β_4 expression also appears to be increased on astrocytes within malignant astrocytomas, suggesting a common response of astrocytes to inflammatory conditions [129]. Expression of integrin α_2 is increased on oligodendrocytes in experimental demyelinated lesions, which can be modulated by TNFα [128]. In active lesions select integrin expression is also decreased on endothelial cells (e.g., β_1 or β_4 integrins [129, 130]).

In the development of chronic inflammatory lesions leukocyte integrin receptor expression and adhesion are also altered. For the acute cellular inflammatory response, adhesion of leukocytes to the endothelial cell counter-receptors involves the expression of PSGL-1 and β_2-integrins on PMN leukocytes [131, 132]. In murine EAE, adhesion of lymphocytes to the vascular endothelium is mediated by α_4 integrins (e.g., β_1 and β_7) [133]. This mechanism does not appear to operate in malignant lesions of the CNS [130], but is common to other lymphocyte adhesive interactions where the endothelial cell receptor VCAM-1 is required [27].

Conclusions

Integrin expression by microvascular cells, glial cells, and neurons has been variously described in the intact CNS and in cell culture, and can be altered during ischemia and inflammatory processes. Rapidly following MCA:O, alterations in the expression of integrin-matrix constituents occur which include integrin receptors on endothelial cells and astrocyte end-feet, and the loss of their matrix ligands. These coincide exactly with clear evidence of neuron injury. In addition, select MMPs are generated in the ischemic zone acutely from microvascular and parenchymal cells. In parallel, u-PA and PAI-1, but not t-PA, appear in the ischemic core within 1–2 h following MCA:O. The stimuli for the alterations in matrix and integrin expression are unknown and their mechanisms uncertain, although protease digestion is likely. The demonstration that leukocytes and platelets (through their respective integrin receptors) interact with select microvessels and appear to generate VEGF transcripts as early as 1–2 h following MCA:O indicates that microvascular and leukocyte activation are overlapping events coincident with neuron injury. The appearance of integrin antigens (e.g., integrin $\alpha_V\beta_3$) in the face of increased endothelial cell PMN leukocyte adhesion receptor expression indicates (i) the viability of microvascular endothelial cells during ischemia, (ii) the rapid responsiveness to injury of endothelial cells in proximity to injured neurons, and (iii) their active participation in the transition from ischemia to the cellular inflammatory phase of brain infarction. The coincidence in time and distribution of the rapid down-regulation of both microvascular and astrocyte integrins, and the appearance of neuron injury following MCA:O underscores, but does not prove, a potential interaction of the two cell types in the setting of ischemia. The situation with integrin expression during the development of demyelinating lesions of the CNS is likely to be complex, and serves also to focus attention on the relation of early microvascular and neuronal events.

Acknowledgement

The work described in this manuscript is supported in part by grants RO1 NS 26945 and NS 38710 of the National Institutes of Neurological Disorders and Stroke. This is manuscript 13861-MEM of The Scripps Research Institute.

References

1   Haring H-P, Akamine P, Habermann R, Koziol JA, del Zoppo GJ (1996) Distribution of the integrin-like immunoreactivity on primate brain microvasculature. *J Neuropathol Exp Neurol* 55: 236–245

2   del Zoppo GJ, Copeland BR, Harker LA, Waltz TA, Zyroff J, Hanson SR, Battenberg E (1986) Experimental acute thrombotic stroke in baboons. *Stroke* 17: 1254–1265

3   Okada Y, Copeland BR, Mori E, Tung M-M, Thomas WS, del Zoppo GJ (1994) P-selectin and intercellular adhesion molecule-1 expression after focal brain ischemia and reperfusion. *Stroke* 25: 202–211

4   Haring H-P, Berg EL, Tsurushita N, Tagaya M, del Zoppo GJ (1996) E-selectin appears in non-ischemic tissue during experimental focal cerebral ischemia. *Stroke* 27: 1386–1392

5   Abumiya T, Fitridge R, Mazur C, Copeland BR, Koziol JA, Tschopp JF, del Zoppo GJ (2000) An integrin $\alpha_{IIb}\beta_3$ inhibitor preserves microvascular patency in experimental acute focal cerebral ischemia. *Stroke* 31: 1402–1410

6   Hamann GF, Okada Y, Fitridge R, del Zoppo GJ (1995) Microvascular basal lamina antigens disappear during cerebral ischemia and reperfusion. *Stroke* 26: 2120–2126

7   Hamann GF, Okada Y, del Zoppo GJ (1996) Hemorrhagic transformation and microvascular integrity during focal cerebral ischemia/reperfusion. *J Cereb Blood Flow Metab* 16: 1373–1378

8   del Zoppo GJ, Haring H-P, Tagaya M, Wagner S, Akamine P, Hamann GF (1996) Loss of $\alpha_1\beta_1$ integrin immunoreactivity on cerebral microvessels and astrocytes following focal cerebral ischemia/reperfusion. *Cerebrovasc Dis* 6:9 (Abstract)

9   Wagner S, Tagaya M, Koziol JA, Quaranta V, del Zoppo GJ (1997) Rapid disruption of an astrocyte interaction with the extracellular matrix mediated by integrin $\alpha_6\beta_4$ during focal cerebral ischemia/reperfusion. *Stroke* 28: 858–865

10 del Zoppo GJ, Schmid-Schönbein GW, Mori E, Copeland BR, Chang C-M (1991) Polymorphonuclear leukocytes occlude capillaries following middle cerebral artery occlusion and reperfusion in baboons. *Stroke* 22: 1276–1284

11 Garcia JH, Mitchem HL, Briggs L, Morawetz R, Hudetz AG, Hazelrig JB, Halsey JH Jr, Conger KA (1983) Transient focal ischemia in subhuman primates: Neuronal injury as a function of local cerebral blood flow. *J Neuropathol Exp Neurol* 42: 44–60

12 Ruoslahti E (1991) Integrins. *J Clin Invest* 87: 1–5

13 Luscinskas FW, Lawler J (1994) Integrins as dynamic regulators of vascular function. *FASEB J* 8: 929–938

14 Albelda SM, Buck CA (1990) Integrins and other cell adhesion molecules. *FASEB J* 4: 2868–2880

15 Little JR, Kerr FWL, Sundt TM Jr (1975) Microcirculatory obstruction in focal cerebral ischemia. Relationship to neuronal alterations. *Mayo Clin Proc* 50: 264–270

16 Little JR, Kerr FWL, Sundt TM Jr (1976) Microcirculatory obstruction in focal cerebral ischemia: An electron microscopic investigation in monkeys. *Stroke* 7: 25–30

17 Little JR, Cook A, Cook SA, MacIntyre WJ (1981) Microcirculatory obstruction in focal cerebral ischemia: Albumen and erythrocyte transit. *Stroke* 12: 218–223

18 Mori E, Chambers JD, Copeland BR, Arfors K-E, del Zoppo GJ (1992) Inhibition of polymorphonuclear leukocyte adherence suppresses no-reflow after focal cerebral ischemia. *Stroke* 23: 712–718

19 Thomas WS, Mori E, Copeland BR, Yu J-Q, Morrissey JH, del Zoppo GJ (1993) Tissue factor contributes to microvascular defects following cerebral ischemia. *Stroke* 24: 847–853

20 del Zoppo GJ (1994) Microvascular changes during cerebral ischaemia and reperfusion. *Cerebrovasc Brain Metab Rev* 6: 47–96

21 Lee SJ, Benveniste EN (1999) Adhesion molecule expression and regulation on cells of the central nervous system. *J Neuroimaging* 98: 77–88

22 Archelos JJ, Previtali SC, Hartung HP (1999) The role of integrins in immune-mediated diseases of the nervous system. *Trends Neurosci* 22: 30–38

23 Peters A, Palay BL, Webster HD (1991) *The fine structure of the nervous system. Neurons and their supporting cells.* Oxford University Press, New York

24 Carlson SS, Hockfield S (1996) Central nervous system. In: WD Comper (ed): *Extracellular matrix,* volume 1. Harwood Academic Publishers, Melbourne, 1–23

25 Wright SD, Detmers PA (1988) Adherence promoting receptors on phagocytes. *J Cell Sci* (Suppl) 9: 99–120

26 Springer TA (1990) Adhesion receptors of the immune system. *Nature* 346: 425–433

27 Springer TA (1995) Traffic signals on endothelium for lymphocyte recirculation and leukocyte emigration. *Annu Rev Physiol* 57: 827–872

28 Plow EF, Ginsberg MH (1988) Cellular adhesion: GPIIb/IIIa as a prototype adhesion receptor. *Prog Hemost Thromb* 8: 117–156

29 Plow EF, Pierschbacher MD, Ruoslahti E, Marguerie GA, Ginsberg MH (1985) The effect of Arg-Gly-Asp-containing peptides on fibrinogen and von Willebrand factor binding to platelets. *Proc Natl Acad Sci USA* 82: 8057–8061

30 Shattil SJ (1999) Signaling through platelet integrin $\alpha_{IIb}\beta_3$: Inside-out, outside-in, and sideways. *Thromb Haemost* 82: 318–325

31 Yurchenko PD, Schittny JC (1986) Molecular architecture of basement membranes. *J Biol Chem* 261: 1577–1590

32 Bernstein JJ, Getz R, Jefferson M, Kelemen M (1985) Astrocytes secrete basal lamina after hemisection of rat spinal cord. *Brain Res* 327: 135–141

33 Kusaka H, Hirano A, Bornstein MB, Raine CS (1985) Basal lamina formation by astrocytes in organotypic cultures of mouse spinal cord tissue. *J Neuropathol Exp Neurol* 44: 295–303

34 Tagami M, Yamagata K, Fujino H, Kubota A, Nara Y, Yamori Y (1992) Morphological differentiation of endothelial cells co-cultured with astrocytes on type-I or type-IV collagen. *Cell Tissue Res* 268: 225–232

35 Webersinke G, Bauer H, Amberger A, Zach O, Bauer HC (1992) Comparison of gene expression of extracellular matrix molecules in brain microvascular endothelial cells and astrocytes. *Biochem Biophys Res Commun* 189: 877–884

36 Ard MD, Faissner A (1991) Components of astrocytic extracellular matrix are regulated by contact with axons. *Ann NY Acad Sci* 633: 566–569

37 Kozlova M, Kentroti S, Vernadakis A (1993) Influence of culture substrata on the differentiation of advanced passage glial cells in cultures from aged mouse cerebral hemispheres. *Int J Dev Neurosci* 11: 513–519

38 Nagano N, Aoyagi M, Hirakawa K (1993) Extracellular matrix modulates the proliferation of rat astrocytes in serum-free culture. *GLIA* 8: 71–76

39 Janzer RC, Raff MC (1987) Astrocytes induce blood-brain barrier properties in endothelial cells (Letter). *Nature* 325: 353–355

40   Hurwitz AA, Berman JW, Rashbaum WK, Lyman WD (1993) Human fetal astrocytes induce the expression of blood-brain barrier specific proteins by autologous endothelial cells. *Brain Res* 625: 238–243

41   Minakawa T, Bready J, Berliner J, Fisher M, Cancilla PA (1991) *In vitro* interaction of astrocytes and pericyte with capillary-like structures of brain microvessel endothelium. *Lab Invest* 65: 32–40

42   Estrada C, Bready JV, Berliner JA, Pardridge WM, Cancilla PA (1990) Astrocyte growth stimulation by a soluble factor produced by cerebral endothelial cells *in vitro*. *J Neuropathol Exp Neurol* 49: 539–549

43   Pinkstaff JK, Detterich J, Lynch G, Gall C (1999) Integrin subunit gene expression is regionally differentiated in adult brain. *J Neurosci* 19: 1541–1556

44   Jacques TS, Relvas JB, Nishimura S, Pytela R, Edwards GM, Streuli CH, ffrench-Constant C (1998) Neural precursor cell chain migration and division are regulated through different beta1 integrins. *Development* 125: 3167–3177

45   Einheber S, Schnapp LM, Salzer JL, Cappiello ZB (1996) Regional and ultrastructural distribution of the α_8 integrin subunit in developing and adult rat brain suggests a role in synaptic function. *J Comp Neurol* 370: 105–134

46   Milner R, Huang X, Wu J, Nishimura S, Pytela R, Sheppard D, French-Constant C (1999) Distinct roles for astrocyte $\alpha_V\beta_5$ and $\alpha_V\beta_8$ integrins in adhesion and migration. *J Cell Sci* 112: 4271–4279

47   Milner R (1997) Understanding the molecular basis of cell migration; implications for cliical therapy in multiple sclerosis. *Clin Sci* 92: 113–122

48   Milner R, Edwards G, Streuli C, French-Constant C (1996) A role in migration for the $\alpha_V\beta_1$ integrin expressed on oligodendrocyte precursors. *J Neurosci* 16: 7240–7252

49   Nishimura SL, Boylen KP, Einheber S, Milner TA, Ramos DM, Pytela R (1998) Synaptic and glial localization of the integrin $\alpha_V\beta_8$ in mouse and rat brain. *Brain Res* 791: 271–282

50   Sebire G, Hery C, Peudenier S, Tardieu M (1993) Adhesion proteins on human microglial cells and modulation of their expression by IL1α and TNFα. *Res Virol* 144: 47–52

51   McGeer PL, Zhu SG, Dedhar S (1990) Immunostaining of human brain capillaries by antibodies to very late antigens. *J Neuroimmunol* 26: 213–218

52   Albelda SM (1992) Differential expression of integrin cell-substratum adhesion receptors on endothelium. In: R Steiner, PB Weisz, R Langer (eds): *Angiogenesis: key principles – science – technology – medicine*. Birkhäuser Verlag, Basel, Switzerland, 188–192

53   Paulus W, Baur I, Schuppan D, Roggendorf W (1993) Characterization of integrin receptors in normal and neoplastic human brain. *Am J Pathol* 143: 154–163

54   Grooms SY, Terracio L, Jones LS (1993) Anatomical localization of β_1 integrin-like immunoreactivity in rat brain. *Exp Neurol* 122: 253–259

55   Spinardi L, Ren Y-L, Sanders R, Giancotti FG (1993) The β_4 subunit cytoplasmic domain mediates the interaction of $\alpha_6\beta_4$ integrin with the cytoskeleton of hemidesmosomes. *Mol Biol Cell* 4: 871–884

56   Wegiel J, Wisniewski HM (1994) Rosenthal fibers, eosinophilic inclusions, and anchor-
     age densities with desmosome-like structures in astrocytes in Alzheimer's disease. *Acta
     Neuropathol (Berlin)* 87: 335–361

57   Hynes RO, Bader BL (1997) Targeted mutations in integrins and their ligands: Their
     implications for vascular biology. *Thromb Haemost* 78: 83–87

58   Yang JT, Rayburn H, Hynes RO (1993) Embryonic mesodermal defects in alpha 5 inte-
     grin-deficient mice. *Development* 119: 1093–1095

59   Muller U, Wang D, Denda S, Meneses JJ, Pedersen RA, Reichardt LF (1997) Integrin
     $\alpha_8\beta_1$ is critically important for epithelial-mesenchymal interactions during kideny mor-
     phogenesis. *Cell* 88: 603–613

60   Stephens LE, Sutherland AE, Klimanskaya IV, Andrieux A, Meneses J, Pedersen RA,
     Damsky CH (1995) Deletion of β_1 integrins in mice results in inner cell mass failure and
     peri-implantation lethality. *Genes Dev* 9: 1883–1895

61   Fassler R, Meyer M (1995) Consequences of lack of β_1 integrin gene expression in mice.
     Genes Dev 9: 1896–1908

62   Gimond C, Baudoin c, van der Neut R, Kramer D, Calafat J, Sonnenberg A (1998) Cre-
     loxP-mediated inactivation of the α_{6A} integrin splice variant *in vivo*: Evidence for a spe-
     cific functional role of α_{6A} in lymphocyte migration but not in heart development. *J Cell
     Biol* 143: 253–266

63   Bader BL, Rayburn H, Crowley D, Hynes RO (1998) Extensive vasculogenesis, angio-
     genesis, and organogenesis precede lethality in mice lacking all α_V integrins. *Cell* 95:
     507–519

64   Hamann GF, Okada Y, Fitridge R, del Zoppo GJ (1995) Microvascular basal lamina
     antigens disappear during cerebral ischemia and reperfusion. *Stroke* 26: 2120–2126

65   Okada Y, Copeland BR, Hamann GF, Koziol JA, Cheresh DR, del Zoppo GJ (1996)
     Integrin $\alpha_V\beta_3$ is expressed in selected microvessels following focal cerebral ischemia. *Am
     J Pathol* 149: 37–44

66   Krane SM (1994) Clinical importance of metalloproteinases and their inhibitors. Inhi-
     bition of matrix metalloproteinases: therapeutic potential. *Ann NY Acad Sci* 732: 1–10

67   Levin EG, del Zoppo GJ (1994) Localization of tissue plasminogen activator in the
     endothelium of a limited number of vessels. *Am J Pathol* 144: 855–861

68   Woessner JF Jr (1994) The family of matrix metalloproteinases. *Ann NY Acad Sci* 732:
     11–21

69   Pagenstecher A, Stalder AK, Kincaid CL, Shapiro SD, Campbell IL (1998) Differential
     expression of matrix metalloproteinase and tissue inhibitor of matrix metalloproteinase
     genes in the mouse central nervous system in normal and inflammatory states. *Am J
     Pathol* 152: 729–741

70   Uhm JH, Dooley NP, Oh LY, Yong VW (1998) Oligodendrocytes utilize a matrix met-
     alloproteinase, MMP-9, to extend processes along an astrocyte extracellular matrix.
     GLIA 22 (1): 53–63

71   Wells GM, Catlin G, Cossins JA, Mangan M, Ward GA, Miller KM, Clements JM
     (1996) Quantitation of matrix metalloproteinases in cultured rat astrocytes using the

polymearase chain reaction with a multi-competitor cDNA standard. *GLIA* 18 (4): 332–340

72 Cross AK, Woodroofe MN (1999) Chemokine modulation of matrix metalloproteinase and TIMP production in adult rat brain microglia and a human microglial cell line *in vitro*. *GLIA* 28 (3): 183–189

73 Gottschall PE, Deb S (1996) Regulation of matrix metalloproteinase expressions in astrocytes, microglia and neurons. *Neuroimmunomodulation* 3 (2–3): 69–75

74 Gottschall PE, Yu X, Bing B (1995) Increased production of gelatinase B (matrix metalloproteinase-9) and interleukin-6 by activated rat microglia in culture. *J Neurosci Res* 42 (3): 335–342

75 Bode IO, Fernandez-Catalan C, Grans F, Gomis-Rüth F-X, Nagase H, Tschesche H, Maskos K, Greenwold RA, Zucker S, Golub LM (1999) Insight into MMP-TIMP interactions in inhibition of matrix metalloproteinases. *Ann NY Acad Sci* 878: 73–91

76 Fabunmi RP, Baker AH, Murray EJ, Booth RFG, Newby AC (1996) Divergent regulation by growth factors and cytokines of 95 kDa and 72 kDa gelatinases and tissue inhibitors of metalloproteinases-1, -2, and -3 in rabbit aortic smooth muscle cells. *Biochem J* 315: 335–342

77 Galis ZS, Kranzhöfer R, Fenton JWII, Libby P (1997) Thrombin promotes activation of matrix metalloproteinase-2 produced by cultured vascular smooth muscle cells. *Arterioscler Thromb Vasc Biol* 17: 483–489

78 Murphy G, Reynolds JJ, Bretz U, Baggiolini M (1987) Collagenase is a component of the specific granules of human neutrophil leukocytes. *Biochem J* 162: 195–197

79 Watanabe H, Hattori S, Katsuda S, Nakanishi I, Nagai Y (1990) Human neutrophil elastase: Degradation of basement membrane components and immunolocalization in the tissue. *J Biochem* 108: 753–759

80 Heck LW, Blackburn WD, Irwin MH, Abrahamson DR (1990) Degradation of basement membrane laminin by human neutrophil elastase and cathepsin G. *Am J Pathol* 136: 1267–1274

81 Pike MC, Wicha MS, Yoon P, Mayo L, Boxer LA (1989) Laminin promotes the oxidative burst in human neutrophils via increased chemoattractant receptor expression. *J Immunol* 142: 2004–2011

82 Anthony DC, Ferguson B, Matyzak MK, Miller KM, Esiri MM, Perry VH (1997) Differential matrix metalloproteinase expression in cases of multiple sclerosis and stroke. *Neuropathol Appl Neurobiol* 23: 406–415

83 Hibbs MS, Hasty KA, Seyer JM, Kang AH, Mainardi CL (1985) Biochemical and immunological characterization of the secreted forms of human neutrophil gelatinase. *J Biol Chem* 260: 2493–2500

84 Masos T, Miskin R (1996) Localization of urokinase-type plasminogen activator mRNA in the adult mouse brain. *Brain Res Mol Brain Res* 35: 139–148

85 Tranque P, Naftolin F, Robbins R (1994) Differential regulation of astrocyte plasminogen activators by insulin-like growth factor-I and epidermal growth factor. *Endocrinology* 134: 2606–2613

86 van Hinsbergh VW, van den Berg EA, Fiers W, Dooijewaard G (1990) Tumor necrosis factor induces the production of urokinase-type plasminogen activator by human endothelial cells. *Blood* 75: 1991–1998

87 Nakajima K, Tsuzaki N, Shimojo M, Hamanoue M, Kohsaka S (1992) Microglia isolated from rat brain secrete a urokinase-type plasminogen activator. *Brain Res* 577: 285–292

88 Unemori E, Ferrara N, Bauer E, Amento E (1992) Vascular endothelial growth factor induces interstitial collagenase expression in human endothelial cells. *J Cell Physiol* 153: 557–562

89 Rosenberg GA, Dencoff JE, McGuire PG, Liotta LA, Stetler-Stevenson WG (1994) Injury-induced 92-kilodalton gelatinase and urokinase expression in rat brain. *Lab Invest* 71: 417–422

90 Rosenberg GA, Navratil M, Barone F, Feuerstein G (1996) Proteolytic cascade enzymes increase in focal cerebral ischemia in rat. *J Cereb Blood Flow Metab* 16: 360–366

91 Gashe Y, Fujimura M, Morita-Fujimura Y, Copin J-C, Kawase M, Massengale J, Chan PH (1999) Early appearance of activated matrix metalloproteinase-9 after focal cerebral ischemia in mice: a possible role in blood-brain barrier dysfunction. *J Cereb Blood Flow Metab* 19: 1020–1028

92 Clark AW, Krekoski CA, Bou SS, Chapman KR, Edwards DR (1997) Increased gelatinase A (MMP-2) and gelatinase B (MMP-9) activities in human brain after focal ischemia. *Neurosci Lett* 238: 53–56

93 Fujimura M, Gasche Y, Morita-Fujimura Y, Massengale J, Kawase M, Chan PH (1999) Early appearance of activated matrix metalloproteinase-9 and blood-brain barrier disruption in mice after focal cerebral ischemia and reperfusion. *Brain Res* 842: 92–100

94 Heo JH, Lucero J, Abumiya T, Koziol JA, Copeland BR, del Zoppo GJ (1999) Matrix metalloproteinases increase very early during experimental focal cerebral ischemia. *J Cereb Blood Flow Metab* 19: 624–633

95 Krystosek A, Seeds NW (1986) Normal and malignant cells, including neurons, deposit plasminogen activator on growth substrata. *Exp Cell Res* 166: 31–46

96 Pittman RN (1985) Release of plasminogen activator and a calcium-dependent metalloprotease from cultured sympathetic and sensory neurons. *Dev Biol* 110: 91–101

97 Vincent VA, Lowik CW, Verheijen JH, de Bart AC, Tilders FJ, Van Dam AM (1998) Role of astrocyte-derived tissue-type plasminogen activator in the regulation of endotoxin-stimulated nitric oxide production by microglial cells. *GLIA* 22: 130–137

98 Toshniwal PK, Firestone SL, Barlow GH, Tiku ML (1987) Characterization of astrocyte plasminogen activator. *J Neurol Sci* 80: 277–287

99 Tsirka SE, Rogove AD, Bugge TH, Degen JL, Strickland S (1997) An extracellular proteolytic cascade promotes neuronal degeneration in the mouse hippocampus. *J Neurosci* 17: 543–552

100 Danglet G, Vinson D, Chapeville F (1986) Qualitative and quantitative distribution of plasminogen activators in organs from healthy adult mice. *FEBS Lett* 194: 96–100

101 Matsuo O, Okada K, Fukao H, Suzuki A, Ueshima S (1992) Cerebral plasminogen activator activity in spontaneously hypertensive stroke-prone rats. *Stroke* 23: 995–999

102 Dent MA, Sumi Y, Morris RJ, Seeley PJ (1993) Urokinase-type plasminogen activator expression by neurons and oligodendrocytes during process outgrowth in developing rat brain. *Eur J Neurosci* 5: 633–647

103 Sappino A-P, Madani R, Huarte J, Belin D, Kiss JZ, Wohlwend A, Vassalli J-D (1993) Extracellular proteolysis in the adult murine brain. *J Clin Invest* 92: 679–685

104 Wang YF, Tsirka SE, Strickland S, Stieg PE, Soriano SG, Lipton SA (1998) Tissue plasminogen activator (tPA) increases neuronal damage after focal cerebral ischemia in wild-type and tPA-deficient mice. *Nature Med* 4: 228–231

105 Nagai N, De Mol M, Lijnen HR, Carmeliet P, Collen D (1999) Role of plasminogen system components in focal cerebral ischemic infarction: a gene targeting and gene transfer study in mice. *Circulation* 99: 2440–2444

106 Mackay AR, Corbitt RH, Hartzler JL, Thorgeirsson UP (1990) Basement membrane type IV collagen degradation: evidence for the involvement of a proteolytic cascade independent of metalloproteinases. *Cancer Res* 50: 5997–6001

107 Norton WT, Cammer W, Bloom BR, Gordon S (1978) Neutral proteinases secreted by macrophages degrade basic protein: a possible mechanism of inflammatory demyelination. *Adv Exp Med Biol* 100: 365–381

108 McGuire PG, Seeds NW (1989) The interaction of plasminogen activator with a reconstituted basement membrane matrix and extracellular macromolecules produced by cultured epithelial cells. *J Cell Biochem* 40: 215–227

109 Saksela O, Rifkin DB (1988) Cell-associated plasminogen activation: regulation and physiological functions. *Annu Rev Cell Biol* 4: 93–126

110 Vassalli JD, Sappino AP, Belin D (1991) The plasminogen activator/plasmin system. *J Clin Invest* 88: 1067–1072

111 Chen ZL, Strickland S (1997) Neuronal death in the hippocampus is promoted by plasmincatalyzed degradation of laminin. *Cell* 91: 917–925

112 Kazes I, Delarue F, Hagege J, Bouzhir-Sima L, Rondeau E, Sraer JD, Nguyen G (1998) Soluble latent membrane-type 1 matrix metalloprotease secreted by human mesangial cells is activated by urokinase. *Kidney Int* 54: 1976–1984

113 He CS, Wilhelm SM, Pentland AP, Marmer BL, Grant GA, Eisen AZ, Goldberg GI (1989) Tissue cooperation in a proteolytic cascade activating human interstitial collagenase. *Proc Natl Acad Sci USA* 86: 2632–2636

114 Mazzieri R, Masiero L, Zanetta L, Monea S, Onisto M, Garbisa S, Mignatti P (1997) Control of type IV collagenase activity by components of the urokinase-plasmin system: a regulatory mechanism with cell-bound reactants. *EMBO J* 16: 2319–2332

115 Ahn MY, Zhang ZG, Tsang W, Chopp M (1999) Endogenous plasminogen activator expression after embolic focal cerebral ischemia in mice. *Brain Res* 837: 169–176

116 Pfefferkorn T, Staufer B, Liebetrau M, Bultemeier G, Vosko MR, Zimmermann C, Hamann GF (2000) Plasminogen activation in focal cerebral ischemia and reperfusion. *J Cereb Blood Flow Metab* 20: 337–342

117 Zhang GZ, Chopp M, Goussev A, Lu D, Morris D, Tsang W, Powers C, Ho K-L (1999) Cerebral microvascular obstruction by fibrin is associated with upregulation of PAI-1 acutely after onset of focal embolic ischemia in rats. *J Neurosci* 19: 10898–10907

118 Hosomi N, Lucero J, Heo JH, Koziol JA, Copeland BR, del Zoppo GJ (2001) Rapid differential endogenous plasminogen activator expression after acute middle cerebral artery occlusion. *Stroke* 32: 1341–1348

119 del Zoppo GJ, Wagner S, Haring H-P, Tagaya M (1997) Focal cerebral ischemia produces topographically graded microvascular injury. *Stroke* 28: 247 (Abstract)

120 Abumiya T, Lucero J, Heo JH, Tagaya M, Koziol JA, Copeland BR, del Zoppo GJ (1999) Activated microvessels express vascular endothelial growth factor and integrin $\alpha_v\beta_3$ during focal cerebral ischemia. *J Cereb Blood Flow Metab* 19: 1038–1050

121 Verheul HMW, Jorna AS, Hoekman K, Broxterman HJ, Gebbink MFBG, Pinedo HM (2000) Vascular endothelial growth factor-stimulated endothelial cells promote adhesion and activation of platelets. *Blood* 96: 4216–4221

122 Webb NJ, Myers CR, Watson CJ, Bottomley MJ, Brenchley PE (1998) Activated human neutrophils express vascular endothelial growth factor (VEGF). *Cytokine* 10 (4): 254–257

123 Salven P., Orpana A., Joensuu H (1999) Leukocytes and platelets of patients with cancer contain high levels of vascular endothelial growth factor. *Clin Cancer Res* 5(3): 487–491

124 Scalia R., Booth G, Lefer DJ (1999) Vascular endothelial growth factor attenuates leukocyte-endothelium interaction during acute endothelial dysfunction: Essential role of endothelium-derived nitric oxide. *FASEB J* 13 (9): 1039–1046

125 Garcia JH, Liu KF, Yoshida Y, Lian J, Chen S, del Zoppo GJ (1994) The influx of leukocytes and platelets in an evolving brain infarct (Wistar rat). *Am J Pathol* 144: 188–199

126 Coudhri TF, Hoh BL, Zerwes HG, Prestigiacomo CJ, Kim SC, Connolly E, Sander Jr. E, Kottirsch G, Pinsky DJ (1998) Reduced microvascular thrombosis and improved outcome in acute murine stroke by inhibiting GP IIb/IIIa receptor-mediated platelet aggregation. *J Clin Invest* 102: 1301–1310

127 del Zoppo GJ, Hecker KJ, Hallenbeck JM (2001). Inflammation after stroke: Is it harmful? *Arch Neurol* 58: 669–672

128 Previtali SC, Archelos JJ, Hartung HP (1997) Modulation of the expression of integrins on glial cells during experimental autoimmune encephalomyelitis. A central role for TNF-α. *Am J Pathol* 151: 1425–1435

129 Previtali S, Quattrini A, Nemni R, Truci G, Ducati A, Wrabetz L, Canal N (1996) $\alpha_6\beta_4$ and $\alpha_6\beta_1$ integrins in astrocytomas and other CNS tumors. *J Neuropathol* 55: 456–465

130 Sobel RA, Hinojoza JR, Maeda A, chen M (1998) Endothelial cell integrin laminin receptor expression in multiple sclerosis lesions. *Am J Pathol* 153: 405–415

131 McEver RP (1991) Selectins: Novel receptors that mediate leukocyte adhesion during inflammation. *Thromb Haemost* 65: 223–228

132 McEver RP, Moore KL, Cummings RD (1995) Leukocyte trafficking mediated by selectin-carbohydrate interactions. *J Biol Chem* 270: 11025–11028

133 Kanwar JR, Harrison JE, Wang D, Leung E, Mueller W, Wagner N, Krissansen GW (2000) β_7 integrins contribute to demyelination disease of the central nervous system. *J Neuroimmunol* 103: 146–152

134 Romanic AM, Madri JA (1994) Extracellular matrix-degrading proteinases in the nervous system. *Brain Pathol* 4: 145–156

135 Docagne F, Nicole O, Marti HH, MacKenzie ET, Buisson A, Vivien D (1999) Transforming growth factor-β_1 as a regulator of the serpins/t-PA axis in cerebral ischemia. *FASEB J* 13 (11): 1315–1324

The inflammatory response in focal cerebral ischemia

Daniel C. Morris[1] and Michael Chopp[2]

[1]Department of Emergency Medicine, Henry Ford Health System, Detroit, MI, 48202, USA;
[2]Department of Neurology, Henry Ford Health System, 2799 W. Grand Blvd, Detroit, MI,
48202, USA, and Oakland University, Physics Department, Rochester, MI, 48307, USA

Introduction

Inflammation is the reaction of vascularized living tissue to local injury. Local injury is caused by invading microorganisms, radiation, chemical injuries or ischemia. The inflammatory response serves to destroy or contain the infectious or noxious agent and to trigger a series of complex events that repair or replace the damaged tissue. The inflammatory response of any disease, whether it be infectious or ischemic, is highly controlled and any exacerbation of the response can actually harm the organism. Uncontrolled inflammatory reactions can cause chronic disease or death, as illustrated by rheumatoid arthritis or life-threatening hypersensitivity reactions. Occlusion of an artery in the brain causes cerebral ischemic which provokes a well coordinated inflammatory response. The inflammatory response is hypothesized to limit or contain hypoxic damage to a small area. However, as in other inflammatory diseases, the inflammatory response to cerebral ischemia promotes secondary injury to surrounding viable cerebral tissue commonly referred to as the penumbra. This secondary injury or response occurs because of molecular adhesive events, platelet activation, fibrin deposition and cytokine production which occur early after ischemia and reperfusion [1–5].

The initial inflammatory response in the brain after ischemia is expression of adhesion molecules and associated receptors on platelets, neutrophils and endothelial cells [5, 6, 7–10]. Adhesion molecules promote cell-cell interaction which causes release of growth factors, chemoattractants, proteases and free radicals. This triad of interaction between platelets, neutrophils and endothelial cells promotes further hemostasis. Thus cerebral ischemia induces a procoagulant state exacerbating secondary inflammatory injury. This chapter will describe the inflammatory response in cerebral ischemia as it relates to thrombosis in secondary injury. We propose that preservation of the penumbra can be accomplished only by inhibiting the interaction between platelets, neutrophils and endothelial cells after cerebral ischemia.

Inflammation and Stroke, edited by Giora Z. Feuerstein
© 2001 Birkhäuser Verlag Basel/Switzerland

Infiltration of leukocytes in cerebral tissue after ischemia

After stroke, leukocytes accumulate in brain microvascular *via* the interaction of adhesion molecules on leukocytes, platelets and endothelial cells [11–15]. The initial event in leukocyte recruitment is that of selectin mediated leukocyte rolling [16]. Expression of the integrin Mac-1 on the neutrophil is upregulated by chemoattractant molecules such as IL-1 and monocyte chemoattractant protein-1 (MCP-1) [17, 18]. Expression of intercellular adhesion molecule-1 (ICAM-1) then binds the integrin and causes firm adhesion of the leukocytes to the endothelium [11, 10]. The temporal profile of leukocyte accumulation in experimental focal cerebral ischemia has been demonstrated in numerous models. Neutrophil influx occurs earlier after transient ischemia than after permanent ischemia and the peak numbers of neutrophils occur at 24 h after transient ischemia and at 48 h after permanent ischemia [11, 12, 19]. Permanent MCA occlusion results in smaller inflammatory response and intraparenchymal migration of neutrophils than after transient ischemia. Leukocytes are present in the cerebral microvessels at 1 h of middle cerebral occlusion (MCA) and in the parenchyma at 1 h of reperfusion after 2 h of MCA occlusion. However, at 24 h after permanent MCA occlusion, neutrophils were found only within blood vessels and were not observed throughout the infarcted tissue. Reperfusion promotes earlier leukocyte infiltration into the parenchyma than permanent MCA occlusion.

Proposed mechanisms of injury mediated by leukocyte accumulation after stroke include reduction of perfusion by direct mechanical obstruction of the microvasculature and cell damage caused by oxygen radicals, proteases and cytokines released by the leukocytes. Neutropenia in animal stroke models has shown reduction of infarction volume and neuronal injury [20–22]. Therefore, it is reasonable that therapies that reduce neutrophil adhesion and accumulation will reduce ischemic cell damage and ultimately improve outcome in stroke.

Expression of the selectins after onset of cerebral ischemia

The selectin family consists of three adhesive receptors that mediate leukocyte-endothelial cell and leukocyte-platelet adhesive interactions: L-selectin (CD62L), E-selectin (CD62E) and P-selectin (CD62P). P-selectin and E-selectin are expressed on activated endothelial cells while only P-selectin is expressed on activated platelets. L-selectin is constitutively expressed on circulating leukocytes, except for a subpopulation of lymphocytes. The selectins are required for polymorphonuclear leukocytes (PMNs) to roll on and adhere to the vascular endothelial cells, which is a first and necessary step for the transmigration of PMNs into the damaged parenchyma [23]. The expression of P- and E- selectins is regulated. P-selectin is a glycoprotein, composed of a single polypeptide chain with a molecular weight of

140 kDa and it is stored in the Weibel-Palade bodies of the vascular endothelium and the alpha-granules of the platelet [24]. After stimulation by thrombin, histamine and/or complement activation, P-selectin is rapidly translocated to the cell surface. E-selectin is not stored, so its expression is regulated by transcription activation by cytokines, such as tumor necrosis factor-α (TNFα) or interleukin (IL)-1β [25, 26].

Zhang et al. observed rapid P-selectin expression on the surface of endothelial cells after cerebral ischemia using three different stroke models: suture model with reperfusion after 2 h, injection of thrombin in the middle cerebral artery (MCA) to produce thrombosis and injection of a fibrin clot in the MCA [5]. Partial reperfusion due to endogenous fibrinolysis has been observed at 6 h in thrombotic model while in the embolic model, reperfusion was not detected until 24 h after the MCA occlusion. Therefore, these models represent a range of transient and permanent occlusion. In all three models, expression of P-selectin as measured by immunohistochemistry occurred in two phases after middle cerebral artery (MCA) occlusion in the rat. An early phase of expression occurs within 15 min and then decreases to control levels at 1 hour. Late phase of expression occurs at 2 h and peaks at 6 h. Expression lasted up to 96 h in all three models. In contrast, Suzuki et al. found differences in the duration of P-selectin expression between transient and permanent occlusion using the suture rat model [27]. The expression was diminished by 1 day of permanent occlusion and 3 days of reperfusion. Persistent upregulation of P-selectin of at least 24 h was also observed on precapillary arterioles and postcapillary venules in a baboon model of MCA occlusion [9].

In contrast to the early expression of P-selectin, E-selectin expression on the endothelial cells was first observed at zero to 2 h of reperfusion; it peaked at 4 and 10 h of reperfusion and decreased after 72 h [28]. Zhang et al. demonstrated that E-selectin mRNA was detected at 2 h of reperfusion and peaked between 10 and 22 h of reperfusion. After 46 h, E-selectin mRNA was undetectable. Wang et al. observed that expression of E-selectin mRNA differs between transient and permanent MCA occlusion [29, 30]. E-selectin mRNA increased at 6 h in permanent MCA occlusion, peaked at 12 h and persisted for greater than 48 h. The expression of E-selectin mRNA occurs earlier after transient than after permanent ischemia. Neutrophils accumulate more rapidly in transient ischemia than in permanent, suggesting that reperfusion upregulates transcription factors for E-selectin mRNA production and that E-selectin plays a pivotal role in neutrophil recruitment. The differences between transient and permanent ischemia in experimental models cannot be overlook when extrapolating experimental results to humans.

Pretreatment with anti-P-selectin antibody reduced infarction volume and hemorrhage in both reperfusion and permanent MCA occlusion models in the rat [31–33]. In these studies, pretreatment with an IgG murine anti-rat antibody reduced infarction volume but post-treatment failed to reduce infarction volume. The number of infiltrating leukocytes were reduced in the pretreatment models but not in the reperfusion models. Regional blood flow was also improved in the pretreatment models. Connolly et al. using transgenic P-selectin deficient mice with a 45 min MCA occlusion time followed by 22 h of reperfusion demonstrated decreased infarction volumes and reduced neutrophil accumulation in the ischemic cortex [34]. In addition, reduced neutrophil influx was accompanied by greater postischemic cerebral reflow as measured by laser Doppler in null P-selectin mice. However, Soriano et al. using transgenic mice with both P- and E-selectin gene knockouts and a 3-h occlusion time followed by 21 h of reperfusion showed no difference in infarct volumes from nontransgenic littermates indicating that other mechanisms mediate ischemic cell damage after a prolonged period of transient focal ischemia [35]. Collectively, these results demonstrate that P-selectin is acting within the first 2 h after onset of ischemia to predispose the brain to petechial hemorrhage and to promote increase in infarction volume.

The selectins have a calcium-dependent lectin domain and bind to carbohydrate ligands such as sialyl-Lewis (Sle). This selectin-carbohydrate interaction can be blocked *in vitro* by synthetic oligopeptides targeting the lectin domain of selectin. Zhang et al. demonstrated a beneficial effect of a novel sialyl Lewis-containing oligosaccharide analog (CY-1503), which blocks both E- and P-selectin function [28, 36]. CY-1503 was administered to rats upon reperfusion 2 h after onset of MCA occlusion. Treatment of the ischemic animals with CY-1503 significantly reduced infarct volume and significantly reduced myeloperoxidase (MPO) reactive cells in the ischemic lesion by 60%.

Studies involving the use of L-selectin in acute stroke are few. Bednar et al. tested a humanized anti-L-selectin nonoclonal antibody DREG200 in a rabbit model of acute stroke. This study compared DREG200 with and without tPA [8]. DREG200 was administered 3 h after clot embolization, followed immediately by a 2-h intravenous infusion of t-PA. A moderate reduction in infarction volume and improvement in cerebral blood flow was observed but no efficacy was demonstrated in the group receiving DREG200 without concomitant t-PA therapy.

Integrin expression after onset of cerebral ischemia

Integrins are a family of cell surface adhesion receptors that are expressed on a wide variety of cells [37]. Integrins mediate important cell-to-cell contacts as well as attachment to extracellular matrices. All integrins are α/β heterodimers. The α subunits vary in size between 120 and 180 kDa and are each noncovalently associated with a β subunit ranging in size from 90–100 kDa. Both subunits of integrins are transmembrane glycoproteins each with a single hydrophobic transmembrane segment.

Neutrophil-platelet contact and adhesion depends on the interaction of P-selectin and the leukocyte β_2 (CD18) integrin family which consists of three distinct α

chains: α_L (CD11a), α_M (CD11b) and α_X (CD11c) [38]. The CD11a/CD18, CD11b/CD18, and CD11c/CD18 integrins are also called lymphocyte function-associated antigen-1 (LFA-1), Mac-1 and p150.95, respectively. The ligands for these integrins are the immunoglobulin superfamily member, ICAM (intracelluar adhesion molecule), fibrinogen and complement fragments (iC3b).

Inhibition of Mac-1 in animal models of cerebral ischemia has been well studied by numerous groups. Antibodies against both the α and β subunits of Mac-1 have been used with similar results. Using the rat suture model, Chen et al. demonstrated that administration of anti-CD11b (1B6c) antibody resulted in a dose-dependent, significant functional improvement and reduction in lesion volume after 2 h of MCA occlusion followed by 22 h of reperfusion [39]. In this study, the anti-CD11b antibody was administered twice, once at onset of and at 22 h of reperfusion. Rats were sacrificed at 48 h from onset of MCA occlusion. In a similar study, Chopp et al. observed in the same rat suture model that administration of 1B6c 1 h after onset of reperfusion resulted in significant reduction in lesion volume and intraparenchymal neutrophils. In a more elaborate study designed to extend the therapeutic window of anti-Mac-1 therapy, Zhang et al. showed that use of 1B6 or an anti-CD18 monoclonal antibody (CL26) reduced infarction volume when administered 2 h after reperfusion, i.e. 4 h after stroke. Anti-CD11b treatment significantly inhibited the increase of MPO activity in the ischemic hemisphere. In this study, the therapeutic window [40] intervention to reduce ischemic cell damage in this model was at least 4 h from the onset of MCA occlusion. Yenari et al. used a rabbit model to show reduced ischemic neuronal damage using humanized monoclonal antibody Hu23F2G administered 20 min after middle cerebral, anterior cerebral and internal carotid arteries occlusion using aneurysm clips [41]. After 2 h, the clips were removed followed by 6 h of reperfusion before sacrifice. Neutrophil infiltration was also significantly reduced.

Using the embolic stroke model in which a fibrin clot is placed in the MCA, Zhang et al. showed that combination therapy with rt-PA and anti-CD18 antibody significantly reduced infarction volume and improved neurological deficits after 2 h of MCA occlusion [42]. However, administration of anti-CD18 antibody alone did not reduce infarction volume or neurological deficits. A similar result regarding differences in transient vs. permanent ischemia stroke models was also observed by Prestigiacomo et al. Using a transgenic CD18 knockout murine stroke model, Prestigiacomo et al. found that after 45 min of MCA occlusion followed by reperfusion, infarction volumes were reduced as well as accumulation of PMNs [43]. However, transgenic CD18 knockout mice and wild type CD18 mice subjected to permanent ischemia showed no change in infarction volume or accumulation of PMNs. Similar results in using two different stroke models confirm differences of the inflammatory response in transient and permanent ischemia. Prolonged ischemia may override any potential beneficial effects of antiadhesion molecule therapy. In addition, the temporal profile of inflammatory response is dependent on the duration of ischemia. As mentioned earlier, migration of leukocytes is delayed after permanent ischemia compared with transient ischemia and that ischemic cell damage may be complete even before neutrophils accumulate. Soriano et al. used a CD18 transgenic knockout murine model with a 3-h MCA occlusion time followed by 21 h reperfusion period [44]. Infarction volumes were reduced in the CD18 knockout mice although no differences in neutrophil accumulation or regional blood flow were found. Using different stroke models and antibodies to Mac-1, these studies demonstrate that Mac-1 plays an important role in ischemic cell damage in reperfusion injury, although its role in permanent ischemia is less clear.

GP IIb/IIIa expression after onset of cerebral ischemia

The integrin glycoprotein GP IIb/IIIa is the most abundant platelet receptor which acts as the final common pathway for platelet aggregation [45]. Accumulation of platelets in the cerebral microvasculature after MCA occlusion has been observed in numerous stroke models. Platelets play a role in the development and progression of cell damage after focal cerebral ischemia. An evolving hypothesis is that activated platelets accumulate in the microvasculature forming thrombi that contribute to infarct progression irrespective of the initial occluding clot. Indeed, Ames et al. made an important observation that after experimental stroke, cerebral tissue is hypoperfused producing a low-flow or no-flow state [46]. Tissue perfusion is reduced, even if the primary occluded vessel is opened. Therefore, numerous studies have focused on inhibiting the GPIIb/IIIa receptor on the activated platelets to improve microvascular perfusion after MCA occlusion. Choudhri et al. demonstrated that pre-administration of an inhibitor of the glycoprotein IIb/IIIa receptor, SDZ GPI 562 reduced platelet and fibrin accumulation by 48% and 47%, respectively, in a suture murine model of cerebral ischemia [47]. A dose-dependent reduction of infarction volumes as well as improvement in postischemic cerebral blood flow was observed. When SDZ GPI 562 was given at reperfusion after 45 min of MCA occlusion, infarction volumes were reduced by 70% supporting the hypothesis that platelet aggregation in the microcirculation contributes to postischemic hypoperfusion even after recanalization of the MCA. Intracerebral hemorrhage (ICH) was not significantly increased at therapeutic doses. Using a baboon model of cerebral ischemia, Abumiya, et al. demonstrated increased microvascular patency using the GP IIb/IIIa inhibitor TP9201 after 3 h of MCA occlusion and 1 h of reperfusion [48].

Platelets are normally activated at sites of vascular injury by a combination of collagen exposure, local thrombin generation and the release of ADP from damaged cells and other activated platelets. The primary ligand for GP IIb/IIIa is fibrinogen which acts as a bridge when platelets aggregate. Components of the extracellular matrix fibronectin and vitronectin bind to GP IIb/IIIa. VonWillebrand factor, an adhesive glycoprotein on endothelial cells also binds GP IIb/IIIa promoting platelet/endothelial interactions [49]. Zhang et al. demonstrated fibrin deposition and platelet aggregation in the microcirculation in an embolic rat model of cerebral ischemia [1]. Three-dimensional analysis revealed that intravascular fibrin deposition directly blocks microvascular plasma perfusion. Vascular plugs contained erythrocytes, polymorphonuclear leukocytes and platelets enmeshed in fibrin. Microvascular plasma perfusion deficit and fibrin deposition expanded concomitantly from the subcortex to the cortex during 1 and 4 h of embolic MCA occlusion. These findings support the hypothesis that intravascular fibrin deposition contributes to progressive cerebral microvascular perfusion deficits after MCA occlusion

In agreement with other studies [50, 51], Zhang et al. demonstrated accumulation of platelets in downstream cerebral microvessels 4 h after ischemia [52]. However, the pure fibrin clot used to occlude the MCA showed increases in platelets and plasminogen activator inhibitor 1 (PAI-1). In addition, fibrin deposition was also observed in the parenchyma, suggesting that the vascular wall was compromised. Diffuse abnormal loss of type IV collagen, a major component of the microvasculature wall, was associated with platelet GP IIb/IIIa at 1 h after MCA occlusion and complete loss of type IV collagen at 4 h. Matrix metalloproteinases (MMPs), a group of zinc-dependent enzymes that degrade components of the extracellular matrix (ECM), are increased in acute ischemic stroke [53, 54]. MMPs are secreted in a soluble proenzyme form and require activation for proteolytic activity. MMP2 (gelatinase A) and MMP9 (gelatinase B) cleave a wide range of substrates *in vitro*, including type IV collagen. The appearance of proform of MMP9 at 4 h and a significant increase in both pro and active forms of MMP9 at 24 h of MCA occlusion [52] are consistent with previous studies of increases in MMP9 activity in ischemic brains in the rat and mouse [53, 54]. Platelet accumulation coincided with increases in MMP9, loss of collagen IV in microvessels and parenchymal fibrin deposition. Taken together, these results support the hypothesis that activated platelets and fibrin deposition form aggregates *via* GP IIb/IIIa which promotes cerebral microvascular perfusion deficits. Secondly, this platelet aggregation is related to loss of integrity of cerebral microvessels in which MMPs may play significant role in microvascular degradation.

Fibrinogen is a common ligand for both Mac-1 and GP IIb/IIIa. The interaction between Mac-1 (neutrophil) and GP IIb/IIIa (platelet) has not been explored in cerebral ischemia. Weber and Springer, in an elegant study using a parallel flow chamber, demonstrated that neutrophil accumulation in flow involves interactions of Mac-1 with fibrinogen presented by GPIIb/IIIa on platelets with activation by platelet activating factor (PAF) [55]. Transient interactions of neutrophils with platelets that were ICAM-2 and L-selectin dependent occurred at low shear stresses. The arrest and adhesion strengthening on platelets in flow appeared to be mainly stimulated by PAF. Minimal interactions were observed in the presence of GPIIb/IIIa inhibitors suggesting that unidentified ligands may contribute to neutrophil arrest and adhesion strengthening on activated platelets. However, a model of neutrophil and platelet interactions described by Coller involves initial neutrophil attachment and rolling by P-selectin expressed on activated platelets [49]. In this model, binding of P-selectin with its ligand activates Mac-1 with possible involvement and/or activation of PAF by binding to its receptor. Fibrinogen binding to GP IIb/IIIa and finally the firm attachment of neutrophils to platelets is facilitated *via* the fibrinogen bridge to Mac-1.

Intracellular adhesion molecule (ICAM) expression in cerebral ischemia

The ICAMs are members of the immunoglobulin superfamily that are consitutively expressed on the endothelial cells. Neutrophil emigration is mediated by adhesion proteins that are highly expressed on the endothelial surface during inflammatory processes in the brain. ICAM-1 is an inducible glycoprotein adhesion molecule that binds to the leukocyte CD11/CD18 integrins and facilitates neutrophil adhesion and transendothelial migration [56]. Numerous stroke models have demonstrated upregulation of ICAM-1. Blocking ICAM-1 reduces neutrophil infiltration into the tissue and thereby reduces infarction volume and ischemic cell damage. Wang et al. demonstrated that ICAM-1 mRNA level was significantly elevated in the ischemic cortex at 3 h, peaked at 6 to 12 h and remained elevated up to 5 days after permanent MCA occlusion in SHR rats [30]. Using a reperfusion model, they showed that the expression of ICAM-1 mRNA level was significantly increased at 1 h of reperfusion, peaked at 12 h and persisted to 5 days of reperfusion after 160 min after MCA occlusion. Zhang et al. demonstrated that administration of an anti-ICAM monoclonal antibody (1A29) at reperfusion after 2 h of MCA occlusion resulted in a 41% reduction in infarction volume and PMN infiltration [57]. In a second study designed to describe the temporal relationship of ICAM expression in cerebral ischemia, Zhang et al. showed that ICAM-1 mRNA was detected 1 h after MCA occlusion. ICAM mRNA maximized at 10 h of reperfusion (after 2 h of MCA occlusion) and persisted out to 1 week of reperfusion. ICAM-1 significantly increased in microvascular endothelial cells at 2 h of reperfusion, maximized at 46 h and persisted out to 1 week of reperfusion [58].

The transient and permanent MCA occlusion models show great differences in infarction volume and ischemic cell damage. Zhang et al. conclusively demonstrated that anti-ICAM-1 antibody reduces ischemic cell damage after transient MCA occlusion but not after not permanent MCA occlusion [58]. One group of rats was subjected to 2 h of MCA occlusion followed by 1 h of reperfusion before administration of 1A29 while a separate group of rats was subjected to permanent MCA occlusion. After 1 week, the rats were sacrificed. Significant reductions in both infarction volume (44%) and weight loss were found in the transient ischemic group. In contrast, the permanent MCA occlusion group showed no differences in infarction volume or weight loss when compared to controls. Earlier studies by Bowes et al. and Clark et al. using rabbit models of multiple brain emboli with or without reperfusion demonstrated similar differences between transient and permanent ischemic models [59-61].

Because of the potential for complex antibody-antigen interactions that may skew results, transgenic ICAM-1 knockout mice were investigated during MCA occlusion. Soriano et al. subjected transgenic ICAM-1 knockout mice to 3 h of MCA occlusion followed by a 21- or 45-h reperfusion period [62]. When compared to wild-type controls, the ICAM-1 deficient group demonstrated a 5.6-fold and 7.8-fold reduction in infarction volume after 48 h. Neutrophil infiltration at 21 h was reduced in the ICAM-1 deficient group, but no differences in infiltration existed in the 45 h group. A later study by the same group observed that the ICAM-1 deficient group showed less cellular necrosis but the level of apoptosis was similar. Although ICAM-1 deficiency resulted in a milder form of ischemic injury, apoptotic cell death was not inhibited implying other ischemic mediated mechanisms act on the vunerable hypoxic neurons [63]. Likewise, *in vitro* studies revealed that progression to apoptosis or necrosis depends on the intensity of the ischemic insult. Kitagawa et al. observed similar results in ICAM-1 deficient mice, however they compare infarction volume and neutrophil infiltration in both transient and permanent stroke models [64]. The transient stroke model consisted of 30 or 45 min of MCA occlusion followed reperfusion for 6 h to 48 h. Infarction volume was significantly reduced in the ICAM-1 deficient mice, however no differences in infarction volumes between transient and permanent were observed. In addition, the number of infiltrating neutrophils were similar in both the wild type and ICAM-1 deficient mice, however depletion of granulocytes by use of a monoclonal antibody, further reduced infarction volume in the transient ischemia ICAM-1 deficient mice. Microcirculation was reduced after ischemia but was better preserved in the ICAM-1 deficient mice. These authors concluded that inhibition of ICAM-1 alone was not enough to suppress the aggravating role of neutrophils since depletion of the neutrophils further reduced the size of the infarction. They also concluded ICAM-1 plays a role in reducing perfusion in the microcirculation. An interesting observation was that in ICAM-1 deficient mice no differences in infarction volume were seen when compared to transient and permanent stroke models. The explanation was felt to be related to the trangenic model, because deficiency of ICAM-1 in knockout mice was a more effective suppressor of ICAM-1 function than the monoclonal antibody. The Enlimomab Acute Stroke Trial involved administration of a murine anti-ICAM (human) antibody to acute stroke victims within 6 h of symptom onset [65]. Doses were administered out to 72 h. However, this study showed no benefit in outcome because design of the study was flawed, as reperfusion in humans is difficult to determine.

It estimated that at least 50% of human stroke victims exhibit no reperfusion, so administration of anti-ICAM antibodies to non-reperfused stroke will inevitably fail as demonstrated by previous animal data [66]. Zhang et al. clearly demonstrated that administration of anti-ICAM antibody with rt-PA may be beneficial. Using the embolic stroke rat model, administration of rt-PA at 1 h after embolization resulted in a significant reduction of immunoreactivity for P-selectin and E-selectin at 6 h and for ICAM-1 at 24 h when compared to controls [67]. Rats treated with rt-PA and anti-ICAM-1 antibody at 4 h after embolization showed a significant reduction in ischemic lesion volume and neutrophil infiltration when compared with rats treated with rt-PA treatment alone. Therefore, reperfusion is needed when attempting to treat ischemic stroke with an anti-ICAM antibody.

Neutrophil inhibitors

Neutrophil inhibitory factor is a hookworm-derived 41-kDa glycoprotein ligand of the integrin CD11b/CD18 that inhibits human neutrophil function in the brain and other organs. rNIF blocks the adhesion of activated human neutrophils to vascular endothelium cells, as well as the release of H_2O_2 from activated neutrophils. Using the suture rat model, Jiang et al. demonstrated a significant reduction in infarction volume and neurological outcome when rNIF was administered up to 4 h, or reperfusion after 2 h of MCA occlusion [68, 69]. As described in previous studies, no beneficial effect was seen in permanent ischemia models. Infarction volumes were measured out to 7 days and continuous treatment with rNIF was required to maintain the protective effect.

The extracellular matrix contributes to the cell adhesion process during inflammation. Whereas the β_2 subunits (CD18) are largely involved in cell-cell interacts as previously described, the β_1 subunits (CD29) integrins mediate adhesion to extracellular matrix constituents, specifically, fibronectin and laminin. The interaction of β_1 and extracellular constituents may play a role in the recruitment of leukocytes from the blood to the parenchyma. Thus inhibitors of β_1 may reduce neutrophil infiltration in the brain parenchyma and reduce ischemic cell damage. Synthetic peptides derived from domains of fibronectin and laminin were administered to rats undergoing 1 h of MCA occlusion followed by 48 h of reperfusion. Yanaka et al. administered three different fibronectin-derived polypeptides, RGD domain, the alternatively spliced connecting segment CS-1 and a nonoverlapping sequence corresponding to the FN-C/H region [70–73]. Results of these studies showed a reduction of infarction of volume after 48 h and improved neurological outcome. In addition, the number of infiltrating neutrophils as measured by the MPO assay, was reduced. FN-C/H-V could be given up to 3 h of reperfusion with beneficial effect, but not at 6 h. A permanent ischemia model was not tested.

Transcription factor nuclear factor κB

Nuclear factor κB (NF-κB) is a protein transcription factor that is required for maximal transcription of a wide array of pro-inflammatory molecules involved in acute inflammation [74]. Hypoxia, reactive oxygen species, IL-1α and TNFα activate NF-κB in focal ischemia. In turn, NF-κB is a transcription activator of many genes involved in the pathogenesis of cerebral ischemia such as cytokines, cell adhesion molecules, interferons and hematopoietic growth factors [75]. NF-κB is a DNA binding protein that binds to the enhancing domain of target genes in the configuration of a dimer of two members of the subunits composed RelA (p65), RelB, c-Rel, p50 (NF-κB$_1$) and p52 (NF-κB$_2$). The classical dimer is composed of p50 and RelA [76]. RelA contains a transcription domain that is required for activation of transcription. Under unstimulated conditions, these subunits reside in the cytoplasm as inactive forms complexed to a member of the IκB family that mask their nuclear localization signal. There are six members of the IκB family IκBα, IκBβ, IκBγ, Bcl-3, p100 and p105. p100 and p50 are the precursors for p50 and p52, respectively [77]. Under stimulation, IκB is phosphorylated, polyubiquinated and proteolytically degraded by the 26S proteasome causing translocation of NF-κB homodimers and heterodimers of the different subunits to be translocated to the nucleus [78]. NF-κB has been found to be pro or anti apoptotic and has been examined in many different animal and cell culture models under various conditions, however its exact role is unclear.

NF-κB is activated in transient cerebral ischemia in the rat. Carroll et al. observed activation of NF-κB 15 to 30 min after the beginning of reperfusion after 2 h of MCA occlusion [79]. After 60 min the levels of NF-κB, consisting of p65 and p50 Rel proteins, as measured by electrophoretic mobility shift assay (EMSA) returned to baseline. An inhibitor of NF-κB, N-acetylcysteine (NAC) was administered to rats 1 h prior to the end of occlusion and at 24 h post occlusion. The rats were sacrificed at 48 h and a significant reduction of infarction volume was observed. NAC was also administered 1 h after reperfusion (after the NF-κB peak) and a smaller but still significant reduction in infarction volume was observed. Functional outcome was not measured in this study. Oxygen radicals and oxidative stress are strong inducers of NF-κB activation and its inhibition by NAC was expected, however the lasting effect of NAC was not expected leading to the conclusion that the antioxidant properties of NAC dissociated from its effects on NF-κB. This study did not identify the cell types that expressed NF-κB.

Gabriel et al. observed enhancement of NF-κB binding activity at 1, 4 and 7 days after MCA occlusion, but in contrast to Carroll et al., no binding activity was seen less than 24 h [80]. The rat model in Gabriel et al. study had only 1 h of MCA occlusion vs. 2 h in Carroll et al. Gabriel et al. also observed 1 day post-ischemia selective induction of p65 (Rel A) in neurons located in the penumbra as measured by immunohistochemistry, however, no binding activity at this time point was observed. At 4 days post ischemia, p65 vastly increased along with NF-κB binding activity. Reactive astrocytes and microglia/marcophages were the predominant cell type showing the NF-κB binding. These results suggested that delayed activation of NF-κB after ischemia occurs in reactive glia and involves *de novo* synthesis of p65. In contrast, Stephenson et al. observed exclusive immunoreactivity of p50 and p65 in the nuclei of cortical and striatal neurons in the ischemic hemisphere at 2, 6 and 12 h of reperfusion [81]. The rat model used in this study involved 2 h of MCA occlusion followed by reperfusion. At these time points, NF-κB immunoreactivity was not observed in other cell types. In addition, the presence of p50 and p65 in the nucleus and not the cytoplasm, corresponded to active NF-κB binding as measured by EMSA. This study also tested the antioxidant LY341122 administered prior to MCA occlusion. No siginificant NF-κB binding was observed supporting the hypothesis that neuroprotective antioxidants may inhibit neuronal death by preventing the activation of NF-κB. The contralateral nonischemic hemisphere showed no nuclear NF-κB immunoreactivity.

Investigating the role of NF-κB in neuronal cell death, Schneider et al. demonstrated NF-κB binding activity in a murine model of stroke [82]. After 2 h of MCA occlusion, nuclear translocation of NF-κB occurred in the striatum at 20 h of reperfusion and in the cortex after 72 h of reperfusion as measured by immunohistochemistry. The neurons expressed the p65 exclusively. NF-κB binding of p50 and p65 was observed beginning at 2 h of reperfusion extending out to 72 h. To further delineate the role of NF-κB activity, transgenic p50 knockout mice were compared to wild-type controls after 2 h of MCA occlusion and 20 h of reperfusion. The absence of the p50 subunit of NF-κB resulted in a significant reduction in infarct size in parts of the vascular territory of the MCA, but not in the hippocampus and the upper thalamus. In this murine model, the hippocampus and upper thalamus constituted part of the ischemic penumbra, the main area at risk for delayed neuronal death. The conclusions in this study was that NF-κB promotes a cell death-promoting role in focal ischemia, but the mechanism was unclear.

NF-κB expression and activity was explored in permanent focal ischemia in two separate studies. Irving et al. investigated NF-κB activity at 3, 6, 24 h post-MCA occlusion following permanent focal cerebral ischemia in rats [83]. This study demonstrated an initial trend to increased NF-κB activity 3 h post-MCA occlusion which predominantly occurred in the core infarction. Over time, NF-κB activity decreased in contrast to the transient ischemia models. The authors speculated that because NF-κB binding activity is reduced within regions in which cell death is imminent, that the reduced binding itself is involved in the mechanisms underlying ischemic cell death. A second study by Seegers et al. used magnetic resonance imaging (MRI) and immunohistological techniques in a permanent focal ischemia rat model [84]. They observed NF-κB activation 7 h after MCA occlusion. At this 7 h time point, the animals were sacrificed. The activation was exclusively observed at the periphery of the ischemic lesion, at the level of the penumbra area. In addition to the staining for p65, HSP70 expression, a marker for stressed but intacted neurons, was also measured. The NF-κB activation occurred in dying neurons of the penumbra area devoid of any HSP70 neuronal immunoreactivity. These authors also concluded that NF-κB activation may play a role in neuronal cell death and that MCA occlusion alone, and not reperfusion is sufficient to cause NF-κB activation. Both these studies should be viewed as preliminary because of the small sample sizes used. In addition, Seeger et al. only measured p65 by immunohistological staining and did not use the EMSA technique to determine binding activity.

Finally, Phillips et al. administered a proteasome inhibitor, PS519, which blocks activation of NF-κB by preventing the degradation of IκBα [85]. Rats were subjected to 2 h of MCA occlusion followed by 22 h or 70 h of reperfusion. PS519 was administered as a single bolus at reperfusion or at 4 and 6 h after MCA occlusion. Dose-response analysis at 24 h showed that infarct volume was reduced up to 60% with improvement of neurological outcome. This protection lasted out to 4 h post MCA occlusion. In addition, significant reduction of neutrophil infiltration was achieved with PS519. These results demonstrated administration of a proteasome inhibitor in transient ischemia reduction ischemic cell damage by possibly reducing neutrophil invasion. This study however did not measure NF-κB binding activity.

Taken together, the above studies demonstrate that NF-κB is expressed and activated in both transient and permanent focal ischemic models. NF-κB appears to be limited to the neurons and its activation probably plays a role in cell damage and death. The time frame of expression and binding activity is variable but it appears that blocking its activation by PS519 or administering antioxidants reduces ischemic cell damage. However, many fine details concerning the mechanisms of NF-κB and its time frame of expression need to be more throughly investigated.

Conclusions

The inflammatory response in stroke occurs after the initial embolic or thrombotic event. Receptors are expressed on endothelial cells, platelets and neutrophils which enhance cell to cell contact and interaction. The studies described above suggest that antibodies to the adhesion receptors or ligands administered in transient ischemic stroke may reduce ischemic cell damage by inhibiting neutrophil/platelet, neutrophil/endothelial or platelet/neutrophil adhesion. Inhibiting these interactions ultimately prevent neutrophil infiltration to the parenchyma. An important concept from the studies described in this chapter is that many therapies used to block these interactions can only occur in reperfused cerebral tissue. The inflammatory response is exacerbated in reperfusion and not in permanent ischemia. Failures of numerous neuroprotective agents in human stroke trials may be attributed to the fact that reperfusion is easily controlled in animal models but not in human trials. Many of these human studies neglected to determine the reperfusion status of the infarction.

The inflammatory response in cerebral ischemia promotes coagulation after the initial insult. Expression of the integrins, Mac-1 and GP IIb/IIIa on neutrophils and platelets promotes aggregation and adhesion in the microcirculation causing propagation of the infarction. In addition, intravascular fibrin deposition contributes to progressive cerebral microvascular perfusion deficits after MCA occlusion by bridging Mac-1 to GP IIb/IIIa. The aggregation of the platelets promotes release of the MMPs which most likely destroys vessel integrity and exposure of the underlying extracellular matrix. Components of the extracellular matrix fibronectin and vitronectin also bind to GP IIb/IIIa. VonWillebrand factor, an adhesive glycoprotein on endothelial cells also binds GP IIb/IIIa promoting platelet/endothelial interactions. An important observation in experimental stroke models is that inhibiting the inflammatory response with anti-adhesion molecule antibody after rt-PA infusion may improve outcome to a greater degree than with rt-PA alone and may extend the therapeutic window. Moreover, reducing platelet and neutrophil adhesion to the endothelium may prevent MMP mediated destruction of the microvasculature thereby reducing hemorrhagic transformation.

Finally, inhibition of NF-κB may provide a novel therapeutic action by inhibiting the transcriptional signals of inflammation. Rather than inhibiting many adhesion receptors, perhaps inhibiting the master controlling gene of inflammation will prevent the procoagulational state in cerebral ischemia. Further studies are needed to explore this important possibility.

References

1   Zhang ZG, Chopp M, Goussev A, Lu D, Morris D, Tsang W, Powers C, Ho KL(1999) Cerebral microvascular obstruction by fibrin is associated with upregulation of PAI-1 acutely after onset of focal embolic ischemia in rats. *J Neurosci* 19: 10898–10907

2   Zhang ZG, Chopp M, Gautam S, Zaloga C, Zhang RL, Schmidt HH, Pollock JS, Forstermann U (1994) Upregulation of neuronal nitric oxide synthase and mRNA, and selective sparing of nitric oxide synthase-containing neurons after focal cerebral ischemia in rat. *Brain Res* 654: 85–95

3   Zhang ZG, Chopp M, Bailey F, Malinski T (1995) Nitric oxide changes in the rat brain after transient middle cerebral artery occlusion. *J Neurol Sci* 128: 22–27

4   Zhang ZG, Zhang L, Jiang Q, Zhang R, Davies K, Powers C, Bruggen N, Chopp M (2000) VEGF enhances angiogenesis and promotes blood-brain barrier leakage in the ischemic brain. *J Clin Invest* 106: 829–838

5   Zhang R, Chopp M, Zhang Z, Jiang N, Powers C (1998) The expression of P- and E-selectins in three models of middle cerebral artery occlusion. *Brain Res* 785: 207–214

6   Kim JS, Chopp M, Chen H, Levine SR, Carey JL, Welch KM (1995) Adhesive glycoproteins CD11a and CD18 are upregulated in the leukocytes from patients with ischemic stroke and transient ischemic attacks. *J Neurol Sci* 128: 45–50

7   Suzuki H, Abe K, Tojo S, Morooka S, Kimura K, Mizugaki M, Itoyama Y (1997) Expressions of P-selectin- and HSP72-like immunoreactivities in rat brain after transient middle cerebral artery occlusion. *Brain Res* 759: 321–329

8   Bednar MM, Gross CE, Russell SR, Fuller SP, Ellenberger CL, Schindler E, Klingbeil C, Vexler V (1998) Humanized anti-L-selectin monoclonal antibody DREG200 therapy in acute thromboembolic stroke. *Neurol Res* 20: 403–408

9   Okada Y, Copeland BR, Mori E, Tung MM, Thomas WS, Del Zoppo GJ (1994) P-selectin and intercellular adhesion molecule-1 expression after focal brain ischemia and reperfusion. *Stroke* 25: 202–211

10   Zhang RL, Chopp M, Zaloga C, Zhang ZG, Jiang N, Gautam SC, Tang WX, Tsang W, Anderson DC, Manning AM (1995) The temporal profiles of ICAM-1 protein and mRNA expression after transient MCA occlusion in the rat. *Brain Res* 682: 182–188

11   Zhang RL, Chopp M, Chen H, Garcia JH (1994) Temporal profile of ischemic tissue damage, neutrophil response, and vascular plugging following permanent and transient (2H) middle cerebral artery occlusion in the rat [published erratum appears in *J Neurol Sci* 1994 Oct; 126 (1): 96]. *J Neurol Sci* 125: 3–10

12   Garcia JH, Liu KF, Yoshida Y, Lian J, Chen S, Del Zoppo GJ (1994) Influx of leukocytes and platelets in an evolving brain infarct (Wistar rat). *Am J Pathol* 144: 188–199

13   Barone FC, Hillegass LM, Price WJ, White RF, Lee EV, Feuerstein GZ, Sarau HM, Clark RK, Griswold DE (1991) Polymorphonuclear leukocyte infiltration into cerebral focal ischemic tissue: Myeloperoxidase activity assay and histologic verification. *J Neurosci Res* 29: 336–345

14   Patarroyo M, Prieto J, Rincon J, Timonen T, Lundberg C, Lindbom L, Asjo B, Gahmberg CG (1990) Leukocyte-cell adhesion: a molecular process fundamental in leukocyte physiology. *Immunol Rev* 114: 67–108

15   Hallenbeck JM, Dutka AJ, Tanisima T, Kochanek PM, Thompson CB, Obrenovitch TP, Contreras TJ (1986) Polymorphonuclear leukocyte accumulation in brain regions with low blood flow during the early postischemic period. *Stroke* 17: 246–253

16   Norman KE, Moore KL, Mcever RP, Ley K (1995) Leukocyte rolling *in vivo* is mediated by P-selectin glycoprotein ligand-1. *Blood* 86: 4417–4421

17   Kim JS, Gautam SC, Chopp M, Zaloga C, Jones ML, Ward PA, Welch KM (1995) Expression of monocyte chemoattractant protein-1 and macrophage inflammatory protein-1 after focal cerebral ischemia in the rat. *J Neuroimmunol* 56: 127–134

18   Zhang Z, Chopp M, Goussev A, Powers C (1998) Cerebral vessels express interleukin 1beta after focal cerebral ischemia. *Brain Res* 784: 210–217

19   Zhang Z G, Chopp M (1997) Myeloperoxidase immunoreactive cells inischemic brain after transient middle cerebral artery occlusion in the rat. *Neurosci Res Comm* 20: 85–91

20   Bednar MM, Raymond S, Mcauliffe T, Lodge PA, Gross CE (1991) The role of neutrophils and platelets in a rabbit model of thromboembolic stroke. *Stroke* 22: 44–50

21   Chen H, Chopp M, Bodzin G (1992) Neutropenia reduces the volume of cerebral infarct

after transient middle cerebral artery occlusion in the rat. *Neurosci Res Comm* 11: 93–99

22 Matsuo Y, Onodera H, Siga Y, Shozuhara H, Ninomiya M, Kihara T, Tamatani T, Miyasaka M, Kogure K (1994) Role of cell adhesion molecules in brain injury after transient middle cerebral artery occlusion in the rat. *Brain Res* 656: 344–352

23 Seekamp A, Till GO, Mulligan MS, Paulson JC, Anderson DA, Miyasaka M, Ward PA (1994) Role of selectins in local and remote tissue injury following ischemia and reperfusion. *Am J Pathol* 144: 592–598

24 Mcever RP, Beckstead JH, Moore KL, Marshall-Carlson L, Bainton DF (1989) GMP-140, a platelet alpha-granule membrane protein, is also synthesized by vascular endothelial cells and is localized in Weibel-Palade bodies. *J Clin Invest* 84: 92–99

25 Altavilla D, Francesco S, Patrizia C, Mariapatrizia I, Giuseppe M C, Giovanni S, Antonino S, Achille PC (1995) Tumor necrosis factor induces E-selectin production in splanchnic artery occlusion shock. *Am J Physiol* 268: H1412–H1417

26 Abbassi O, Kishimoto TK, Mcintire LV, Anderson DC, Smith CW (1993) E-selectin supports neutrophil rolling *in vitro* under conditions of flow. *J Clin Invest* 92: 2719–2730

27 Suzuki H, Abe K, Shinichiro T, Kimura K, Mizugaki M, Itoyama Y (1998) A change of P-selectin immunoreactivity in rat brain after transient and permanent middle cerebral artery occlusion. *Neurol Res* 20: 463–469

28 Zhang RL, Chopp M, Zhang ZG, Phillips ML, Rosenbloom CL, Cruz R, Manning A (1996) E-selectin in focal cerebral ischemia and reperfusion in the rat. *J Cereb Blood Flow Metab* 16: 1126–1136

29 Wang X, Feuerstein GZ (1995) Induced expression of adhesion molecules following focal brain ischemia. *J Neurotrauma* 12: 825–832

30 Wang X, Yue TL, Barone FC, Feuerstein GZ (1995) Demonstration of increased endothelial-leukocyte adhesion molecule-1 mRNA expression in rat ischemic cortex. *Stroke* 26: 1665–1668; discussion 1668–1669

31 Goussev AV, Zhang Z, Anderson DC, Chopp M (1998) P-selectin antibody reduces hemorrhage and infarct volume resulting from MCA occlusion in the rat. *J Neurol Sci* 161: 16–22

32 Suzuki H, Abe K, Tojo S J, Kitagawa H, Kimura K, Mizugaki M, Itoyama Y (1999) Reduction of ischemic brain injury by anti-P-selectin monoclonal antibody after permanent middle cerebral artery occlusion in rat. *Neurol Res* 21: 269–276

33 Suzuki H, Hayashi T, Tojo S J, Kitagawa H, Kimura K, Mizugaki M, Itoyama Y, Abe K (1999) Anti-P-selectin antibody attenuates rat brain ischemic injury. *Neurosci Lett* 265: 163–166

34 Connolly ES Jr, Winfree CJ, Prestigiacomo CJ, Kim SC, Choudhri TF, Hoh BL, Naka Y, Solomon RA, Pinsky DJ (1997) Exacerbation of cerebral injury in mice that express the P-selectin gene: identification of P-selectin blockade as a new target for the treatment of stroke. *Circ Res* 81: 304–310

35 Soriano SG, Wang YF, Wagner DD, Frenette PS (1999) P- and E-selectin-deficient mice are susceptible to cerebral ischemia-reperfusion injury. *Brain Res* 835: 360–364

36 Lefer DJ, Flynn DM, Phillips ML, Ratcliffe M, Buda AJ (1994) A novel sialyl Lewis' analog attenuates neutrophil accumulation and myocardial necrosis after ischemia and reperfusion. *Circulation* 90: 2390–2401

37 Hynes RO (1992) Integrins: versatility, modulation, and signaling in cell adhesion. *Cell* 69: 11–25

38 Kishimoto TK, Larson RS, Corbi AL, Dustin ML, Staunton DE, Springer TA (1989) The leukocyte integrins. *Adv Immunol* 46: 149–182

39 Chen H, Chopp M, Zhang RL, Bodzin G, Chen Q, Rusche JR, Todd RF 3rd (1994) Anti-CD11b monoclonal antibody reduces ischemic cell damage after transient focal cerebral ischemia in rat. *Ann Neurol* 35: 458–63

40 Chopp M, Zhang RL, Chen H, Li Y, Jiang N, Rusche JR (1994) Postischemic administration of an anti-Mac-1 antibody reduces ischemic cell damage after transient middle cerebral artery occlusion in rats. *Stroke* 25: 869–875; discussion 875–876

41 Yenari MA, Kunis D, Sun GH, Onley D, Watson L, Turner S, Whitaker S, Steinberg GK (1998) Hu23F2G, an antibody recognizing the leukocyte CD11/CD18 integrin, reduces injury in a rabbit model of transient focal cerebral ischemia. *Exp Neurol* 153: 223–233

42 Zhang RL, Zhang ZG, Chopp M (1999) Increased therapeutic efficacy with rt-PA and anti-CD18 antibody treatment of stroke in the rat. *Neurology* 52: 273–279

43 Prestigiacomo CJ, Kim SC, Connolly ES Jr, Liao H, Yan SF, Pinsky DJ (1999) CD18-mediated neutrophil recruitment contributes to the pathogenesis of reperfused but not nonreperfused stroke. *Stroke* 30: 1110–1117

44 Soriano SG, Coxon A, Wang YF, Frosch MP, Lipton SA, Hickey PR, Mayadas TN (1999) Mice deficient in Mac-1 (CD11b/CD18) are less susceptible to cerebral ischemia/reperfusion injury. *Stroke* 30: 134–139

45 Vorcheimer DA, Badimon JJ, Fuster V (1999) Platelet glycoprotein IIb/IIIa receptor antagonists in cardiovascular disease. *JAMA* 281: 1407–1414

46 Ames A, Wright RL, Kowada M, Thurston JM, Majno G (1968) Cerebral ischemia II The no-flow phenomenon. *Am J Pathol* 52: 437–453

47 Choudhri TF, Hoh BL, Zerwes HG, Prestigiacomo CJ, Kim SC, Connolly ES Jr, Kottirsch G, Pinsky DJ (1998) Reduced microvascular thrombosis and improved outcome in acute murine stroke by inhibiting GP IIb/IIIa receptor-mediated platelet aggregation. *J Clin Invest* 102: 1301–1310

48 Abumiya T, Fitridge R, Mazur C, Copeland BR, Koziol JA, Tschopp JF, Pierschbacher MD, Del Zoppo GJ (2000) Integrin alpha(IIb)beta(3) inhibitor preserves microvascular patency in experimental acute focal cerebral ischemia. *Stroke* 31: 1402–1409; discussion 1409–1410

49 Coller BS (1999) Binding of abciximab to alpha V beta 3 and activated alpha M beta 2 receptors: with a review of platelet-leukocyte interactions. *Thromb Haemost* 82: 326–336

50 Dietrich WD, Dewanjee S, Prado R, Watson BD, Dewanjee MK (1993) Transient platelet accumulation in the rat brain after common carotid artery thrombosis. An In-labeled platelet study. *Stroke* 24: 1534–1540

51 Obrenovitch TP, Hallenbeck JM (1985) Platelet accumulation in regions of low blood flow during the postischemic period. *Stroke* 16: 224–234

52 Zhang ZG, Zhang L, Tsang L, Goussev A, Morris DC, Powers C, Smyth S, Coller BS, Chopp M (2001) Dynamic platelet accumulation at the site of the occluded middle cerebral atrtery and in downstream microvessels is associated with loss of microvascular integrity after embolic middle cerebral artery occlusion. *Brain Res; in press*

53 Romanic AM, White RF, Arleth AJ, Obhlstein EH, Barone FC (1998) Matrix metalloproteinase expression increases after cerebral focal ischemia in rats: inhibition of matrix metalloproteinase-9 reduces infarct size. *Stroke* 29: 1020–1030

54 Rosenberg GA, Navratil M, Barone F, Feuerstein GZ (1996) Proteolytic cascade enzymes increase in focal cerebral ischemia in rat. *J Cereb Blood Flow Metab* 16: 360–366

55 Weber C, Springer TA (1997) Neutrophil accumulation on activated, surface-adherent platelets in flow is mediated by interaction of Mac-1 with fibrinogen bound to alphaI-Ibbeta3 and stimulated by platelet-activating factor. *J Clin Invest* 100: 2085–2093

56 Springer TA (1995) Traffic signals on endothelium for lymphocyte recirculation and leukocyte emigration. *Annu Rev Physiol* 57: 827–872

57 Zhang RL, Chopp M, Li Y, Zaloga C, Jiang N, Jones ML, Miyasaka M, Ward PA (1994) Anti-ICAM-1 antibody reduces ischemic cell damage after transient middle cerebral artery occlusion in the rat. *Neurology* 44: 1747–1751

58 Zhang RL, Chopp M, Jiang N, Tang WX, Prostak J, Manning AM, Anderson DC (1995) Anti-intercellular adhesion molecule-1 antibody reduces ischemic cell damage after transient but not permanent middle cerebral artery occlusion in the Wistar rat. *Stroke* 26: 1438–1442; discussion 1443

59 Bowes MP, Zivin JA, Rothlein R (1993) Monoclonal antibody to the ICAM-1 adhesion site reduces neurological damage in a rabbit cerebral embolism stroke model. *Exp Neurol* 119: 215–219

60 Bowes MP, Rothlein R, Fagan SC, Zivin JA (1995) Monoclonal antibodies preventing leukocyte activation reduce experimental neurologic injury and enhance efficacy of thrombolytic therapy. *Neurology* 45: 815–819

61 Clark WM, Madden KP, Rothlein R, Zivin JA (1991) Reduction of central nervous system ischemic injury in rabbits using leukocyte adhesion antibody treatment. *Stroke* 22: 877–883

62 Soriano SG, Lipton SA, Wang YF, Xiao M, Springer TA, Gutierrez-Ramos JC, Hickey PR (1996) Intercellular adhesion molecule-1-deficient mice are less susceptible to cerebral ischemia-reperfusion injury. *Ann Neurol* 39: 618–624

63 Soriano SG, Wang YF, Lipton SA, Dikkes P, Gutierrez-Ramos JC, Hickey PR (1998) ICAM-1 dependent pathway is not involved in the development of neuronal apoptosis after transient focal cerebral ischemia. *Brain Res* 780: 337–341

64 Kitagawa K, Matsumoto M, Mabuchi T, Yagita Y, Ohtsuki T, Hori M, Yanagihara T (1998) Deficiency of intercellular adhesion molecule 1 attenuates microcirculatory dis-

turbance and infarction size in focal cerebral ischemia. *J Cereb Blood Flow Metab* 18: 1336–1345

65   Degraba TJ (1998) The role inflammation after acute stroke Utility of pursuing anti-adhesion molecule therapy. *Neurology* 51: S62–S68

66   Feuerstein GZ, Barone FC (1995) Editorial comment. *Stroke* 26: 1443

67   Zhang RL, Zhang ZG, Chopp M (1999) Thrombolysis with tissue plasminogen activator alters adhesion molecule expression in the ischemic rat brain. *Stroke* 30: 624–629

68   Jiang N, Chopp M, Chahwala S (1998) Neutrophil inhibitory factor treatment of focal cerebral ischemia in the rat. *Brain Res* 788: 25–34

69   Jiang N, Moyle M, Soule HR, Rote WE, Chopp M (1995) Neutrophil inhibitory factor is neuroprotective after focal ischemia in rats. *Ann Neurol* 38: 935–942

70   Yanaka K, Camarata PJ, Spellman SR, Mccarthy JB, Furcht LT, Low WC (1997) Antagonism of leukocyte adherence by synthetic fibronectin peptide V in a rat model of transient focal cerebral ischemia. *Neurosurgery* 40: 557–563; discussion 563–564

71   Yanaka K, Camarata PJ, Spellman SR, Mccarthy JB, Furcht LT, Low WC, Heros RC (1996) Neuronal protection from cerebral ischemia by synthetic fibronectin peptides to leukocyte adhesion molecules. *J Cereb Blood Flow Metab* 16: 1120–1125

72   Yanaka K, Camarata P J, Spellman SR, Mccarthy JB, Furcht LT, Low WC, Heros RC (1996) Synthetic fibronectin peptides and ischemic brain injury after transient middle cerebral artery occlusion in rats. *J Neurosurg* 85: 125–130

73   Yanaka K, Camarata PJ, Spellman SR, Skubitz AP, Furcht LT, Low WC (1997) Laminin peptide ameliorates brain injury by inhibiting leukocyte accumulation in a rat model of transient focal cerebral ischemia. *J Cereb Blood Flow Metab* 17: 605–611

74   Baeuerle PA (1991) The inducible transcription activator, NF-κB: regulation by distinct protein subunits. *Biochim Biophys Acta* 1072: 63–80

75   Collins T (1993) Endothelial nuclear factor-κB and the initiation of the atherosclerotic lesion. *Lab Invest* 68: 499–508

76   Mercurio F, Manning AM (1999) Multiple signals converging on NF-κB. *Curr Opin Cell Biol* 11: 226–232

77   Baeuerle PA (1998) IkappaB-NF-kappaB structures: at the interface of inflammation control. *Cell* 95: 729–731

78   Palmonbella VJ, Rando OJ, Goldberg AL, Maniatis T (1994) The ubiquitin-proteasome pathway is required for processing the NF-κN1 precursor protein and the activation of NF-κB. *Cell* 274: 773–785

79   Carroll JE, Howard EF, Hess DC, Wakade CG, Chen Q, Cheng C (1998) Nuclear factor-kappa B activation during cerebral reperfusion: effect of attenuation with N-acetyl-cysteine treatment. *Brain Res Mol Brain Res* 56: 186–191

80   Gabriel C, Justicia C, Camins A, Planas AM (1999) Activation of nuclear factor-κB in the rat brain after transient focal ischemia. *Mol Brain Res* 65: 61–69

81   Stephenson D, Yin T, Smalstig E B, Hsu M A, Panetta J, Little S, Clemens J (2000) Transcription factor nuclear factor-kappa B is activated in neurons after focal cerebral ischemia. *J Cereb Blood Flow Metab* 20: 592–603

82 Schneider A, Martin-Villalba A, Weih F, Vogel J, Wirth T, Schwaninger M (1999) NF-kappaB is activated and promotes cell death in focal cerebral ischemia. *Nat Med* 5: 554–559

83 Irving EA, Hadingham SJ, Roberts J, Gibbons M, Chabot-Fletcher M, Roshak A, Parsons AA (2000) Decreased nuclear factor-kappaB DNA binding activity following permanent focal cerebral ischaemia in the rat. *Neurosci Lett* 288: 45–48

84 Seegers H, Grillon E, Trioullier Y, Vath A, Verna JM, Blum D (2000) Nuclear factor-kappa B activation in permanent intraluminal focal cerebral ischemia in the rat. *Neurosci Lett* 288: 241–245

85 Phillips JB, Williams AJ, Adams J, Elliott PJ, Tortella FC (2000) Proteasome inhibitor PS519 reduces infarction and attenuates leukocyte infiltration in a rat model of focal cerebral ischemia. *Stroke* 31: 1686–1693

Chronic neuronal perturbation mediated by RAGE, a receptor for β-sheet fibrils and S100/calgranulins

Shi Du Yan, Ann Marie Schmidt and David M. Stern

Departments of Pathology, Surgery, Medicine and Physiology and Cellular Biophysics of Columbia University College of Physicians and Surgeons, 630 West 168th Street, New York, NY 10032, USA

Introduction

Many studies have addressed means through which the vasculature responds to acute stress, such as changes in environmental oxygen concentration in ischemia/reperfusion injury and exposure to toxic bacterial products, while elucidation of mechanisms underlying chronic vascular dysfunction has been more difficult. Although more sustained changes in vascular properties could simply reflect the persistent action of mediators associated with the acute vascular response, such as elaboration of cytokines, there are also likely to be factors related to the chronic disease process which drive pathogenicity. Our current concept of atherogenesis provides an example of this viewpoint [1]. Accumulation of modified lipoproteins in the vessel wall leads to activation of vascular cells, especially endothelium and smooth muscle, causing them to recruit mononuclear phagocytes and lymphocytes to a lesional site which becomes a chronic inflammatory focus [1]. This view suggests the relevance of a two-hit model underlying such chronic vascular processes in which an underlying perturbant, such as modified lipoproteins, provides a first hit which then perpetuates an exaggerated host response to subsequent environmental challenges.

Two types of chronic vascular disease in which pathogenic mechanisms are less clear concern diabetic vasculopathy [2] and amyloid angiopathy [3, 4]. While the salient features of these disease states clearly differentiates them from normal vasculature, namely the presence of hyperglycemia (for diabetes) [2] and deposition of β-sheet fibrils (for amyloid angiopathy) [3, 4], the actual mechanisms leading to persistent vascular cell dysfunction and vasculopathy have not been fully elucidated. In diabetes, while hyperglycemia is transient, and may or may not be accompanied by insulin resistance, accelerated macrovascular disease (atherosclerosis) is persistent suggesting the involvement of factors other than immediate plasma glucose levels. Exposure of aldoses to free amino groups starts the process of nonenzymatic glycoxidation whereby macromolecules in the vessel wall are modified with the initial formation of reversible early glycation endproducts and the later formation of

Inflammation and Stroke, edited by Giora Z. Feuerstein

advanced glycation endproducts (AGEs) [5–8]. The most abundant AGE *in vivo*, (carboxymethyl)lysine adducts [7], accumulates in the tissues and vasculature of patients with diabetes, and is also associated with disorders characterized by sustained oxidant stress, such as renal failure and chronic inflammation. Our studies have led to the recognition of a cell surface receptor (termed RAGE) capable of interacting with AGEs, such as (carboxymethyl)lysine, and mediating their effects on critical cellular targets in the vessel wall and tissues [9–11].

Receptor for advanced glycation endproducts (RAGE) is a multiligand member of the immunoglobulin superfamily of cell surface molecules comprised of an extracellular domain with three immunoglobulin-like regions; one V-type followed by two C-type regions [9, 12]. The N-terminal V-type portion appears to be most critical for interaction with the ligands, especially (carboxymethyl)lysine adducts [11]. There is a single transmembrane spanning domain and a short cytosolic tail, the latter apparently devoid of motifs which suggest how the receptor engages cytosolic signalling mechanisms. However, the importance of this cytosolic tail for RAGE-mediated cellular activation is exemplified by the dominant-negative properties of a variant of the receptor from which the cytosolic portion has been deleted [13, 14]. Although ligand binds to dominant-negative (tail-deleted) and wild-type receptor virtually identically, occupancy of the truncated receptor does not result in cellular activation (phosphorylation of mitogen activated protein kinases, cytokine expression, etc.). Furthermore, expression of tail-deleted RAGE in cells which endogenously express wild-type receptor results in a dominant-negative phenotype; i.e., on subsequent exposure to ligands, RAGE-dependent cellular activation does not occur [13, 14]. Although a comprehensive view of RAGE-dependent activation of signaling pathways remains to be elucidated, a broad engagement of transduction mechanisms occurs; generation of oxidants [15], activation of p21[ras] and phophatidylinositol 3'-kinase [16, 17], and activation of rac and cdc42 [18] have been identified. These more proximal changes lead to phosphorylation of mitogen-activated protein kinases (erk1/2, SAPK and p38) [14], cell migration and elaboration of cellular processes [14, 19–21], nuclear translocation of nuclear factor (NF)-κB [14, 15, 22], and other signaling events. In view of the multitude of pathways activated by engagement of RAGE, it is evident that blocking ligand-receptor interaction is likely to be the most effective means of preventing RAGE-dependent cellular effects. However, it will also be essential to delineate the linker/adapter molecules which couple the signal of ligand occupancy to signaling mechanisms as this might provide another means of blocking RAGE-mediated activation of cellular processes.

RAGE has properties of a multiligand receptor, being able to interact with AGEs (such as [carboxymethyl]lysine adducts) [9, 11], amphoterins [21], members of the S100/calgranulin family [13], and β-sheet fibrils [23, 24]. Though these ligands are clearly diverse with respect to their chemical composition and situations in which they occur in tissues, there must be structural common denominators allowing them to interact with RAGE. This suggests that RAGE may share, at least in biologic terms, features with "pattern receptors", such as those involved in innate immunity [25, 26]. In this context, RAGE and the type A macrophage scavenger receptor (the latter a member of the group of receptors considered to be involved in innate immunity) [27] share ligands, such as AGEs and amyloid fibrils [9, 11, 23, 24, 28, 29]. A key feature of RAGE biology is the induction of receptor expression at sites where ligand is found [30]. For example, although RAGE is present only at low levels in normal vasculature, the deposition of AGEs in diabetes is accompanied by an increase in the expression of RAGE in both endothelium and smooth muscle. In the case of RAGE ligands, such as (carboxymethyl)lysine adducts which activate NF-κB in a receptor-dependent manner [11]), one target of RAGE activation would appear to be two NF-κB sites in the RAGE promoter itself [31]. Thus, one consequence of RAGE-induced cellular activation is upregulation of the receptor potentially initiating a positive feed-back loop in which increased levels of receptor magnify the effects of RAGE ligands by amplifying RAGE-dependent cellular activation.

This overview of RAGE biology provides a basis for considering how RAGE-amyloid interaction may contribute to cellular activation in vasculature and brain parenchyma accompanying amyloidoses such as Alzheimer's disease (AD).

RAGE and the amyloidoses

During the course of studies to analyze mechanisms of chronic vascular perturbation in diabetes (described above), our laboratory also set out to identify a receptor which might mediate the interaction of amyloid with the blood vessel wall. Amyloid angiopathy is another chronic vascular disorder, most frequently associated with AD, but also with other amyloidoses [3, 4, 32]. To our initial surprise, the results of studies in which amyloid-beta peptide (Aβ) was employed as the ligand to screen tissue extracts (especially lung, in view of its rich vasculature) for potential receptors was RAGE (23). The extracellular domain of RAGE interacted with $A\beta_{1-40}$, $A\beta_{1-42}$ and $A\beta_{25-35}$, whether the latter peptides were freshly prepared (and, presumably most in random conformation) or incubated under conditions which promote fibril formation. In contrast, scrambled peptides of the same composition did not bind to RAGE. Further studies [24] have shown that fibrils composed of amyloid A, prion-derived peptide, or amylin also bind to RAGE with a similar affinity as fibrillar Aβ (kDa in the 50–150 nM range) (Fig. 1). In the case of prion-derived peptide or amylin, when these ligands were presented to the receptor in random conformation, no binding occurred [33]. These data suggest that RAGE interacts broadly with β-sheet fibrils. The apparent specificity of this binding is suggested the failure of RAGE to interact with collagen or elastin fibrils, and the lack of RAGE binding to erabutoxin B, a protein with extensive β-sheet structure which does not form fibrils [34]. The greater propensity with which Aβ assembles into fibrillar structures, compared with the other monomers, also appears to be consistent with the hypothesis

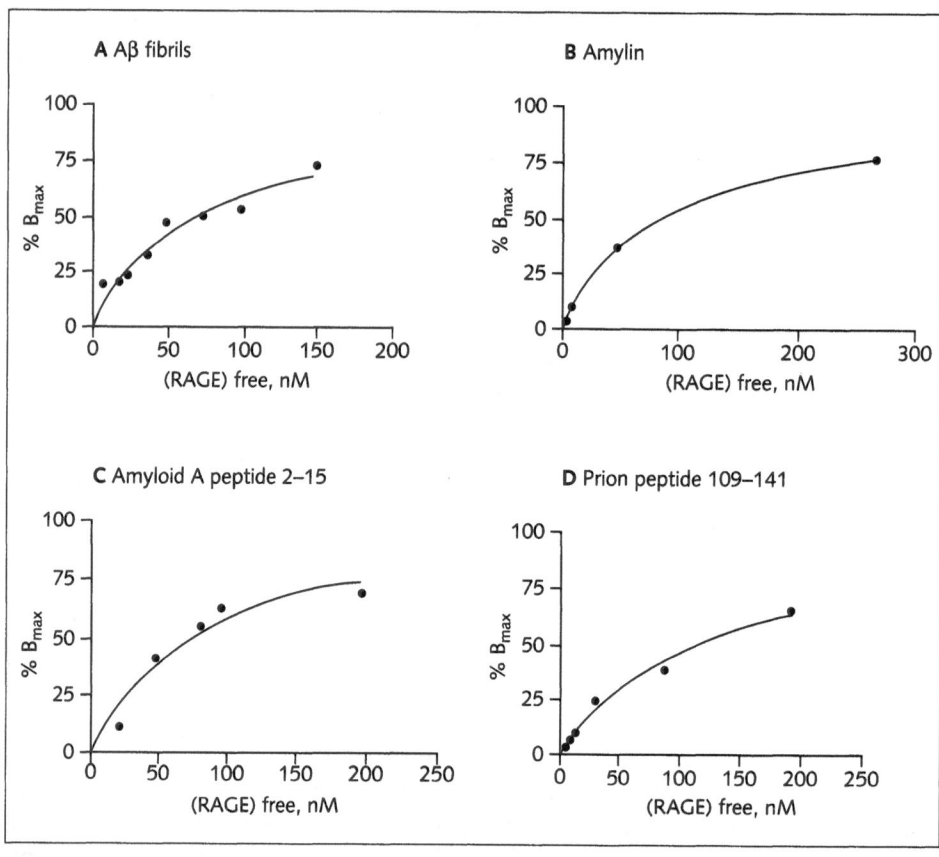

Figure 1

Binding of RAGE to fibrils composed of Aβ, serum amyloid A, amylin and prion derived peptide. Adapted from [24].

that RAGE interacts with fibrils. However, it is difficult to be certain of the structure of ligand actually binding to the receptor, and it could be a small fibril, dimer or multimer of Aβ or other subunits.

Expression of RAGE in the brain follows a biphasic time-course. Early in development, RAGE is expressed at high levels in most neurons [21]. Under these conditions, the brain is rich in amphoterin, another ligand of RAGE, previously identified based on its capacity to induce neurite outgrowth [20, 21, 35]. Transcripts and antigen for amphoterin and RAGE could be colocalized in developing rat brain, consistent with the hypothesis that there might be a physiological interaction of receptor and ligand [21]. As animals mature, RAGE expression decreases dramatically with only occasional neurons and vasculature displaying continued receptor expression

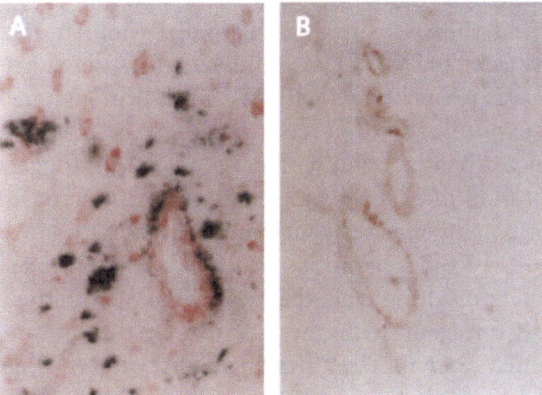

Figure 2

Immunohistochemical analysis of RAGE in vasculature from a patient with AD (A) and an apparently normal age-matched control (B). Samples were immunostained with antibody to RAGE. Similar studies of the same samples with antibody to Aβ showed abundant Aβ in vasculature from the patient with AD, but barely detectable levels in the control sample. Adapted from [23].

[23, 36]. With the occurrence of a disease process involving deposition of RAGE ligand, then receptor expression increases strongly. In AD brain, RAGE is expressed in vasculature rich in Aβ (Fig. 2), as well as in neurons and microglia proximal to plaques [23]. Thus, the brain of patients with AD represents a situation in which the effects of RAGE-mediated cellular activation on Aβ-rich vasculature and brain parenchyma (especially neurons and microglia) can be analyzed.

Using RAGE-bearing PC12 cells as a model system [23], we have found that incubation with nanomolar levels of Aβ (corresponding to those which increase occupancy of the receptor) results in activation of mitogen-activated protein kinases, including erk1/2, and nuclear translocation of NF-κB. These data clearly indicate that RAGE has the ability to transmit and magnify the effects of low concentrations of Aβ on cells, though it is difficult to draw conclusions from such *in vitro* experiments as to whether the outcome will be cytoprotective or cytotoxic. Activation of NF-κB has been observed in AD brain [37], and can be associated with expression of a number of mediators, especially those related to the inflammatory response [38]. For example, we have observed that expression of macrophage-colony stimulating factor (M-CSF) in AD brain can be colocalized, at least in part, with neurons expressing RAGE [39]. In cell culture, the interaction of Aβ with RAGE-bearing neuroblastoma cells resulted in NF-κB-dependent expression of M-CSF. While neurons do not express the receptor for M-CSF (termed c-fms), and, therefore are inert with respect to its biologic effects, microglia respond potently to M-CSF [40, 41].

This cytokine/growth factor has been shown to induce microglial proliferation, migration, differentiation and activation [42, 43]. In addition, when the transformed microglial line of BV-2 cells was preincubated with M-CSF, it demonstrated enhanced viability on subsequent exposure to toxic concentrations of Aβ [39]. These data suggest a scenario in which Aβ interaction with neuronal RAGE triggers a series of events resulting in elaboration of M-CSF and recruitment of microglia. The latter microglia undergo activation and enhanced survival in the vicinity of Aβ deposits, due in part to the effects of M-CSF. In contrast, neurons become increasingly immersed in a hostile environment resulting from the presence of Aβ and toxic products released from microglia. Consistent with these results in cell culture, ELISA of cerebrospinal fluid obtained *post mortem* from patients with AD has demonstrated increased levels of M-CSF [39].

These data suggest that RAGE contributes to Aβ-induced cell stress, at the level of *in vitro* studies and immunohistochemical analysis of AD brain. To gain insight into the possible applicability of this hypothesis *in vivo*, two types of experiments have been designed; studies in a model of systemic amyloidoses [24], where RAGE can be blocked with anti-RAGE antibody fragments (F[ab']$_2$) or by administration of soluble (s) RAGE, and experiments in genetically manipulated mice. Mice treated with a regimen of amyloid enhancing factor (AEF) and silver nitrate (SN) develop amyloid in the spleen over a period of 4–5 days composed of amyloid A [44, 45]. This model has been used to test agents such as sulphonates for their ability to prevent amyloid accumulation [44]. Concomitant with amyloid deposition, activation of NF-κB and expression of target genes (such as heme oxygenase type 1, M-CSF and interleukin (IL)-6) in the spleen has been observed [24]. These results and the relatively brief time frame of these experiments (less than a week) led us to analyze the effects of blocking RAGE by administration of either sRAGE, a truncated form of the receptor comprised of only the ligand binding domain which functions as a decoy to prevent ligands from engaging cell surface RAGE [46], or anti-RAGE F(ab')$_2$. In each case, RAGE blockade suppressed activation of NF-κB and expression of target genes in the spleen and accumulation of amyloid (note that the high levels of amyloid A in the plasma of AEF/SN treated animals was not affected by either regimen of RAGE blockade) [24]. Controls, for example animals treated with nonimmune F(ab')$_2$, did not show a similar effect. Immunoprecipitation of sRAGE from the plasma of animals treated with AEF/SN demonstrated the presence of complexes of soluble receptor with amyloid A [24]. The latter included immunoreactive species of serum amyloid A migrating at ≈9 and ≈14 kDa. The truncated form of amyloid A (9 kDa) is associated with cleavage of the intact molecule (14 kDa) in the tissues at the site of amyloid deposition. The results of these studies are consistent with the concept that RAGE interaction with amyloid A contributes both to amyloid deposition and amyloid-induced cellular perturbation *in vivo*.

Experiments are now underway to test the contribution of RAGE to Aβ-induced cellular perturbation in the context of the brain. For these studies, expression of

RAGE will be modulated employing genetically manipulated mice. For example, full-length or dominant-negative RAGE can be upregulated in neurons using the platelet-derived growth factor B-chain promoter [47]. Furthermore, homozygous RAGE null mice are devoid of the receptor in all cell types. Crossbreeding of these mice with animals overexpressing a mutant form of amyloid precursor protein (APP) associated with familial AD and increased production of Aβ provides a model system with genetically altered RAGE expression in an Aβ-rich environment. Our first preliminary studies have used mice with targeted overexpression of full-length RAGE in neurons and transgenic mice with a mutant hAPP transgene [48]. Double transgenic mice, overexpressing both RAGE and mutant hAPP displayed enhanced activation of NF-κB, as well as expression of M-CSF and IL-6 by 3–5 months of age. Furthermore, immunoreactivity of synaptophysin and microtubule-associated protein 2, associated with the density of synapses and dendrites, respectively, was suppressed in double transgenic mice compared with single transgenics and nontransgenic littermate controls [48]. These pilot data are consistent with the hypothesis that RAGE contributes to Aβ-induced cell stress *in vivo*, though firm conclusions must await the completion of studies with the different types of mice with genetically manipulated RAGE expression described above.

RAGE and the S100/calgranulins

It seemed unlikely that a receptor would have evolved solely to interact with ligands such as AGEs and amyloid. Thus, our group set out to identify endogenous ligands of RAGE. In view of the high levels of RAGE expression in the lung, this tissue seemed to be a logical starting point for isolation of endogenous ligands. Two polypeptides were identified based on screening tissue extracts and, subsequently, chromatographic fractions for RAGE binding activity; a member of the S100/calgranulin family termed EN-RAGE (also known as S100A12) [13] and amphoterin [21]. The identification of amphoterin as promoter of neurite outgrowth expressed especially early in development has been mentioned above. More recently, amphoterin has also been proposed as a late mediator of endotoxin-induced toxicity [49].

S100/calgranulins comprise a family of about 15 closely related polypeptides that have been associated with a range of acute and chronic inflammatory processes [50]. Our studies have demonstrated that RAGE serves as a receptor for S100/calgranulins on endothelium, macrophages and lymphocytes [13]. In view of the expression of S100/calgranulins in Alzheimer's disease [51] and other chronic disorders [50], it is possible that several RAGE ligands might coexist in tissues simultaneously. For example, β-sheet fibrils and S100/calgranulins in AD, and AGEs and S100/calgranulins in diabetic vasculature. In such a situation, the effects of receptor engagement by one ligand might be reinforced and magnified by interaction with a second ligand.

Consequences of RAGE binding to S100/calgranulins have been shown in models of inflammation. For example, in delayed-type hypersensitivity induced in mice by methylated albumin, blockade of RAGE suppressed recruitment of inflammatory cells and tissue swelling [13]. Inhibition of RAGE-ligand interaction prevented activation of NF-κB in the footpads of mice subject to the delayed-type hypersensitivity protocol, as well as expression of tumor necrosis factor-α and IL-2. These observations suggest that blocking RAGE interaction with its ligands suppresses the inflammatory response at an early stage (at the level of expression of proinflammatory mediators, prior to the occurrence of actual tissue damage). Consistent with this view, colitis in IL-10 null mice was also inhibited by administration of sRAGE; in parallel, the influx of inflammatory cells, NF-κB activation and levels of tumor necrosis factor-alpha in serum were blocked by administration of the soluble receptor [13].

Experiments are in progress to determine the mechanism through which interception of RAGE-ligand interaction suppresses the ongoing inflammatory response. While it is likely that S100/calgranulins are the ligands most relevant in these situations, further studies will be required to determine whether other RAGE ligands are also present. The power of these mechanisms is emphasized by our recent preliminary studies indicating that blockade of RAGE can also inhibit collagen-induced arthritis.

Hypothesis

Based on the data presented above, we propose that RAGE is a receptor which propagates cell stress in a range of pathophysiologically relevant situations. By functioning as a multiligand receptor capable of interacting with species as diverse as AGEs, β-sheet fibrils and S100/calgranulins, RAGE promotes and maintains cellular activation functioning as a "first hit" in a two-hit model of cellular dysfunction. The "second hit" is the cellular response to ischemic, inflammatory (as reflected by an intercurrent infection) or atherogenic (accumulation of modified lipoproteins) stimuli. In the presence of underlying RAGE-mediated cellular activation, the "second hit" causes exaggerated cellular responses promoting tissue destruction rather than restitution of homeostasis. Although further experiments will be required to prove the validity of this hypothesis in different *in vivo* models, our findings, thus far, suggest that RAGE may be a therapeutic target in a wide spectrum of disorders.

Acknowledgements
This work was supported by grants from the USPHS, Juvenile Diabetes Foundation, Burroughs Wellcome Trust, and the Surgical Research Fund.

References

1   Ross R (1999) Atherosclerosis – an inflammatory disease. *New Engl J Med* 340: 115–126

2   King G, Brownlee M (1996) The cellular and molecular mechanisms of diabetic complications. *Endocrin Metabol Clin N Am* 25: 255–270

3   Glenner GG, Henry JH, Fujiwara S (1981) Congophilic angiopathy in the pathogenesis of Alzheimer's degeneration. *Ann Pathol* 1: 120–129

4   Ghiso J, Wisniewski T, Frangione B (1994) Unifying features of systemic and cerebral amyloidosis. *Molec Neurobiol* 8: 49–63

5   Brownlee M (1995) Advanced glycosylation in diabetes and aging. *Ann Rev Med* 46: 223–234

6   Dyer D, Dunn J, Thorpe S, Bailie K, Lyons T, McCance D, Baynes J (1993) Accumulation of Maillard products in skin collagen in diabetes and aging. *J Clin Invest* 91: 2463–2469

7   Reddy S, Bichler J, Wells Knecht K, Thorpe S, Baynes J (1995) Carboxymethyllysine is a dominant AGE antigen in tissue proteins. *Biochem* 34: 10872–10878

8   Grandhee S, Monnier VM (1991) Mechanisms of formation of the Maillard protein crosslink pentosidine: ribose, glucose, fructose and ascorbate as pentosidine precursors. *J Biol Chem* 266: 11649–11653

9   Schmidt AM, Vianna M, Gerlach M, Brett J, Ryan J, Kao J, Esposito C, Hegarty H, Hurley W, Clauss M et al (1992) Isolation and characterization of binding proteins for advanced glycosylation endproducts from lung tissue which are present on the endothelial cell surface. *J Biol Chem* 267: 14987–14997

10 Schmidt AM, Hori O, Brett J, Yan SD, Wautier JL, Stern DM (1994) Cellular receptors for AGEs. *Arterioscler Thromb* 14: 1521–1528

11 Kislinger T, Fu C, Qu W, Yan S-D, Hofmann M, Yan S-F, Pischetsrieder M, Stern D, Schmidt AM (1999) N(epsilon)-(carboxymethyl)lysine adducts of proteins are ligands for RAGE that activate cell signalling pathways and modulate gene expression. *J Biol Chem* 274: 31740–31749

12 Neeper M, Schmidt AM, Brett J, Yan SD, Wang F, Pan YC, Elliston K, Stern DM, Shaw A (1992) Cloning and expression of RAGE: a cell surface receptor for advanced glycosylation end products of proteins. *J Biol Chem* 267: 14998–15004

13 Hofmann M, Drury S, Caifeng F, Qu W, Lu Y, Avila C, Kambhan N, Slattery T, McClary J, Nagashima M et al (1999) RAGE mediates a novel proinflammatory axis: the cell surface receptor for S100/calgranulin polypeptides. *Cell* 97: 889–901

14 Taguchi A, DelToro G, Canet A, Lee D, Tanji N, Lu Y, Ingram M, Lalla E, Hofmann M, Fu J et al (2000) Blockade of RAGE/amphoterin suppresses tumor growth and metastases. *Nature* 405: 354–360

15 Yan SD, Schmidt AM, Anderson GM, Zhang J, Brett J, Zou YS, Pinsky D, Stern D (1994) Enhanced cellular oxidant stress by the interaction of AGEs with their receptors/binding proteins. *J Biol Chem* 269: 9889–9897

16 Lander H, Tauras J, Ogiste J, Moss R, Schmidt AM (1997) Activation of RAGE triggers a MAP kinase pathway regulated by oxidant stress. *J Biol Chem* 272: 17810–17814

17 Deora A, Win T, Vanhaesebroeck B, Lander H (1998) A redox-triggered Ras-effector interaction: recruitment of phosphatidylinositol 3'-kinase to Ras by redox stress. *J Biol Chem* 273: 29923–29928

18 Huttunen H, Fages C, Rauvala H (1999) RAGE-mediated neurite outgrowth and activation of NF-kB require the cytoplasmic domain of the receptor but different downstream signaling pathways. *J Biol Chem* 274: 19919–19924

19 Schmidt AM, Yan S-D, Brett J, Mora R, Nowygrod R, Stern DM (1993) Regulation of human mononuclear phagocyte migration by cell surface binding proteins for AGEs. *J Clin Invest* 91: 2155–2168

20 Rauvala H, Merenmies J, Pihlaskari R, Korkolainen M, Huhtala J, Panula P (1987) The adhesive and neurite-promoting molecule p30: analysis of the amino terminal sequence and production of antipeptide antibodies that detect p30 at the surface of neuroblastoma cells and of brain neurons. *J Cell Biol* 107: 2293–2305

21 Hori O, Brett J, Nagashima M, Nitecki D, Morser J, Stern DM, Schmidt AM (1995) RAGE is a cellular binding site for amphoterin: mediation of neurite outgrowth and co-expression of RAGE and amphoterin in the developing nervous system. *J Biol Chem* 270: 25752–25761

22 Schmidt A-M, Hori O, Chen J-X, Li J-F, Crandall J, Zhang J, Cao R, Yan S-D, Brett J, Stern D (1995) Advanced glycation endproducts interacting with their endothelial receptor induce expression of VCAM-1 in cultured human endothelial cells and in mice. *J Clin Invest* 96: 1395–1403

23 Yan S-D, Chen X, Chen M, Zhu H, Roher A, Slattery T, Zhao L, Nagashima M, Morser J, Migheli A et al (1996) RAGE and amyloid-beta peptide neurotoxicity in Alzheimer's disease. *Nature* 382: 685–691

24 Yan S-D, Zhu H, Zhu A, Golabek A, Roher A, Yuv, Soto C, Schmidt A-M, Stern DM, Kindy M (2000) Receptor-dependent cell stress and amyloid accumulation in systemic amyloidosis. *Nat Med* 6: 643–651

25 Krieger M, Abrams J, Lux A, Steller H (1957) Molecular flypaper, atherosclerosis, and host defense: structure and function of the macrophage scavenger receptor. *Cold Spring Harb Symp Quant Biol* 57: 605–609

26 Platt N, da Silva R, Gordon S (1998) Recognizing death: the phagocytosis of apoptotic cells. *Trends Cell Biol* 8: 365–372

27 Krieger M, Herz J (1994) Structures and functions of multiligand lipoprotein receptors: macrophage scavenger receptors and LDL receptor-related protein. *Ann Rev Biochem* 63: 601–637

28 Khoury J, Thomas C, Loike J, Hickman S, Cao L, Silverstein S (1994) Macrophages adhere to glucose-modified basement membrane *via* their scavenger receptors. *J Biol Chem* 269: 10197–10200

29 El Khoury J, Hickman S, Thomas C, Cao L, Silverstein S, Loike J (1996) Scavenger receptor-mediated adhesion of microglia to beta-amyloid fibrils. *Nature* 382: 716–719

30   Schmidt A-M, Yan S-D, Stern DM (1995) The dark side of glucose. *Nature Med* 1: 1002–1004

31   Li J, Schmidt A-M (1997) Characterization and functional analysis of the promoter of RAGE. *J Biol Chem* 272: 16498–16506

32   Castano EM, Prelli F, Soto C, Beavis R, Matsubara E, Shoji M, Frangione B (1987) The length of amyloid-beta in hereditary cerebral hemorrhage with amyloidosis, Dutch type. *Proc Natl Acad Sci USA* 84: 5991–5994

33   Sell D, Monnier VM (1989. Structure elucidation of senescence cross-link from human extracellular matrix: implication of pentoses in the aging process. *J Biol Chem* 264: 21597–21602

34   Kimball M, Sato A, Richardson J, Rosen L, Low B (1979) Molecular conformation of erabutoxin b: atomic coordinates at 2.5 A resolution. *Biochem Biophys Res Comm* 88: 950–956

35   Rauvala H, Pihlaskari R (1987) Isolation and some characteristics of an adhesive factor of brain that enhances neurite outgrowth in central neurons. *J Biol Chem* 262: 16625–16635

36   Brett J, Schmidt A-M, Zou Y-S, Yan S-D, Weidman E, Pinsky DJ, Neeper M, Przysiecki M, Shaw A, Migheli A, Stern DM (1993) Tissue distribution of the receptor for advanced glycation endproducts (RAGE): expression in smooth muscle,cardiac myocytes,and neural tissue in addition to vasculature. *Am J Pathol* 143: 1699–1712

37   Yan S-D, Yan S-F, Chen X, Fu J, Chen M, Kuppusamy P, Smith M, Perry G, Godman G, Nawroth P et al (1995) Nonenzymatically glycated tau in Alzheimerís disease induces neuronal oxidant stress resulting in cytokine gene expression and release of amyloid beta-peptide. *Nature Med* 1: 693–699

38   Lendard M, Baltimore D (1988) NF-κB: a pleiotropic mediator of inducible and tissue-specific gene control. *Cell* 58: 227–229

39   Yan SD, Zhu H, Fu J, Yan S-F, Roher A, Tourtellotte WW, Rajavashisth T, Chen X, Godman GC, Stern D, Schmidt AM (1997) Amyloid beta peptide-receptor for advanced glycation endproduct interaction elicits neuronal expression of macrophage-colony stimulating factor: a proinflammatory pathway in Alzheimer disease. *Proc Natl Acad Sci USA* 94: 5296–5301

40   Hume D, Yue X, Ross I, Favot P, Lichanska A, Ostrowski M (1997) Regulation of CSF-1 receptor expression. *Mol Reprod Dev* 46: 46–52

41   Hamilton J (1997) CSF-1 signal transduction. *J Leukoc Biol* 62: 145–155

42   Stanley E, Berg K, Einstein D, Lee P, Pixley F, Wang Y, Yeung Y (1997) Biology and action of colony stimulating factor-1. *Mol Reprod Dev* 46: 4–10

43   Fixe P, Praloran V (1998) M-CSF: haematopoietic growth factor or inflammatory cytokine? *Cyto* 10: 32–37

44   Kisilevsky R, Lemieux J, Fraser P, Kong X, Hultin P, Szarek W (1995) Arresting amyloidosis *in vivo* using small molecule anionic sulphonates or sulphates: implications for Alzheimer's disease. *Nature Med* 1: 143–148

45 Kindy M, Rader D (1998) Reduction in amyloid A amyloid formation in apolipoprotein-E-deficient mice. *Am J Pathol* 152: 1387–1395

46 Park L, Raman K, Lee K, Lu Y, Ferran L, Chow W-S, Stern D, Schmidt A-M (1998) Suppression of accelerated diabetic atherosclerosis by sRAGE. *Nat Med* 4: 1025–1031

47 Sasahara M, Fries J, Raines E, Gown A, Westrum L, Frosch M, Bonthron D, Ross R, Collins T (1991) PDGF B-chain in neurons of the central nervous system, posterior pituitary and in a transgenic model. *Cell* 64: 217–227

48 Stern D, Zhu Y, Zhu A, Du H, Schmidt A, Yan S-D (2000) Enhanced neuronal stress in double transgenic mice with targeted overexpression of RAGE and mutant APP. *Soc Neurosci (Abstr.)* Part I: 1319

49 Wang H, Bloom O, Zhang M, Vishnubhakat J, Ombrellino M, Che J, Frazier A, Yang H, Ivanova S, Borokikova L et al (1999) HMG1 as a late mediator of endotoxin lethality in mice. *Science* 285: 248–251

50 Schafer B, Heizmann C (1996) The S100 family of EF-hand calcium-binding proteins: functions and pathology. *TIBS* 21: 134–140

51 Sheng J, Mrak R, Rovnaghi C, Kozlowska E, Van Eldik L, Griffin W (1996) Human brain S100 beta and S100 beta mRNA expression increases with age: pathogenic implications for Alzheimer's disease. *Neurobiol Aging* 17: 359–363

Mediators of inflammation and blood-brain barrier permeability in cerebral ischemia

Danica B. Stanimirovic

Institute for Biological Sciences, National Research Council of Canada, Montreal Road Campus, Bldg. M-54, Ottawa, ON, K1A 0R6, Canada

Secondary ischemic brain damage

Secondary brain damage is tissue injury that is not apparent immediately after an insult, but develops after a delay of hours or days and has typically been observed after ischemia, trauma or subarachnoidal haemorrhage [1]. Secondary ischemic brain damage develops as a consequence of: (a) brain edema, (b) post-ischemic microvascular stasis and vasomotor/hemodynamic deficits leading to hypoperfusion, and (c) post-ischemic inflammation involving activation of microglia and brain infiltration of peripheral inflammatory cells [1–3]. It is believed that damage to the tissues surrounding the ischemic core, known as the penumbra, can be reduced by therapeutic measures designed to prevent or minimize molecular events contributing to the development of secondary brain damage [3].

Cerebral endothelial cells (CEC) play a pivotal role in orchestrating events involved in the development of secondary brain damage. CEC have distinct morphological and functional properties that are essential for maintaining strict control over the exchange of water and nutrients between blood and brain; this function of CEC is known as the blood-brain barrier (BBB) [4]. CEC also restrict immune interactions of peripheral blood cells with brain cells, and secrete an array of mediators involved in vasomotor, metabolic and BBB permeability changes in the cerebral microvascular bed [5, 6].

Inflammatory mediators of blood-brain barrier opening

Nosologically, brain edema has been divided into cytotoxic and vasogenic edema. However, both components are functionally linked and jointly contribute to the phasic disruption of the BBB seen in cerebral ischemia [2]. During the onset of ischemic brain edema, the BBB undergoes morphological reorganization including the opening of tight junctions and changes in endothelial cell membrane fluidity [2]. Whereas in the ischemic core the BBB is disintegrated due to the necrotic death of endothelial cells and tissue in general, vasogenic edema in the penumbra is the result

Inflammation and Stroke, edited by Giora Z. Feuerstein

of biochemical opening of the BBB, involving mediators released by both parenchymal and endothelial cells, or produced by polymorphonuclear leukocytes (PMNs) (Tab. 1). Ischemic brain edema can be viewed as an integral part of the ischemic inflammation as many ischemic inflammatory mediators are also capable of increasing the BBB permeability [5, 6].

Cytokines

During cerebral ischemia, inflammatory cytokines are released by various cell types, including microglia, astroglia and CEC [5]. Cytokines IL-1β and TNFα have been shown to induce both adhesion molecules, including ICAM-1, VCAM-1 and E-selectin in human CEC [5, 7] and neutrophil adhesion to CEC monolayers [7]. Cytokines have also been shown to influence the transport of compounds into the brain by opening the BBB [6, 8]. *In vitro* studies have shown that the tightness of CEC monolayers is decreased by TNFα, IL-1 and IL-6 [6, 8]. *In vivo* studies demonstrated enhanced uptake of albumin, and increased number of leukocytes in the CSF after intracisternal or intracerebroventricular injections of TNFα or IL-1β [9, 10].

Transmitters

Serotonin

A correlation between 5-HT accumulation, inhibition of Na-K-ATPase, and brain water content has been observed during brain ischemia [11]. In addition, substances that inhibit 5-HT synthesis or release were shown to reduce ischemic brain swelling [11]. In addition to depolarization-triggered neuronal relase, 5-HT is also released from serotonergic vascular nerves, platelets, endothelium and mast cells [12], i.e., cellular components either present in or involved in the formation of vascular clots. Human CEC have been shown to express $h5-HT_{1D}$ and $5-HT_7$ receptors linked to cAMP production [13], and are likely targets and effectors of microvascular responses to 5-HT, including BBB permeability.

Histamine

Histamine is vasodilator of cerebral microvessels and has been shown to increase transendothelial transport and BBB permeability *in vitro* and *in vivo* [14]. Histamine-induced BBB permeabilization appears to be mediated *via* H_2 receptors coupled to cAMP production in CEC [14, 15]. Histamine is also readily released from aggregated platelets and can induce endothelial permeability, the expression of E- and P-selectins, and neutrophil rolling [14] by acting from the luminal side of vessels during ischemia.

Table 1 - Inflammatory mediators reported to increase blood-brain barrier permeability

Arachidonic acid and metabolites	Arachidonic acid, leukotriene C_4, prostaglandins, platelet activating factor
Cytokines	Interleukins (IL-1α, IL-1β, IL-2), tumor necrosis factor α, chemokines (interleukin-8), macrophage inflammatory proteins (MIP-1, MIP-2)
Transmitters	Histamine, 5-hydroxytriptamine (5-HT)
Peptides	Bradykinin, calcitonin gene related peptide (CGRP), endothelins
Neutrophil-derived mediators	Free radicals, leukotrienes, metalloproteinases (gelatinase-B), elastases

Peptides

Bradykinin is a member of the kalikrein-kinin system and has been shown to induce permeabilization of CEC monolayers in *in vitro* BBB models [6], as well as extravasation of sodium fluorescein after cortical superfusion *in vivo* [15]. Subsequent studies implicated signaling responses elicited *via* B_2 receptor, including activation of phospholipase A_2, release of arachidonic acid and production of free radicals in causing BBB permeabilization [6, 15]. Bradykinin is upregulated in the ischemic brain tissue and the B_2 receptor antagonist, HOE 140, was shown to partially reduce ischemia-induced BBB opening [15].

Endothelins

Endothelins are potent vasoactive peptides that can also act as modulators of CEC permeability and inflammatory phenotype [16]. We have shown that ET-1 can promote inflammatory responses in human CEC including the upregulation of ICAM-1, VCAM-1 and E-selectin expression [16] and the stimulation of arachidonic acid and prostaglandin release [16, 17]. These events are mediated *via* ET_A-triggered signaling pathway(s) and have been shown to increase CEC permeability *in vitro* [16]. Interestingly, the anti-inflammatory glucocorticoid dexamethasone, often used in clinical practice to alleviate brain edema, was able to suppress ET-1-induced inflammatory responses in human CEC by downregulating ET_A receptor expression [17].

CGRP

Recently, we have shown that human CEC express receptors for calcitonin gene-related peptide (CGRP) and adrenomedullin [18], the peptides shown to be induced in ischemic brain. CGRP has long been considered an immunomodulatory peptide in peripheral tissues where it has been shown to stimulate the expression and release of chemokine IL-8 and prostaglandins, and to cause plasma extravasation [19]. Although immunomodulatory function of CGRP in the brain remains to be confirmed, we have recently reported that CGRP increases the permeability of the *in vitro* BBB model [20].

Neutrophil-dependent opening of the blood-brain barrier

In addition to soluble mediators produced in brain parenchyma and microvascular compartment during ischemic inflammation, neutrophil-mediated endothelial cytotoxicity is now believed to be a key player in the ischemic BBB disruption (Fig. 1).

Leukocytes are selectively recruited into the ischemic brain *via* complex interactions with CEC mediated by adhesion molecules [21]. Mediators produced in ischemic brain, including cytokines, neuropeptides, and free redicals [5, 16, 22], and *in vitro* hypoxia [5, 6] have been shown to induce or upregulate the expression of adhesion molecules in human CEC [5, 16, 22]. Oxygen-glucose deprivation (OGD)-induced upregulation of ICAM-1 in human CEC [5, 6] causes avid ICAM-1/CD18-dependent adhesion of freshly isolated human neutrophils to CEC [6].

However, the molecular events that follow neutrophil-CEC adhesion and lead to the commonly observed transient opening of the BBB and subsequent neutrophil transmigration into the brain are poorly understood. Several putative mediators released by activated neutrophils including free radicals, metalloproteinases, and eicosanoids have been implicated in CEC injury, disruption of the basement membrane and transient permeabilization of the BBB.

Free radicals

Neutrophils activated with agonists that stimulate oxidative burst, such as phorbol ester, have been shown to damage and kill endothelial cell monolayers [23]. On the other hand, neutrophil adhesion to endothelial cells is a potent inducer of neutrophil oxidative burst [23] and antibodies against adhesion molecules were also shown to prevent endothelial cell damage by neutrophils [23]. Activated neutrophils interacting with peripheral microvascular endothelial cells have been shown to release elastase that converts endothelial xanthine dehydrogenase into xanthine oxidase, leading to the intra-endothelial generation of superoxide radicals [23].

Oxygen radicals have been shown to alter the reactivity of cerebral vessels to physiological regulators and to increase permeability of the BBB for micro- and macromolecules *in vitro* and *in vivo* [2, 15]. Lipid-dependent, membrane attached enzymes rich in thiol groups, such as the ionic pump Na,K-ATPase are prime targets for free radicals. Na,K-ATPase is distributed predominantly on the abluminal

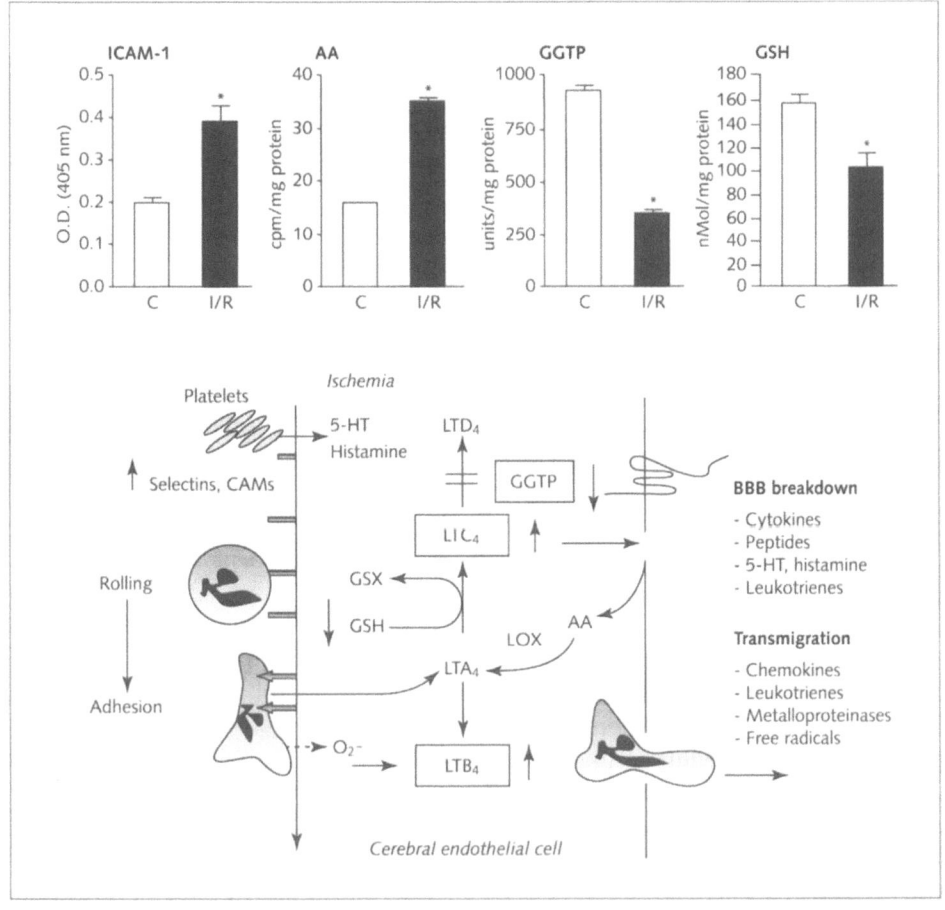

Figure 1
A model of molecular mechanisms/events involved in the blood-brain barrier (BBB) break-down and neutrophil infiltration (i.e., rolling, adhesion, transmigration) into the brain during stroke.

side of the cerebral endothelium [4] and is critically involved in water and ion exchange at the BBB. Free radicals have been shown to inhibit Na,K-ATPase in isolated cerebral microvessels and in CEC *in vitro* [28]. Free radical-mediated loss of sodium pump activity is caused by lipid peroxidation of CEC membranes and is followed by increased "leakiness" of CEC monolayers for small molecules [28].

Hypoxia makes endothelial cells vulnerable to free radicals by exhausting endogenous endothelial anti-oxidative defenses. We found that *in vitro* OGD significantly depletes reduced glutathione (GSH) and increases the activity of the peroxide quenching enzymes, glutathione peroxidase (GPHx) and glutathione S-transferase (GST) in human CEC [29]. Decreased GSH levels have been shown to increase the sensitivity of immortalized CEC to oxidants [26]. Interestingly, redox imbalance in endothelial cells has also been shown to facilitate neutrophil-endothelial cell adhesion by up-regulating expression of endothelial adhesion molecules [27].

Leukotrienes

Leukotrienes (LTs) are bioactive pro-inflammatory compounds generated by the 5-lipoxygenation of arachidonic acid. Arachidonic acid is released from brain phospholipids during ischemia and is a major source of free radicals and mediators of BBB disruption [15]. The first product of the leukotriene cascade, LTA_4, is either enzymatically hydrolyzed to a potent neutrophil chemoattractant, LTB_4, or is conjugated with GSH to yield inflammatory and permeabilizing LTC_4 [28]. The breakdown of LTC_4 into LTD_4 is catalyzed by γ-glutamyl-transpeptidase (GGTP), an enzyme selectively enriched in CEC [29].

Neutrophils are enriched in 5-lipoxygenase, a key enzyme of leukotriene biosynthetic pathway. On the other hand, CEC appear to lack 5-lipoxygenase, since they are not capable of producing LTA_4 from arachidonic acid [30]. However, it has been shown that neutrophils and endothelial cells when placed in close proximity *in vitro* can initiate a transcellular leukotriene biosynthetic pathway [31]. Activated neutrophils adhering to endothelial cells release LTA_4 which is then "taken up" and converted into LTC_4 by endothelial cells and platelets, but not by fibroblasts or smooth muscle cells [31]. In peripheral tissues, LTC_4 produced by these interactions will act as a permeabilizing agent causing plasma leakage and neutrophil migration. However, the role of leukotrienes in mediating BBB permeability and brain edema is still controversial. A correlation between LTC_4 content and BBB breakdown has been shown in human brain tumors [32] and increases in BBB permeability were observed when low doses of LTC_4 were administered after focal cerebral ischemia [33], but not in normal brain tissues, suggesting that leukotrienes act as mediators of BBB opening only in the presence of other condition(s) injurious to the BBB.

Two perturbations imparted to CEC by hypoxia, oxidative stress and the depletion of the enzymatic barrier against leukotrienes, GGTP, have been shown to increase CEC vulnerability to permeabilizing actions of LTC_4 [25]. OGD followed by reoxygenation depletes GGTP activity in human CEC by 70–80% [25]. In parallel, LTC_4 increases the permability of *in vitro* BBB model only when GGTP activity of CEC is reduced by the inhibitor acivicin or by the OGD [25].

LTB_4 is a potent PMN chemotaxin that also induces neutrophils to degranulate, generate superoxide, and adhere to vascular endothelium [28]. Therefore, the leukotriene cascade triggered by CEC/neutrophil adhesion during ischemia can generate compounds which simultaneously act to permeabilize endothelial cells (LTC$_4$, free radicals), facilitate neutrophil chemotaxis (LTB$_4$), and maintain the adhesion process by re-inducing adhesion molecule expression and neutrophil activation (LTC$_4$, LTB$_4$).

Neutrophil transmigration

A transient breakdown of the BBB that follows neutrophil/CEC adhesion is necessary but not sufficient to cause neutrophil transmigration across the BBB. Chemoattractant stimuli are essential for directional movement of neutrophils to the site of injury [34, 35].

Chemokines are a family of 8–12 kDa peptides that mediate selective leukocyte recruitment at inflammation sites [34]. Increased levels of monocyte chemoattracting protein-1 (MCP-1), macrophage inflammatory protein-1 (MIP-1) and IL-8 have been detected in the ischemic brain [35], and systemic administration of anti-IL-8 antibody has been shown to reduce cerebral edema, BBB permeability, and infarct size in experimental models of stroke [36]. Both human CEC and human astrocytes upregulate and secrete IL-8, MCP-1, and other neutrophil chemoattractants when exposed to IL-1β or OGD [37]. IL-8 is the principal neutrophil chemoattractant released by hypoxic human CEC since neutrophil chemotaxis induced by hypoxic CEC-conditioned media is prevented by IL-8 blocking antibody [37].

Neutrophil chemotaxis across the BBB also requires the disruption of the CEC basement membrane and movement through the extracellular matrix (ECM) of brain tissue. A part of this process is thought to be mediated by a group of enzymes known as matrix metalloproteinases (MMPs). MMPs are a gene family of zinc and calcium-dependent endopeptidases that cleave components of the ECM [38]. Gelatinase A (MMP-2) and gelatinase B (MMP-9), also known as type IV collagenases, degrade essential components of the CEC basement membrane, type IV collagen, fibronectin, and gelatin. MMP-2 and MMP-9 have been implicated in neurological disorders associated with the disruption of the BBB [38]. Both neutrophils and endothelial cells have been shown to express and store various MMPs [38]. Degranulation of preformed neutrophil gelatinase B is rapidly (< 30 min) induced by IL-8 or other CXC chemokines [39]. Moreover, soluble factors released from neutrophils have been shown to activate endothelial cell MMP-2 [39].

It has been observed that the ECM microenvironment itself elicits remarkable changes in leukocyte molecular make-up and behavior as cells adhere to and migrate across endothelial barrier [21]. In parallel, leukocyte migration effects a profound endothelial tissue remodeling. Redistribution and then a loss of the tight junction proteins occludin and zonnula occludens-1 from CEC have been shown *in vivo* during neutrophil-induced BBB breakdown [40]. Adherent neutrophils have been shown to induce endothelial calcium transients resulting in the activation of endothelial contractile apparatus and paracellular gap formation [41]. Intraendothelial signaling elicited by neutrophil adhesion then modulates endothelial VE-cadherin/catenin complexes in a locally restricted fashion to loosen the barrier [41].

It is clear that rather than being a passive target for neutrophil-mediated toxicity, ischemic CEC play an active and in many cases decisive role in first capturing circulating leukocytes and then establishing functional communications between the two cell types that allows neutrophils to access the brain (Fig. 1). The common consequences of these interactions are the BBB disruption and the development of brain edema and inflammation.

References

1 Siesjo BK, Siesjo P (1996) Mechanisms of secondary brain injury. *Eur J Anaesth* 13: 247–268

2 Rosenberg GA (1999) Ischemic brain edema. *Prog Cardiovasc Dis* 42: 209–216

3 Feuerstein GZ, Wang X, Barone FC (1997) Inflammatory gene expression in cerebral ischemia and trauma. Potential new therapeutic targets. *Ann NY Acad Sci* 825: 179–193

4 Betz AL, Firth JA, Goldstein GW (1980) Polarity of the blood brain barrier: distribution of enzymes between luminal and antiluminal membranes of brain capillary endothelial cells. *Brain Res* 192: 17–28

5 Stanimirovic D and Satoh K (2000) Inflammatory mediators of cerebral endothelium: A role in ischemic brain inflammation. *Brain Pathology* 10: 113–126

6 Abbott NJ (2000) Inflammatory mediators and modulation of blood-brain barrier permeability. *Cell Mol Neurobiol* 20: 131–147

7 Stanimirovic DB, Shapiro A, Wong J, Hutchison J, Durkin JP (1997) The induction of ICAM-1 in human cerebromicrovascular endothelial cells (HCEC) by ischemia-like conditions promotes enhanced neutrophil/HCEC adhesion. *J Neuroimmunol* 76: 193–205

8 de Vries HE, Blom-Roosemalen MC, van Oosten M, de Boer AG, van Berkel TJ, Breimer DD, Kuiper J (1996) The influence of cytokines on the integrity of the blood-brain barrier *in vitro*. *J Neuroimmunol* 64: 37–43

9 Kim KS, Wass CA, Cross AS, Opal SM (1992) Modulation of blood-brain barrier permeability by tumor necrosis factor and antibody to tumor necrosis factor in the rat. *Lymphokine Cytokine Res* 11: 293–298

10 Holmin S, Mathiesen T (2000) Intracerebral administration of interleukin-1beta and induction of inflammation, apoptosis, and vasogenic edema. *J Neurosurg* 92: 108–120

11 Kumami K, Yamamoto T, Villacara A, Mrsulja BB, Spatz M (1990) Ischemic cerebral edema. 5-Hydroxytryptamine receptors and the physical state of synaptosomal membranes. *Adv Neurol* 52: 47–56

12 Mannaioni PF, Di Bello MG, Masini E (1997) Platelets and inflammation: role of platelet-derived growth factor, adhesion molecules and histamine. *Inflamm Res* 46: 4–18

13   Cohen Z, Bouchelet I, Villemure J-G, Ball R, Stanimirovic D, Hamel E (1999) Multiple microvascular and astroglial 5-hydroxytryptamine receptor subtypes in human brain: Molecular and pharmacological characterization. *J Cerebral Blood Flow Metab* 19: 908–917

14   Joo F (1993) The role of histamine in brain oedema formation. *Funct Neurol* 8: 243–250

15   Schilling L, Wahl M (1999) Mediators of cerebral edema. *Adv Exp Med Biol* 474: 123–141

16   Spatz M, Stanimirovic D, McCarron RM (1995) Endothelin as a mediator of blood-brain barrier function. In: J Greenwood et al (eds): *New concepts of a blood-brain barrier*. Plenum Press, New York, 47–61

17   Stanimirovic DB, McCarron RM, and Spatz M (1994) Dexamethasone down-regulates endothelin receptors in human cerebromicrovascular endothelium. *Neuropeptides* 26: 145–152

18   Moreno M, Stanimirovic D, Ball R, Hamel E (1999) Functional calcitonin gene-related peptide (CGRP) type 1 and adrenomedullin receptors in human trigeminal ganglia, brain vessels, cerebromicrovascular and astroglial cells in culture. *J Cerebral Blood Flow Metab* 19: 1270–1278

19   Schaffer M, Beiter T, Becker HD, Hunt TK (1998) Neuropeptides: mediators of inflammation and tissue repair? *Arch Surg* 133: 1107–1116

20   Moreno MJ, Ball R, Stanimirovic D, Hamel E (1999) CGRP modulates permeability of human brain endothelial cell cultures. *J Cerebral Blood Flow Metab* 19 (Suppl 1): S259

21   Kishimoto TK, Rothlein R (1994) Integrins, ICAMs, and selectins: role and regulation of adhesion molecules in neutrophil recruitment to inflammatory sites. *Adv Pharmacol* 25: 117–169

22   Merrill JE, Murphy SP (1997) Inflammatory events at the blood brain barrier: regulation of adhesion molecules, cytokines, and chemokines by reactive nitrogen and oxygen species. *Brain Behav Immun* 11: 245–263

23   Lentsch AB, Ward PA (2000) Regulation of inflammatory vascular damage. *J Pathol* 190: 343–348

24   Stanimirovic DB, Wong J, Ball R, Durkin JP (1995) Free radical-induced endothelial membrane dysfunction at the site of blood brain barrier: relationship between lipid peroxidation, Na,K-ATPase activity and ^{51}Cr release. Neurochem Res 20: 1417–1427

25   Muruganandam A, Smith C, Ball R, Stanimirovic DB (2000) Glutathione homeostasis in human blood-brain barrier endothelial cells subjected to *in vitro* ischemia. *Acta Neurochirurgica (Suppl)* 76: 29–34

26   Hurst RD, Heales SJ, Dobbie MS, Barker JE, Clark JB (1998) Decreased endothelial cell glutathione and increased sensitivity to oxidative stress in an *in vitro* blood-brain barrier model system. *Brain Res* 802: 232–240

27   Kokura S, Wolf RE, Yoshikawa T, Granger DN, Aw TY (1999) Molecular mechanisms of neutrophil-endothelial cell adhesion induced by redox imbalance. *Circ Res* 84: 516–524

28 Funk CD (1993) Molecular biology in the eicosanoid field. *Prog Nucl Acid Res Mol Biol* 45: 67–98

29 Frey A (1993) Gamma-glutamyl transpeptidase: molecular cloning and structural and functional features of a blood-brain barrier marker protein. In: WM Pardridge (ed): *The blood-brain barrier cellular and molecular biology.* Raven Press, New York, 339–368

30 Lindgren JA, Karnushina I, and Clesson. H-E. (1989) Role of brain microvessels and choroid plexus in cerebral metabolism of leukotrienes. *Ann NY Acad Sci 559*: 112–120

31 Claesson H-E, Haeggstrom J (1988) Human endothelial cells stimulate leukotriene synthesis and convert granulocyte released leukotriene A_4 into leukotrienes B_4, C_4, D_4, and E_4. *Eur J Biochem* 173: 93–100

32 Baba T, Chio C-C, Black KL (1992) The effect of 5-lipoxygenase inhibition on blood-brain barrier permeability in experimental brain tumors. *J Neurosurg* 77: 403–406

33 Baba T, Black KL, Ikezaki K, Chen K, Becker DP (1991) Intracarotid infusion of leukotriene C_4 selectively increases blood-brain barrier permeability after focal ischemia in rats. *J Cerebral Blood Flow Metab* 11: 638–643

34 Baggiolini M (1998) Chemokines and leukocyte traffic. *Nature* 392: 565–568

35 Glabinski AR, Ransohoff RM (1999) Sentries at the gate: chemokines and the blood-brain barrier. *J Neurovirol 5*: 623–634

36 Matsumoto T, Ikeda K, Mukaida N, Harada A, Matsumoto Y, Yamashita J, Matsushima K (1997) Prevention of cerebral edema and infarct in cerebral reperfusion injury by an antibody to interleukin-8. *Lab Invest* 77: 119–125

37 Zhang W, Smith C, Shapiro A, Monette R, Hutchison J, Stanimirovic DB (1999) Increased expression of bioactive chemokines in human cerebromicrovascular endothelial cells and astrocytes subjected to simulated ischemia *in vitro. J Neuroimmunol* 101: 148–160

38 Lukes A, Mun-Bryce S, Lukes M, Rosenberg GA (1999) Extracellular matrix degradation by metalloproteinases and central nervous system diseases. *Mol Neurobiol* 19: 267–284

39 Schwartz JD, Monea S, Marcus SG, Patel S, Eng K, Galloway AC, Mignatti P, Shamamian P (1998) Soluble factor(s) released from neutrophils activates endothelial cell matrix metalloproteinase-2. *J Surg Res* 76: 79–85

40 Bolton SJ, Anthony DC, Perry VH (1998) Loss of the tight junction proteins occludin and zonula occludens-1 from cerebral vascular endothelium during neutrophil-induced blood-brain barrier breakdown *in vivo. Neuroscience* 86: 1245–1257

41 Garcia JGN, Verin AD, Herenyiova M, English D (1998) Adherent neutrophils activate endothelial myosin light chain kinase: role in transendothelial migration. *J Appl Physiol* 84: 1817–1821

Inflammatory proteases and oxygen radicals in stroke

The role of metalloproteinases on blood-brain barrier breakdown after ischemic stroke

Yvan Gasche[1,2], Jean-Christophe Copin[1,2] and Pak H. Chan[1]

[1]Neurosurgical Laboratories, Departments of Neurosurgery, Neurology and Neurological Sciences, and Program in Neurosciences, Stanford University, Stanford, California 94305, USA; [2]Divisions of Surgical and Medical Critical Care, Departments of Medicine, Anesthesiology, Pharmacology and Surgical Critical Care Medicine, Geneva University Hospital, 1211 Geneva 14, Switzerland

Introduction

The role of the blood-brain barrier (BBB) is to preserve the neuronal microenvironment, which is essential for the normal function of the brain. As a functional entity, BBB includes several cell types and the extracellular matrix (ECM). Microvascular endothelial cells coupled by tight junctions and featuring only a very few endocytotic vesicles are responsible for the permeability properties of the BBB [1]. Although in discontinuous contact with endothelial cells through their end feet, astrocytes seem also to actively participate in BBB phenotype [2]. Similarly, pericytes have been shown to change endothelial behavior [3–5]. Finally, the endothelial basal lamina represents the non-cellular component of BBB. Produced by endothelial cells, the basal lamina is a specialized ECM composed of type IV collagen, fibronectin, laminin and various proteoglycans [6]. The ECM components are connected to endothelial cells *via* integrins and may regulate distinct biological events such as cellular differentiation, survival, morphology, adhesion and gene expression [7–10]. When BBB integrity is lost, inflammatory cells and fluid penetrate the brain, causing vasogenic edema and cell death [11, 12]. BBB permeability properties are challenged in various brain pathologies including ischemic stroke and several mechanisms of BBB disruption have been considered, involving bradykinin [13] other proinflammatory mediators [14] and oxygen free radicals [15, 16].

Evidence of proteolytic BBB disruption during stroke

Several proteases have been shown to increase BBB permeability [17]. Intracerebral injection of type IV collagenase [18], elastase [19] and plasmin induces BBB disruption and multi-focal hemorrhage [18, 19]. During cerebral ischemia-reperfusion, the ECM is disrupted. Major components of the endothelial basal lamina such as

Inflammation and Stroke, edited by Giora Z. Feuerstein

laminin, type IV collagen and fibronectin start to disappear as soon as 2 h after the onset of ischemia [20]. Consistently, the first signs of BBB leakage are observed between 2 to 8 h after the onset of ischemia [21–24]. By 24 h of ischemia-reperfusion, dissolution of microvascular structures leads to clear interruption of microvessels [20, 25] and local hemorrhage [25]. Thus, proteolysis seems to be a critical process of stroke-related BBB disruption. Although, the precise mechanism of BBB disruption during ischemic stroke is still debated, experimental evidence suggests that matrix metalloproteinases play a key role in this process.

The role of MMPs on BBB disruption during brain ischemia

All endothelial basal lamina components can be digested by MMPs, which are proteolytic enzymes (Zn^{2+}-endopeptidases) secreted as zymogen and cleaved to their fully active form in the interstitial space. MMPs are involved in the remodeling of the ECM in a variety of physiological and pathophysiological conditions [26–28]. Among MMPs, gelatinases are expressed by neurons [29, 30], astrocytes [31], microglial cells [32], endothelial cells [33] and oligodendrocytes [34]. Gelatinase A (MMP-2) and gelatinase B (MMP-9) specifically digest type IV collagen in the basal lamina. Several in vivo studies, investigating the role of MMP in stroke, have shown that gelatinase expression was induced during experimental focal ischemia (Tab. 1). Early studies, conducted in spontaneously hypertensive rats, brought some doubt regarding the role of MMP in early BBB disruption, since they could not show any upregulation or activation of the enzymes during the first hours after permanent middle cerebral artery occlusion (pMCAO) [33, 35]. Later studies, using permanent or transient models of MCAO in mice, showed that gelatinase B was already upregulated 1 to 2 h after ischemia [22, 36]. This upregulation was rapidly followed by the appearance of the active form of gelatinase B [22, 37]. One study, conducted in baboons, showed an early upregulation of gelatinase A [38]. These discrepancies can be explained by methodological particularities of the experimental models with variations in MMP measurement techniques and species related specificities. Two studies, carried out in humans, confirmed that MMP-9 expression after stroke is mainly increased in acute ischemic lesions (less than 1 week after stroke onset) while MMP-2 and matrilysin (MMP-7) are increased in chronic lesions (more than 1 week after stroke onset) [39, 40]. Although MMPs form a growing family, only gelatinases have been consistently studied in stroke. One study has examined the expression of MMP-1 and MMP-3 (by Western blotting) after pMCAO, but no expression of these proteins was detected [33].

MMP activation is a tightly regulated and complex process. Gelatinase B can be activated in vitro by other metalloproteinases such as Gelatinase A [41], MMP-3 [42], and MMP-7 or other enzymes such as trypsin. The natural inhibitor of MMP-9 (TIMP-1) prevents its activation. No modification of TIMP-1, at the protein level,

Table 1 - Time-course of MMP-2 and MMP-9 protein expression/activation in ischemic regions after focal cerebral ischemia.

Model/species	Gelatinase expression during stroke	Refs.
pMCAO/SH rat	ProMMP-2: Constitutive expression; ↑ at 5 days	[35]
	ProMMP-9: 0 in controls or at 3 h; ↑ at 12 h, 24 h	
tMCAO/SH rat	ProMMP-2: Constitutive expression; ↑ at 5 days	[24]
	ProMMP-9: (↑) 15 h, significant ↑ at 48 h	
tMCAO/SH rat	ProMMP-2: 0 in controls; ↑ at 24 h → 5 days;	[33]
	MMP-9 ↑ at 5 days	
	ProMMP-9: 0 in controls; MMP-9 ↑ at 12 h → 5 days	
pMCAO/CD-1 mouse	ProMMP-2: Constitutively expressed; ↑ at 24 h;	[22]
	ProMMP-9: + in controls; ↑ at 2 h, 4 h, 24 h;	
	MMP-9 ↑ at 4 h, 24 h	
tMCAO/CD-1 mouse	ProMMP-2: Constitutively expressed; ↑ at 24 h;	[37]
	ProMMP-9: + in controls; ↑ at 24 h.	
	MMP-9 detected at 4 h, 24 h	
Baboon	ProMMP-2: ↑ at 1 h → 7 days	[38]
	ProMMP-9: ↑ in hemorrhagic transformation	
tMCAO/CD-1 mouse	ProMMP-2: 0 in controls; ↑ 12 h, 24 h;	[36]
	ProMMP-9: 0 in controls; ↑ at 1 h, 2 h, 6 h, 24 h;	
	MMP-9 ↑ at 12 h, 24 h	

Abbreviations: pMCAO, permanent cerebral artery occlusion; tMCAO, transient middle cerebral artery occlusion; SH, spontaneously hypertensive.
Brain extract was used in all studies but one to measure MMPs by zymography. In the study by Gasche et al. [22], an affinity-based purification of MMPs was used before zymographic analysis.

has been observed during the first 24 h following experimental stroke [22, 24, 33, 35, 38]. MMP-2 activation is specifically mediated by a membrane associated MMP (MT-MMP). TIMP-2, the natural inhibitor of MMP-2, plays a dual role in its interaction with the gelatinase. Indeed, when TIMP-2 complexes with proMMP-2, cell surface-mediated activation of the enzyme is facilitated, whereas interaction of TIMP-2 with the active enzyme results in inhibition [43–47].

Recently, Rosenberg et al. confirmed the responsibility of MMPs in BBB disruption by demonstrating the ability of the non-selective MMP inhibitor BB-1101 (British Biotechnology, UK) to reduce the early BBB leakage following transient focal ischemia [24]. The possible mechanism of MMP-related BBB alteration is explained by the disruption of the endothelial basal lamina, that prevents the

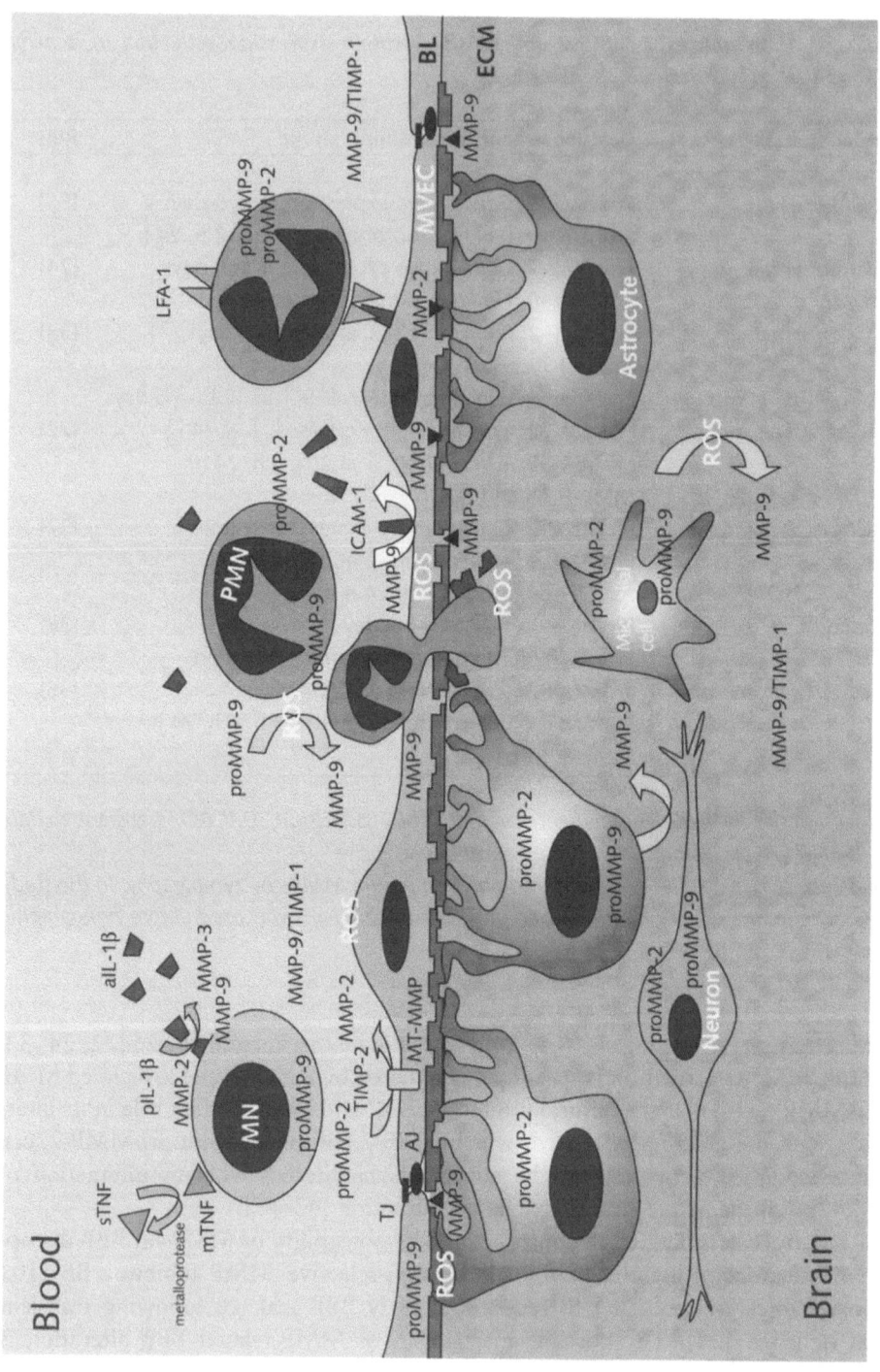

anchorage of the endothelial cells onto the ECM. This will result in the loosening of the tight junctions and eventually to selective endothelial cell death. Indeed several studies have demonstrated that the loss of connection between endothelial cells and the ECM leads to endothelial apoptosis and vascular involution [9, 10, 48]. MMPs may also indirectly affect BBB permeability by interfering with inflammatory pathways triggered by ischemia-reperfusion. Interleukin-1β (IL-1β) is an essential mediator of inflammation and plays a significant role in ischemic brain injury [49–52] and vasogenic edema [53]. From *in vitro* studies, we know that MMPs can process IL-1β into its biologically active form. While MMP-2 activates IL-1β in 24 h, MMP-3 takes 1 h and MMP-9 only a few minutes to process the cytokine. Thus, MMPs may promote inflammatory processes, which will in a positive feedback loop increase MMP production by resident or migrating cells. Eventually, MMPs will also contribute to the increase of endothelial permeability induced by tumor necrosis factor-α (TNFα) [54]. The fundamental role played by MMPs in the development of vasogenic edema during stroke is further substantiated by the fact that these enzymes mediate the capillary leakage triggered by oxidative stress. It is well established that the oxidative unbalance during focal cerebral ischemia is a major contributor to BBB disruption, secondary brain injury and hemorrhagic transformation [23, 55, 56]. Our laboratory has shown that after traumatic brain injury, gelatinase expression and activation were reduced in mice overexpressing CuZn superoxide dismutase as compared to wild type animals [57]. These results confirm previous *in vitro* data suggesting that oxygen free radicals participate in MMP activity regulation [58]. During focal ischemia-reperfusion, we have observed that oxidative stress associated BBB disruption, was prevented by the inhibition of MMPs (Gasche et al., Society for Neuroscience 2000, personal communication). In this study, MMP-

---

Figure 1

Scheme of the possible mechanisms involved in BBB proteolytic disruption during stroke. Latent gelatinases are produced by cerebral resident cells and migrating leucocytes. Gelatinase A is activated by a membrane bound MMP (MT-MMP) during a complex interaction with its natural inhibitor TIMP-2. Gelatinase A and gelatinase B are activated by reactive oxygen species (ROS). During the early period of ischemia-reperfusion the natural inhibitors of gelatinases, TIMP-2 and TIMP-1 are not upregulated at the protein level. The resulting proteolytic unbalance disrupts the ECM and basal lamina (BL). Neutrophils adhere to the endothelium and eventually migrate across the capillaries. Various pro-inflammatory mediators are released and lead to secondary brain damage.

Abbreviations: pIL-1β, prointerleukin-1β; aIL-1β, active interleukin-1β; sTNF, soluble tumor necrosis factor α; mTNF, membrane TNF α; LFA-1, lymphocyte function associated antigen-1; ICAM-1, intercellular adhesion molecule-1; MN, monocytes; PMN, polymorphonuclear; MVEC, microvascular endothelial cell; TJ, tight junction; AJ, adherent junction.

mediated *in situ* proteolysis, observed at the capillary level, correlated with the local production of oxygen free radicals.

MMPs seem to be essential effectors of proteolytic BBB disruption during stroke (Fig. 1), but the respective role of gelatinases or other MMPs in BBB disruption has not yet been elucidated. Nevertheless, two studies have shown that MMP-9 is an important mediator of secondary brain injury following permanent focal ischemia. In these studies the infarct volume was reduced in mice treated with an anti-MMP-9 antibody [33] or in animals lacking MMP-9 [36] as compared to controls. BBB disruption was studied in a model of transient focal ischemia in MMP-9 knockout mice (Gidday et al., Society for Neuroscience 2000, personal communication). The authors observed a reduced BBB leakage in MMP-9-deficient mice during the first hours following the ischemic insult.

Our understanding of the exact implication of MMPs in the pathophysiological cascade of cerebral ischemia-reperfusion is fragmentary. Further studies, targeting the different enzymes, are needed to unravel the proteolytic mechanisms leading to secondary brain injury and hemorrhage. The reduction of BBB proteolysis might bring forward a new therapeutic strategy destined to increase the therapeutic window between the onset of ischemia and thrombolytic reperfusion.

References

1   Reese TS, Karnowsky MJ (1967) Fine ultrastructural localization of a blood-brain barrier to exogenous peroxidase. *J Cell Biol* 34: 207–217

2   Janzer RC, Raff MC (1987) Astrocytes induce blood-brain barrier properties in endothelial cells. *Nature* 325: 253–257

3   Larson DM, Carson MP, Haudenschild CC (1987) Junctional transfer of small molecules in cultured bovine brain microvascular endothelial cells and pericytes. *Microvasc Res* 38: 184–199

4   Fujimoto K (1995) Pericyte-endothelial gap junctions in developing rat cerebral capillaries. *Anat Rec* 242: 562–565

5   Antonelli-Orlidge A, Saunders K, Smith SR, D'Amor PA (1989) An activated form of transforming growth factor β is produced by cocultures of endothelial cells and pericytes. *Proc Natl Acad Sci USA* 86: 4544–4548

6   Yurchenco PD, Schittny JC (1990) Molecular architecture of basement membranes. *FASEB J* 4: 1577–1590

7   Chen CS, Mrksich M, Huang S, Whitesides GM, Ingber DE (1997) Geometric control of cell life and death. *Science* 276: 1425–1428

8   Maniotis AJ, Chen CS, Ingber DE (1997) Demonstration of mechanical connections between integrins cytoskeletal filaments and nucleoplasm that stabilize nuclear structure. *Proc Natl Acad Sci USA* 94: 849–854

9   Brooks PC, Montgomery AM, Rosenfeld M, Reisfeld RA, Hu T, Klier G, Cheresh DA

(1994) Integrin alpha v beta 3 antagonists promote tumor regression by inducing apoptosis of angiogenic blood vessels. *Cell* 79: 1157–1164

10 Ingber DE, Folkman J (1989) How does extracellular matrix control capillary morphogenesis. *Cell* 58: 803–805

11 Chen H, Chopp M, Bodzin G (1992) Neutropenia reduces the volume of cerebral infarct after transient middle cerebral artery occlusion in the rat. *Neurosci Res Comm* 11: 93–99

12 Fishman RA (1975) Brain edema. *N Engl J Med* 293: 706–711

13 Wahl M, Unterberg A, Baethmann A, Schilling L (1988) Mediators of blood-brain barrier dysfunction and formation of vasogenic brain edema. *J Cereb Blood Flow Metab* 8: 621–634

14 Abbott NJ (2000) Inflammatory mediators and modulation of blood-brain barrier permeability. *Cell Mol Neurobiol* 20: 131–147

15 Chan PH, Fishman RA, Schmidley JW, Chen SF (1984) Release of polyunsaturated fatty acids from phospholipids and alteration of brain membrane integrity by oxygen-derived free radicals. *J Neurosci Res* 12: 595–605

16 Chan PH, Schmidley JW, Fishman RA, Longar SM (1984) Brain injury, edema, and vascular permeability changes induced by oxygen-derived free radicals. *Neurology* 34: 315–320

17 Robert AM, Godeau G (1974) Action of proteolytic and glycolytic enzymes on the permeability of the blood-brain barrier. *Biomedicine* 21: 36–39

18 Rosenberg GA, Kornfeld M, Estrada E, Kelley RO, Liotta LA, Stetler-Stevenson WG (1992) TIMP-2 reduces proteolytic opening of blood brain barrier by type IV collagenase. *Brain Res* 576: 203–207

19 Armao D, Kornfeld M, Estrada EY, Grossetete M, Rosenberg GA (1997) Neutral proteases and disruption of the blood-brain barrier in rat. *Brain Res* 767: 259–264

20 Hamann GF, Okada Y, Fitridge R, Del Zoppo GJ (1995) Microvascular basal lamina antigens disappear during cerebral ischemia and reperfusion. *Stroke* 26: 2120–2126

21 Belayev L, Busto R, Zhao W, Ginsberg MD (1996) Quantitative evaluation of blood-brain barrier permeability following middle cerebral artery occlusion in rats. *Brain Res* 739: 88–96

22 Gasche Y, Fujimura M, Morita-Fujimura Y, Copin JC, Kawase M, Massengale J, Chan PH (1999) Early appearance of activated matrix metalloproteinase-9 after focal cerebral ischemia in mice: a possible role in blood-brain barrier dysfunction. *J Cereb Blood Flow Metab* 19: 1020–1028

23 Kondo T, Reaume AG, Huang TT, Carlson E, Murakami K, Chen SF, Hoffman EK, Scott RW, Epstein CJ, Chan PH (1997) Reduction of CuZn-superoxide dismutase activity exacerbates neuronal cell injury and edema formation after transient focal cerebral ischemia. *J Neurosci* 17: 4180–4189

24 Rosenberg GA, Estrada EY, Dencoff JE (1998) Matrix metalloproteinases and TIMPs are associated with blood-brain barrier opening after reperfusion in rat brain. *Stroke* 29: 2189–2195

25 Hamann GF, Okada Y, Del Zoppo GJ (1996) Hemorrhagic transformation and microvascular integrity during focal cerebral ischemi/reperfusion. *J Cereb Blood Flow Metab* 16: 1373–1378

26 Migita K, Eguchi K, Kawabe Y, Ichinose Y, Tsukada T, Aoyagi T, Nakamura H, Nagataki S (1996) TNF-alpha-mediated expression of membrane-type matrix metalloproteinase in rheumatoid synovial fibroblasts. *Immunology* 89: 553–557

27 Nikkari ST, Hoyhtya M, Isola J, Nikkari T (1996) Macrophages contain 92-kd gelatinase (MMP-9) at the site of degenerated internal elastic lamina in temporal arteritis. *Am J Pathol* 149: 1427–1433

28 Clements JM, Cossins JA, Wells GM, Corkill DJ, Helfrich K, Wood LM, Pigott R, Stabler G, Ward GA, Gearing AJ et al (1997) Matrix metalloproteinase expression during experimental autoimmune encephalomyelitis and effects of a combined matrix metalloproteinase and tumour necrosis factor-alpha inhibitor. *J Neuroimmunol* 74: 85–94

29 Pagenstecher A, Stalder AK, Kincaid CL, Shapiro SD, Campbell IL (1998) Differential expression of matrix metalloproteinase and tissue inhibitor of matrix metalloproteinase genes in the mouse central nervous system in normal and inflammatory states. *Am J Pathol* 152: 729–741

30 Backstrom JR, Lim GP, Cullen MJ, Tokes ZA (1996) Matrix metalloproteinase-9 (MMP-9) is synthesized in neurons of the human hippocampus and is capable of degrading the amyloid-beta peptide (1-40). *J Neurosci* 16: 7910–7919

31 Gottschall PE, Yu X (1995) Cytokines regulate gelatinase A and B (matrix metalloproteinase 2 and 9) activity in cultured rat astrocytes. *J Neurochem* 64: 1513–1520

32 Gottschall PE, Yu X, Bing B (1995) Increased production of gelatinase B (matrix metalloproteinase-9) and interleukin-6 by activated rat microglia in culture. *J Neurosci Res* 42: 335–342

33 Romanic AM, White RF, Arleth AJ, Ohlstein EH, Barone FC (1998) Matrix metalloproteinase expression increases after cerebral focal ischemia in rats: inhibition of matrix metalloproteinase-9 reduces infarct size. *Stroke* 29: 1020–1030

34 Oh LYS, Larsen PH, Krekoski CA, Edwards DR, Donovan F, Werb Z, Yong VW (1999) Matrix metalloproteinase-9/Gelatinase B is required for process outgrowth by oligodendrocytes. *J Neurosci* 19: 8464–8475

35 Rosenberg GA, Navratil M, Barone F, Feuerstein G (1996) Proteolytic cascade enzymes increase in focal cerebral ischemia in rat. *J Cereb Blood Flow Metab* 16: 360–366

36 Asahi M, Asahi K, Jung JC, del Zoppo GJ, Fini ME, Lo EH (2000) Role for matrix metalloproteinase 9 after focal cerebral ischemia: effects of gene knockout and enzyme inhibition with BB-94. *J Cereb Blood Flow Metab* 20: 1681–1689

37 Fujimura M, Gasche Y, Morita-Fujimura Y, Massengale J, Kawase M, Chan PH (1999) Early appearance of activated matrix metalloproteinase-9 and blood-brain barrier disruption in mice after focal cerebral ischemia and reperfusion. *Brain Res* 842: 92–100

38 Heo JH, Lucero J, Abumiya T, Koziol JA, Copeland BR, del Zoppo GJ (1999) Matrix metalloproteinases increase very early during experimental focal cerebral ischemia. *J Cereb Blood Flow Metab* 19: 624–633

39 Anthony DC, Ferguson B, Matyzak MK, Miller KM, Esiri MM, Perry VH (1997) Differential matrix metalloproteinase expression in cases of multiple sclerosis and stroke. *Neuropathol Appl Neurobiol* 23: 406–415

40 Clark AW, Krekoski CA, Bou SS, Chapman KR, Edwards DR (1997) Increased gelatinase A (MMP-2) and gelatinase B (MMP-9) activities in human brain after focal ischemia. *Neurosci Lett* 238: 53–56

41 Fridman R, Toth M, Pena D, Mobashery S (1995) Activation of progelatinase B (MMP-9) by gelatinase A (MMP-2). *Cancer Res* 55: 2548–2555

42 Okada Y, Gonoji Y, Naka K, Tomita K, Nakanishi I, Iwata K, Yamashita K, Hayakawa T (1992) Matrix metalloproteinase 9 (92 kDa gelatinase/type IV collagenase) from HT 1080 human firborsarcoma cells. Purification and activation of the precursor and enzymatic properties. *J Biol Chem* 267: 21712–21719

43 Strongin AY, Marmer BL, Grant GA, Goldberg GI (1993) Plasma membrane-dependent activation of the 72-kDa type IV collagenase is prevented by complex formation with TIMP-2. *J Biol Chem* 268: 14033–14039

44 Strongin AY, Collier Y, Bannikov G, Marmer BL, Grant GA, Goldberg GI (1995) Mechanism of cell surface activation of 72-kDa type IV collagenase. *J Biol Chem* 270: 5331–5338

45 Willenbrock F, Murphy G (1994) Structure-function relationships in the tissue inhibitors of metalloproteinases. *Am J Respir Crit Care Med* 150: S165–S170

46 Goldberg GI, Marmer BL, Grant JA, Eisen AZ, Wilhelm S, He C (1989) Human 72k type IV collagenase forms a complex with a tissue inhibitor of metalloproteinase designed TIMP-2. *Proc Natl Acad Sci USA* 86: 8207–8211

47 Bergmann U, Tuuttila A, Stetler-Stevenson WG, Tryggvason K (1995) Autolytic activation of recombinant human 72 kilodalton type IV collagenase. *Biochemistry* 34: 2819–2825

48 Ingber DE, Madri JA, Folkman J (1986) A possible mechanism for inhibition of angiogenesis by angiostatic steroids: induction of capillary basement membrane dissolution. *Endocrinology* 119: 1768–1775

49 Clark ET, Desai TR, Hynes KL, Gewertz BL (1995) Endothelial cell response to hypoxia-reoxygenation is mediated by IL-1. *????* 58: 675–681

50 Liu T, McDonnell PC, Young PR, White RF, Siren AL, Hallenbeck JM, Barone FC, Feurestein GZ (1993) Interleukin-1 beta mRNA expression in ischemic rat cortex. *Stroke* 24: 1746–1750

51 Liu XH, Kwon D, Schielke GP, Yang GY, Silverstein FS, Barks JD (1999) Mice deficient in interleukin-1 converting enzyme are resistant to neonatal hypoxic-ischemic brain damage. *J Cereb Blood Flow Metab* 19: 1099–1108

52 Yang GY, Liu XH, Kadoya C, Zhao YJ, Mao Y, Davidson BL, Betz AL (1998) Attenuation of ischemic inflammatory response in mouse brain using an adenoviral vector to induce overexpression of interleukin-1 receptor antagonist. *J Cereb Blood Flow Metab* 18: 840–847

53 Holmin S, Mathiesen T (2000) Intracerebral administration of interleukin-1beta and induction of inflammation, apoptosis, and vasogenic edema. *J Neurosurg* 92: 108–120

54 Partridge CA, Jeffrey JJ, Malik AB (1993) A 96-kDa gelatinase induced by TNFα contributes to increased microvascular endothelial permeability. *Am J Physiol* 265: L438–L447

55 Lewen A, Matz P, Chan PH (2000) Free radical pathways in CNS injury. *J Neurotrauma* 17: 871–890

56 Asahi M, Asahi K, Wang X, Lo EH (2000) Reduction of tissue plasminogen activator-induced hemorrhage and brain injury by free radical spin trapping after embolic focal cerebral ischemia in rats. *J Cereb Blood Flow Metab* 20: 452–457

57 Morita-Fujimura Y, Fujimura M, Gasche Y, Copin JC, Chan PH (2000) Overexpression of copper and zinc superoxide dismutase in transgenic mice prevents the induction and activation of matrix metalloproteinases after cold injury-induced brain trauma. *J Cereb Blood Flow Metab* 20: 130–138

58 Weiss SJ, Peppin G, Ortiz X, Ragsdale C, Test ST (1985) Oxidative autoactivation of latent collagenase by human neutrophils. *Science* 227: 747–749

Matrix metalloproteinases and their inhibitors in hypoxia/reoxygenation and stroke

Ariel Miller[1,3,4], Yaara Ben-Yosef[1], Clara Braker[1] and Sarah Shapiro[2]

[1]Neuroimmunlogy and [2]Immunology Research Units, Carmel Medical Center, 7 Michal St., Haifa 34362, Israel; [3]Rappaport Institute for Research in the Medical Sciences, Haifa, Israel, and [4]Faculty of Medicine, Technion – Israel Institute of Technology, Haifa, Israel

Hypoxia and reoxygenation

Hypoxia, resulting from ischemic events, leads to a variety of pathological processes, depending on the duration and severity of the primary insult. The ensuing reoxygenation, resulting from reperfusion, may have opposing effects; either aggravation of the primary hypoxia-induced injury or stimulation of repair processes in an attempt to minimize the tissue damage. Amongst the cells directly exposed to changes in oxygen tension are endothelial cells (ECs), lining the vascular bed, as well as peripheral blood leukocytes (PBL). The response of these cells to hypoxia involves a complex cascade of events including: increased release of thrombolytic factors, increased permeability of the endothelium, immune activation, release of chemokines, cytokines and growth factors, as well as up-regulation of surface adhesion molecules. Includes. Two additional processes are part of the responses to hypoxia: immune cell transvasation and angiogenesis of ECs, processes which are dependent on the activity of enzymes, members of the matrix metalloproteinases (MMPs) family [1–4].

Matrix metalloproteinases (MMPs) and their regulation

Key molecules implicated in hypoxia-mediated effects are the MMPs, proteolytic enzymes, responsible for the remodeling of the extracellular matrix (ECM). This family of zinc-dependent proteases includes to date at least 19 different human proteins [5, 6]. The MMPs are classified into sub-families according to their protein structure and substrate specificity, although considerable substrate overlap exists. The main groups include the collagenases (MMP-1, MMP-8, MMP-13), gelatinases (MMP-2, MMP-9), stromelysins (MMP-3, MMP-10, MMP-11) and membrane-type (MT)-MMPs. Apart from those anchored to the membrane, MMPs are secreted as inactive zymogens requiring activation through proteolysis by serine proteases and members of the MMPs family [5]. Virtually most cell types may potentially secrete MMPs. However, except for MMP-2, the MMPs are generally not constitutively expressed. Growth factors, cytokines and cell-cell interactions involving adhesion molecules play an important role in the regulation of MMPs' activity.

The potential destructive nature of MMPs requires tight control of their transcription as well as their activity. Amongst the multiple levels of MMPs' regulation is the activation of their latent forms, in addition to inhibition through binding to circulating plasma proteins. Example for these proteins include α_1-antiproteinase and α_2-macroglobulin, as well as specific endogenous inhibitors known as tissue inhibitors of MMPs (TIMPs) [5, 7]. Four distinct TIMPs have been identified to date [8, 9]. While most TIMPs react with all activated MMPs, TIMP-2 binds to pro-MMP-2 and TIMP-1 inhibits specifically pro-MMP-9. It is accepted that the balance between MMPs and TIMPs expression at a local microenvironment determines the ECM's integrity or turnover. Where MMP activity is elevated in relation to the level of TIMPs, excessive ECM degradation may result. On the other hand, where expression of excess TIMPs predominates in relation to MMPs, ECM build-up may result. Cytokines can influence expression and processing of MMPs, from their inactive zymogenic form to active enzymes. Alternatively, cytokines (TNFα, TGFβ, IL-1β) membrane-bound cytokine receptors (IL-6R, TNFR) and adhesion molecules (ICAM-1), often serve as substrates for MMPs activity, which may lead to their degradation or shedding from the cell surface [10–14].

MMPs and hypoxia of endothelial cells

Although ECs are considered to be among the cell types most tolerant to changes in oxygen tension, nonetheless, conditions of hypoxia, and specifically if followed by reoxygenation (H/R), have the potential to disrupt the complex homeostatic functions of the endothelium [15]. As mentioned above, the main results of H/R and associated oxidative stress of ECs are the release of pro-coagulant factors, the increased vascular permeability and the pro-inflammatory response that evokes recruitment of immune cells into the target organ [16]. However, divergent response to hypoxia may be the proliferation of ECs and angiogenesis, driven by pro-angiogenic factors. In response to hypoxia immune cells, particularly monocytes, are induced to secrete potent angiogenic factors such as vascular endothelial growth factor (VEGF), which may enhance ECs proliferation and neovascularization. These processes require ECs to loosen inter-endothelial contacts, emigrate from their resident site by penetrating the supporting basal membrane and degrading the surrounding matrix. MMPs, amongst other proteolytic enzymes, facilitate angiogenesis by degrading the ECM and liberating vascular growth factors (VEGF, bFGF and IGF-1) sequestered within it [15]. MMP-2 and MMP-9, which are constitutively expressed and are inducible in primary endothelial cells, seem to be implicated in these processes [17].

Additional crucial molecules modulated by hypoxia are adhesion molecules whose expression increases both on ECs and leukocytes at hypoxic sites. Amongst the elevated adhesion molecules important to MMP activation is the vitronectin receptor, $\alpha_V\beta_3$, which is upregulated by VEGF. $\alpha_V\beta_3$ is involved in the activation of latent pro-MMP-2 to its active form [14], thus contributing to ECM turnover during hypoxia.

The present knowledge of the effects of H/R on the activity of MMPs is still fragmentary. Research has been carried out mainly on ischemic animal models and tissues derived from deceased humans [6, 18]. *In vitro* studies using cell lines are scarce. Studies of post-ischemic tissues have shown elevated activity of the gelatinases, MMP-2 and MMP-9, while TIMP-1 levels were elevated or not changed. We recently examined in human endothelial cells, the *in vitro* effects of acute (3 or 6 h), as opposed to prolonged (24 h) hypoxia on the expression of MMP-2, its physiological activator MT1-MMP, and its inhibitor TIMP-2 [19]. These hypoxic conditions were found to differentially modulate MMPs/TIMPs expression (Fig. 1). Short hypoxia led to a significant decrease in the mRNA of the three genes studied. In contrast prolonged hypoxia led to a significant, 1.6-fold elevation in MMP-2 mRNA level, in comparison to cells under normoxic conditions, while the mRNA levels of MT1-MMP and TIMP-2 remained suppressed. Reoxygenation following short hypoxia led to elevation of MMP-2 mRNA back to normoxic levels while the elevation induced by prolonged hypoxia was sustained. Reoxygenation led also to a normalization in MT1-MMP mRNA level, though the TIMP-2 mRNA remained inhibited. The results, while demonstrating complex modulation of the three molecules examined, support increased pro-proteolytic activity following prolonged hypoxia, and also following reoxygenation, with the potential of promoting ECM degradation. The net final result, whether an attempt beneficial to the tissue through promotion of active angiogenesis, or deleterious effects through endothelial detachment and increased blood vessel wall permeability, appears to be dependent on the duration and probably the severity of oxygen deprivation.

MMPs in blood brain barrier (BBB) eruption and cerebral ischemia

The microenvironment of the CNS is maintained by the blood brain barrier (BBB), a complex cellular system comprising cerebral vascular ECs linked by continuous tight junctions, resting on a basal lamina composed predominantly of collagen type IV, and supported by pericytes and astrocytic foot processes. Direct proof of MMP involvement in BBB eruption is the increase in cerebral capillary permeability following intra-cerebral injection of gelatinases, as well as reversal of this effect by the addition of specific MMP inhibitors, amongst them TIMP-2 [18, 20, 21]. Elevated expression levels of MMPs, have been demonstrated in mice and rat models of focal cerebral ischemia (CI) [22–25]. Moreover systemic administration of MMP-9 neu-

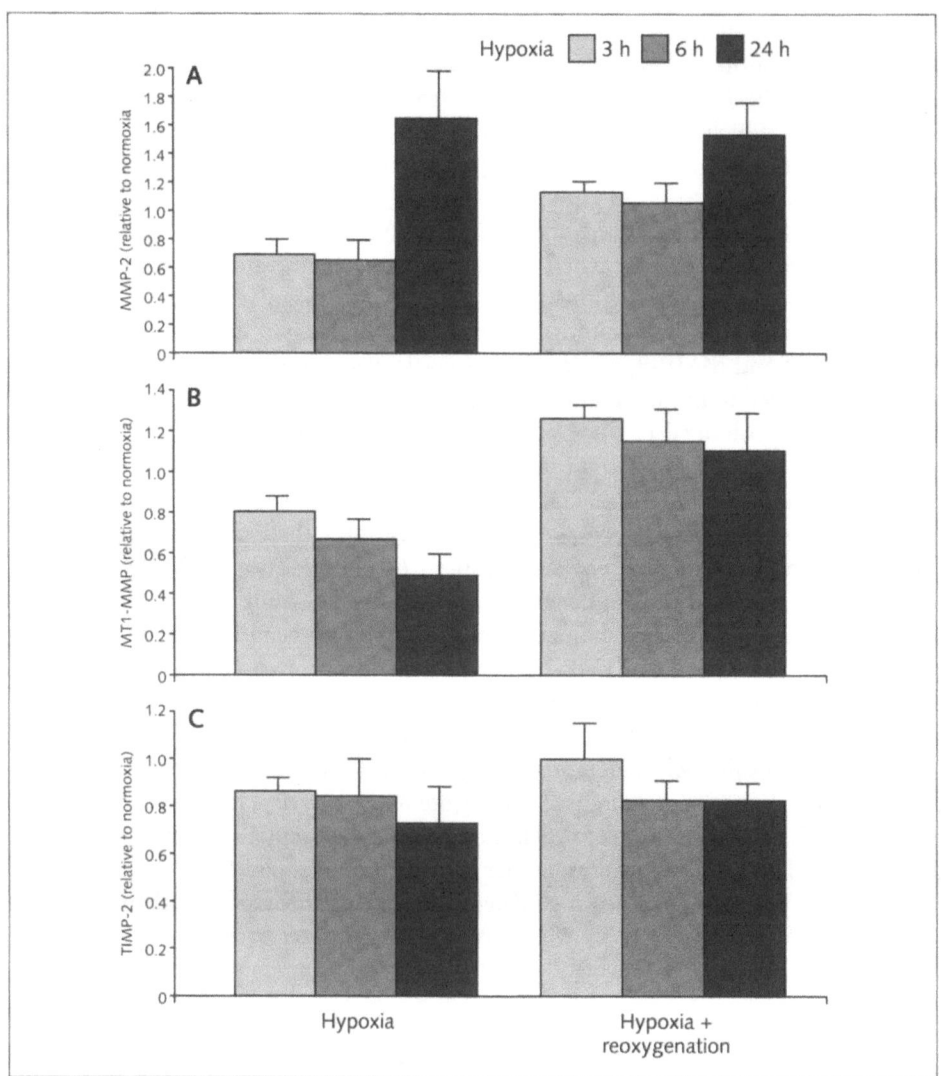

Figure 1

Hypoxia differentially influences the expression of MMP-2, MT1-MMP and TIMP-2. Northern blot analysis was performed to evaluate MMP-2 (A), MT1-MMP (B) and TIMP-2 (C) mRNA level expressed by human endothelial cells (EAhy 926) following exposure to hypoxia (22 mm Hg pO_2) for 3 h, 6 h or 24 h followed by reoxygenation for an additional 24 h in normoxic (158 mm Hg pO_2) conditions. Cells cultured in normoxic conditions for the same length of time served as controls. Expression of 28S rRNA was used to normalize for loading errors. Mean values of ratio between hypoxia to control results ± SD for four experiments are presented.

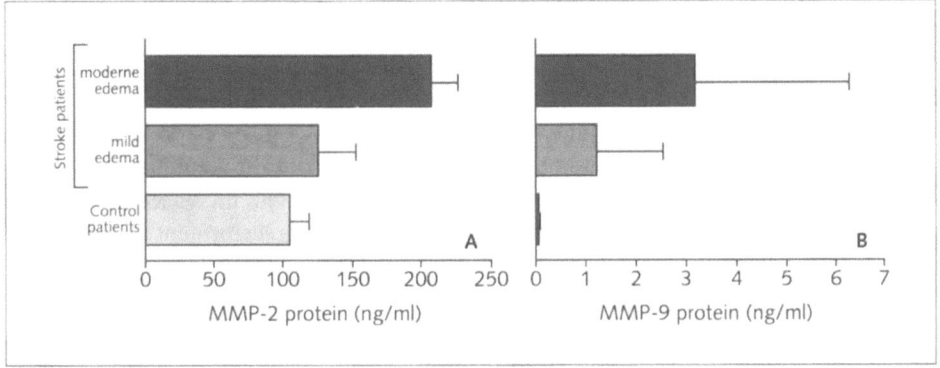

Figure 2
Elevated CSF levels of MMP-2 and MMP-9 correlate with brain edema in stroke patients.
CSF obtained from patients 24–48 h following CVA were evaluated by ELISA for expression
of MMP-2 and MMP-9 and correlated with the degree of brain edema (evaluated by CT).

tralizing antibodies, prevented the increased BBB permeability and reduced infarct size in rats [24]. Studies in non-human primates also demonstrate upregulated expression of MMP-2 and MMP-9 [25]. The results regarding temporal expression of gelatinases in CI have been partially contradictory. Following occlusion of middle cerebral artery in rodents, MMP-9 was reported to appear in the infarct area between 3 to 12 h following ischemia, and related to both endothelial and PMN cells [22–24]. At 24 h post-cerebral ischemic injury, elevated MMP-2 and MMP-9 seemed to be of macrophage origin. Other studies [20–25] showed upregulation primarily of MMP-2 within 3 h, correlating with neuronal damage, while elevated levels of MMP-9 appeared at 48 h and were associated with secondary hemorrhage insult [25]. The differences observed amongst the above mentioned studies may be due either to the methodology employed, as well as to the influence of secondary insults such as hemorrhage.

Studies of MMPs in human cerebral ischemic injury are few. We have recently observed the induction of MMP-9 and an elevation of the constitutively expressed MMP-2, in CSF obtained from stroke patients during the first 24–48 h following the insult [26]. A positive correlation was found between the degree of brain edema (evaluated by CT), and the level of MMP-9 in the CSF (Fig. 2). These findings are supported by studies on brain tissue derived from deceased stroke patients, showing elevated MMP-9 in patients 2 days after CVA, while elevated MMP-2 was observed at a later time and its level was still elevated several months after the ischemic incident [27, 28]. These studies in humans and experimental animal models suggest a central function for gelatinases in the pathogenesis of cerebral infract and perhaps also in the attempt to its resolution.

The primary brain damage resulting from the ischemic injury is often aggravated by an inflammatory wave, also implicating MMPs, leading to secondary cerebral damage. These inflammatory processes include release of pro-inflammatory cytokines such as TNFα [29], known as a potent MMP-9 inducer. MT1-MMP, the MMP-2 activator, is also upregulated by TNFα [30], promoting enhanced cleavage of type IV collagen and other basal lamina components. The increased endothelial permeability may further amplify the CNS injury through recruitment of additional immune cells, leading to neuronal death, by apoptosis or necrosis. Amongst the immune cells infiltrating the CNS, leukocytes and in particular macrophages are major sources of MMPs. Of note, many cellular components of the CNS, including astrocytes, oligodendrocytes, microgeal cells and neurons, have all been shown *in vitro* to be capable of secreting MMPs [6] and are thus capable of being potent participators in the pathogenesis of the ischemic injury. On the other hand, breakdown of the BBB and associated brain edema, which are key features of the primary hypoxic injury as well as being due to either primary or secondary neuroinflammatory conditions, seem to respond to steroid treatment, at least partially, by mechanisms which downregulate MMP-9 [31].

Repair processes following hypoxia, similarly to wound healing processes following injuries of non-hypoxyic etiology, also require ECM remodeling. For example, migration of glial cells in the wound healing process and glial scar formation within the CNS has been associated with MMP secretion [32] as well as with the elevated expression of $\alpha_V\beta_3$ integrin receptor [33], known to promote MMP-2 activity.

Ischemic tolerance and preconditioning

The response of ECs to ischemic stress, in contrast to the induction of pro-inflammatory and pro-coagulatory processes, may lead to molecular responses that protect them against a severe future hypoxic insult, a process referred to as ischemic tolerance or ischemic pre-conditioning (IPC) [34–35]. In fact, brief periods of transient ischemia-reperfusion events and associated repeated H/R have demonstrated effective protection against the deleterious effects of prolonged ischemia. This has been demonstrated in studies of ischemia in a variety of animal models and human organs, including specifically the protective role of recurrent transient ischemic attacks (TIA) against stroke in humans [36]. Preliminary understandings of the molecular mechanism(s) underlying IPC are beginning to be unraveled [2, 34, 35]. A number of signaling pathways have been implicated, amongst them: protein kinase-C, ceramide as well as NF-κB activation [2, 34, 35, 37]. IPC appears to activate "protective genes" which maintain the endothelium in a quiescent phenotype allowing it to retain its barrier and anti-coagulant functions. Amongst the "protective genes" identified is TIMP-1, the elevation of which was reported to correlate with the onset of ischemic tolerance in experimental stroke [38]. Thus, the adaptive response and protective phenomenon involved in IPC seem to include modulation of the MMPs/TIMPs ratio, possibly preventing the endothelium detachment from its basement membrane and thereby preserving its integrity. Additional potential mechanisms contributing to cerebral IPC may include the vascular mechanisms implicated in angiogenesis leading to the generation of collateral circulation, as well as the direct neuroprotective effects of these events.

MMPs and hypoxia associated with brain tumors

Angiogenesis is a key process also as part of the growth of primary tumors and their metastatic dissemination. The relative hypoxia, which is part of the high metabolic demand of the malignant tissue, is considered to be the main trigger for the proliferation of tumoral ECs leading to neovascularization [39, 40]. In addition to the hypoxia-induced expression of vascular growth factors such as VEGF and fibroblast growth factors (FGF), upregulation of certain membrane receptors, such as Tie receptors, essential for intra-tumor angiogenesis, elevated expression of MMP-2, -7 and -9 was found to be associated with the malignancy grade and the invasive capacity of gliomas [41]. Unexpectedly the overexpression of MMPs is often accompanied by elevated expression also of TIMP-1, which may be associated with additional growth-like characteristic of TIMP-1 [9].

Although metastasis of primary brain neoplasia is rare, the CNS is a major destination for disseminating systemic malignant tumors. Tumor cell invasion and metastasis requires degradation of ECM and vascular basement membranes. Accordingly, significant increases in the level of several MMPs have been observed in brain metastasis originating from lung, colon and breast carcinoma [42]. In addition activated MMP-2 and MMP-9, together with VEGF, are overexpressed in the CSF from patients with leptomeningeal metastasis [43]. The elevated expression of these factors may account for the BBB disruption and brain edema associated with brain tumors and metastasis.

Enhanced MMPs accompanied by reduced TIMPs expression associated with hypoxia, as observed in our *in vitro* studies (Fig. 1), may play a key role in hypoxia-mediated processes which promote not only beneficial angiogenesis, but also pathological angiogenesis, enabling tumor growth and dissemination. Thus, suppression of hypoxia-induced angiogenesis, by targeting hypoxia inducible factor (HIF) or the use of MMP antagonists, such as marimastat or tetracyclines [44, 45] are new approaches currently being applied both in experimental models and clinical trails, in attempts to inhibit growth of systemic as well as brain tumors.

In conclusion, the adaptive or pathological response of ECs to H/R appears to lead to an increase in physiological and pathological angiogenesis in the cerebral injured tissue and malignant tumors, respectively. The process of angiogenesis requires ECM remodeling orchestrated by MMPs. Understanding the mechanisms underlying the brain's response to H/R could offer development of therapeutic strategies aimed at alleviating CNS disorders resulting from these injurious conditions. Selective inhibition of hypoxia-mediated pathological angiogenesis of brain tumors or promotion of physiological vasculogenesis, enabling formation of collateral circulation, may be achieved by manipulation of MMPs and TIMPs [46]. Hence, MMPs and TIMPs represent targets for potential therapeutic intervention in CNS disorders such as brain tumors and stroke.

Acknowledgment
This work was supported by funds provided by the Rappaport Institute for Research in the Medical Sciences and the Technion – Israel Institute of Technology, Haifa, Israel.

References

1   Graven K, Farber W (1998) Endothelial cell hypoxic stress proteins. *J Lab Clin Med* 132: 456–463

2   Pohlman TH, Harlan JM (2000) Adaptive responses of the endothelium to stress. *J Surg Res* 98: 85–119

3   Lewis JS, Lee JA, Underwood JCE, Harris AL, Lewis CE (1999) Macrophage responses to hypoxia: relevance to disease mechanisms. *J Leuk Biol* 66: 889–900

4   Faller DV (1999) Endothelial cell responses to hypoxic stress. *Clin Exp Pharmacol Physiol* 26: 74–84

5   Nagase H (1997) Activation mechanisms of matrix metalloproteinases. *Biol Chem* 378: 151–160

6   Yong VW, Krekoski CA, Forsyth PA, Bell R, Edwards DR (1998) Matrix metalloproteinases and diseases of the CNS. *Trends Neurosci* 21: 75–80

7   Borden P, Heller RA (1997) Transcriptional control of matrix metalloproteinases and the tissue inhibitors of matrix metalloproteinases. *Crit Rev Eukaryot Gene Expr* 7: 159–178

8   Henriet P, Blavier L, Declerck YA (1999) Tissue inhibitors of metalloproteinases (TIMP) in invasion and proliferation. *APMIS* 107: 111–119

9   Gomez DE, Alonso DF, Yoshiji H, Thorheirsson UP (1997) Tissue inhibitors of metalloproteinases: structure, regulation and biological functions. *Eur J Cell Biol* 74: 111–122

10 Ito A, Mukaiyama A, Itoh Y, Nagase H, Thogersen IB, Enghild JJ, Sasaguri Y, Mori Y (1996) Degradation of interleukin 1 beta by matrix metalloproteinases. *J Biol Chem* 271: 14657–14660

11 Yu Q, Stamenkovic I (1999) Cell surface-localized matrix metalloproteinase-9 prote-

olytically activates TGF-β and promotes tumor invasion and angiogenesis. *Genes Dev* 14: 163–176

12 Gearing AJH, Beckett, P, Christodoulou M, Churchill M, Clements J, Davidson AH, Drummond AH, Gallaway WA, Gilbert R, Gordon JL et al (1994) Processing of tumor necrosis factor-α percursor by metalloproteinases. *Nature* 370: 555–557

13 Lyons PD, Benveniste EN (1998). Cleavage of membrane-associated ICAM-1 from astrocytes: involvement of metalloproteinase. *Glia* 22: 103–112

14 Lombard MA, Wallace TL, Kubicek MF, Petzold GL, Mitchell MA, Hendges SK, Wolks JW (1998) Synthetic matrix metalloproteinasse inhibitors and tissue inhibitor of metalloproteinase (TIMP)-2 but not TIMP-1 inhibit shedding of tumor necrosis factor-α receptors in a human colon adenocarcinoma (Colo205) cell line. *Cancer Res* 58: 4001–4007

15 Pohlman TH, Harlan JM (2000) Adoptive responses of the endothelium to stress. *J Surg Res* 89: 85–119

16 Hill GE, Whitten CW (1997) The role of the vascular endothelium in inflammatory syndromes, atherogenesis and the propagation of disease. *J Cardiothorac Vasc Anesth* 11: 316–321

17 Belkhiri A, Richards C, Whaley M, McQueen SA, Orr FW (1997) Increased expression of activated matrix metalloproteinase by human endothelial cells after sublethal H_2O_2 exposure. *Lab Invest* 77: 533–539

18 Chandler S Miller KM, Clements JM, Lury J, Corkill D, Anthony DC, Adams SE, Gearing AJ (1997) Matrix metalloproteinases, tumor necrosis factor and multiple sclerosis: an overview. *J Neuroimmunol* 72: 155–161

19 Shapiro S, Lahat N, Finkelstein, Bitterman H, Miller A (1999) Effects of hypoxia, reoxygenation and tumor necrosis factor (TNF)-α on the secretion of MMP-2 by human endothelial cells. *J Neurol* 246 (Suppl 1): 76

20 Rosenberg GA, Estrada Dencoff JE (1998) Matrix metalloproteinases and TIMPs are associated with blood-brain barrier opening after reperfusion in rat brain. *Stroke* 29: 2189–2195

21 Matyszak MK, Perry VH (1996) Delayed-type hypersensitivity lesions in the central nervous system are prevented by inhibitors of matrix metalloproteinases. *J Neuroimmunol* 69: 141–149

22 Gasche Y, Fujimura M, Morita-Fujimora Y, Copin JC, Kawase M, Massengale J, Chan PH (1999) Early appearance of activated matrix metalloproteinase-9 after cerebral ischemia in mice: a possible role in blood-brain barrier dysfunction. *J Cereb Blood Flow Metab* 19: 1020–1028

23 Fujimura M, Gasche Y, Morita-Fujimura Y, Massengale J, Kawase M, Chan PH (1999) Early appearance of activated matrix metalloproteinase-9 and blood-brain barrier disruption in mice after focal cerebral ischemia and reperfusion. *Brain Res* 842: 92–100

24 Romanic AM, White RF, Arleth AJ, Ohlstein EH, Barone FC (1998) Matrix metalloproteinase expression increases after cerebral focal ischemia in rats: inhibition of matrix metalloproteinase-9 reduces infarct size. *Stroke* 29: 1020–1030

25 Heo JH, Lucero J, Abumiya T, Koziol JA, Copeland BR, del Zoppo GJ (1999) Matrix metalloproteinases increase very early during experimental focal cerebral ischemia. *J Cereb Blood Flow Metab* 19: 624–633

26 Braker C, Shapiro S, Lahat N, Honigman S, Miller A (1999) Matrix metalloproteinases (MMPs) and IL-8 CSF levels are correlated with brain edema following cerebral infarction. In: WF List, MM Muller, ASt John (eds): *Advances in critical care testing*. Springer Verlag, Heidelberg, 103–104

27 Clark AW, Krekoski CA, Bou SS, Chapman KR, Edwards DR (1997) Increased gelatinase A (MMP-2) and gelatinase B (MMP-9) activities in human brain after focal ischemia. *Neurosci Lett* 238: 53–56

28 Anthony DC, Ferguson B, Matyzak MK, Miller KM, Esiri MM, Perry VH (1997) Differential matrix metalloproteinase expression in cases of multiple sclerosis and stroke. *Neuropathol Appl Neurobiol* 23: 406–415

29 Muir KW, Weir CJ, Alwan W, Squire IB, Lees KR (1999) C-reactive protein after ischemic stroke. *Stroke* 30: 981–985

30 Rajavashisth TB Xu XP, Jovinge S, Meisel S, Xu XO, Chai NM, Fishbein MC, Kaul S, Cereck B, Sharifi B et al (1999) Membrane type 1 matrix metalloproteinase expression in human artherosclerotic plaques: evidence for activation by proinflamatory mediators. *Circulation* 99: 3103–3109

31 Harkness KA, Adamson P, Sussman JD, Davies-Jones GAB, Geenwood J, Woodroofe MN (2000) Dexamethasone regulation of matrix metalloproteinase expression in CNS vascular endothelium. *Brain* 123: 698–709

32 Uhm JH, Dooley NP, Oh LY, Yong VW (1998) Oligodendrocytes utilize a matrix metalloproteinase, MMP-9, to extend processes along an astrocyte extracellular matrix. *Glia* 22: 53–63

33 Ellison JA, Barone FC, Feuerstein GZ (1999) Matrix remodeling after stroke. *De novo* expression of matrix proteins and integrin receptors. *Ann NY Acad Sci* 890: 204–222

34 Ishida T, Yarimizu K, Gute DC, Korhtuis RJ (1997) Mechanisms of ischemic preconditioning. *Shock* 8: 86–94

35 Yellon DM, Dana A (2000) The preconditioning phenomenon. *Circ Res* 87: 543–550

36 Moncayo J, De Freitas GR, Bogousslavsky J, Altieri M, Melle G (2000) Do transient ischemic attacks have a neuroprotective effect? *Neurology* 54: 2089–2094

37 Ginis I, Schweizer U, Brenner M, Liu J, Azzam N, Spatz M, Hallenbeck JM (1999) TNFα pretreatment prevents subsequent activation of cultured brain cells with TNF-α and hypoxia *via* ceramide. *Am J Physiol* 276: C1171–C1183

38 Wang X, Yaish-Ohad S, Li X, Barone FC, Feurstein GZ (1998) Use of suppression subtractive hybridization strategy for discovery of increased tissue inhibitor of matrix metalloproteinase-1 gene expression in brain ischemic tolerance. *J Cereb Blood Flow Metab* 18: 1173–1177

39 Folkman J (1995) Angiogenesis in cancer, vascular rheumatoid and other disease. *Nature Med* 1: 27–31

40   Plate KH (1999) Mechanisms of angiogenesis in the brain. *J Neuropathol Exp Neurol* 58: 313–320

41   Reijneveld JC, Voest EE, Taphoorn HJB (2000) Angiogenesis in malignant primary and metastatic brain tumors. *J Neurol* 247: 597–608

42   Nakano A, Tani E, Miyazaki K, Yamamoto Y, Furuyama J (1995) Matrix metalloproteinases and tissue inhibitors of metaloproteinases in human gliomas. *J Neurosurg* 83: 298–307

43   Freidberg MH, Glantz MJ, Klempner MS, Cole BF, Perides G (1998) Specific matrix metalloproteinase profiles in the cerebrospinal fluid correlated with the presence of malignant astrocytomas, brain metastases, and carcinomatous meningitis. *Cancer* 82: 923–930

44   Ratcliffe PJ, Pugh CW, Maxwell PH.(2000) Targeting tumors through the HIF system. *Nature Med* 6: 1315–1316

45   Kung AL, Wang S, Klco JM, Kaelin Jr WG, Livingston DM (2000) Suppression of tumor growth through disruption of hypoxia-inducible transcription. *Nature Med* 6: 1335–1340

46   Miller A, Shapiro S, Lahat N, Galboiz Y. Matrix metalloproteinases and their inhibitors in brain injury and repair. In: O Abramsky, A Compston, G Said, A Miller (eds): *Brain disease: Therapeutic strategies and repair*. Martin Dunitz Publishers, London; *in press*

Extracellular matrix-degrading metalloproteinases and neuroinflammation in stroke

Gary A. Rosenberg

Departments of Neurology, Neurosciences, and Cell Biology and Physiology, University of New Mexico Health Sciences Center, Albuquerque, NM 87131, USA

Introduction

Cerebral ischemia initiates a complex cascade of molecular events, culminating in irreversible membrane damage and cell death. Important components of the cascade include the release of glutamate, induction of immediate early genes, and the formation of free radicals and proteases. Lipases attack cell membranes; endonucleases damage DNA, causing apoptosis; and neutral proteases disrupt the extracellular matrix (ECM). The matrix metalloproteinases (MMPs) and serine proteases, including the plasminogen activators (PAs), are two important neutral protease gene families that are involved in the neuroinflammatory response after ischemia. Much is known about the biology of these proteases because of the prominent role that the MMPs and PAs play in cancer and arthritis [1]. Intracerebral injection of activated MMP-2 opens the blood-brain barrier (BBB) [2]. Hemorrhage and ischemia increase gelatinases in the brain [3, 4]. Infiltrating cells are a source of MMPs in injury. Immunohistochemistry shows that brain cells also produce MMPs after an ischemic injury. MMPs are formed as proenzymes, and require activation. Plasmin, which activates several of the MMPs, is formed by the conversion of plasminogen to plasmin through the action of tissue-type and urokinase-type PA [5]. Plasminogen activators act synergistically with the MMPs in many pathological processes, including those involving the central nervous system [6]. In stroke the use of recombinant tissue plasminogen activator (rtPA) has been shown to be an effective treatment when given acutely, but its use increases the risk of intracerebral hemorrhage by tenfold [7]. The unwanted side-effects of rtPA may be related to the presence of plasmin and the activation of the MMPs. Hemorrhagic transformation occurs commonly in stroke in the absence of thrombolytic treatment [8, 9]. Current studies in a number of laboratories are aimed at reducing the impact of ECM degradation and preventing the damage to the BBB that occurs with neuroinflammation. Treatments that control the ECM damage may be useful in reducing the hemorrhagic changes that accompany reperfusion therapy. Several reviews have described the role of the MMPs in neurological diseases [10–13]. The present review will focus on the molecular biology of the MMPs and their role in cerebrovascular diseases.

Inflammation and Stroke, edited by Giora Z. Feuerstein

Table 1 - Substrate-based classification of MMPs

MMP family	Descriptive name	No.	Substrates
Collagenases	Interstitial collagenase	MMP-1	Fibrillar collagen, types I, II, III
	Neutrophil collagenase	MMP-8	
	Collagenase-3	MMP-13	
Gelatinases	Gelatinase A	MMP-2	Nonfibrillar collagens, types IV, V
	Gelatinase B	MMP-9	
Stromelysins	Stromelysin-1	MMP-3	Proteoglycans, laminin,
	Stromelysin-2	MMP-10	Fibronectin, nonfibrillar collagens
	Matrilysin	MMP-7	
	Stromelysin-3	MMP-11	Serine protease inhibitors
Elastase	Metalloelastase	MMP-12	Elastin, nonfibrillar collagen
Membrane-type	MT1-MMP	MMP-14	Progelatinase A

(from Nelson et al. (2000) J Clin Oncol 18: 1135)

Molecular biology of the MMPs

The MMPs are a growing family of neutral proteases of which over twenty members have been identified [1]. They have been grouped according to protein structure and substrate specificity into four main groups (Tab. 1) (see for review [1]). Collagenases, which include interstitial collagenase (MMP-1), neutrophil collagenase (MMP-8) and collagenase-3 (MMP-13), disrupt fibrillary collagens type I, II, and III. Gelatinase A (MMP-2) is constitutively expressed as a latent 72-kDa molecule, and gelatinase B (MMP-9) is a proinflammatory 92-kDa latent enzyme. The gelatinases attack components of the basement membranes, including type IV collagen, fibronectin, lamina, and heparin sulfate. The gelatinases play a major role in the proteolytic opening of the BBB by attacking the basal lamina that surrounds cerebral blood vessels. Stromelysin-1 (MMP-3) attacks multiple components of the ECM, including type IV collagen, fibronectin, laminin, and proteoglycans. In addition to disruption of the ECM glycoproteins, the stromelysins are important in the activation of other MMPs, and have been implicated in cell death in nonbrain tissues [14]. The final group, the membrane-type MMPs activate MMP-2 at the cell surface in the presence of tissue inhibitor for metalloproteinase-2 (TIMP-2) [15].

The MMPs have several domains (Fig. 1). The smallest of the MMPs is matrilysin (MMP-7) which contains only the pre-propeptide and zinc catalytic domains. Addition of a hinge domain attached to a hemopexin domain is found in the stromelysins. The MT-MMPs have both a furin-binding and a transmembrane domain. Gelatinases substitute a fibronectin-binding domain for the furin-binding domain.

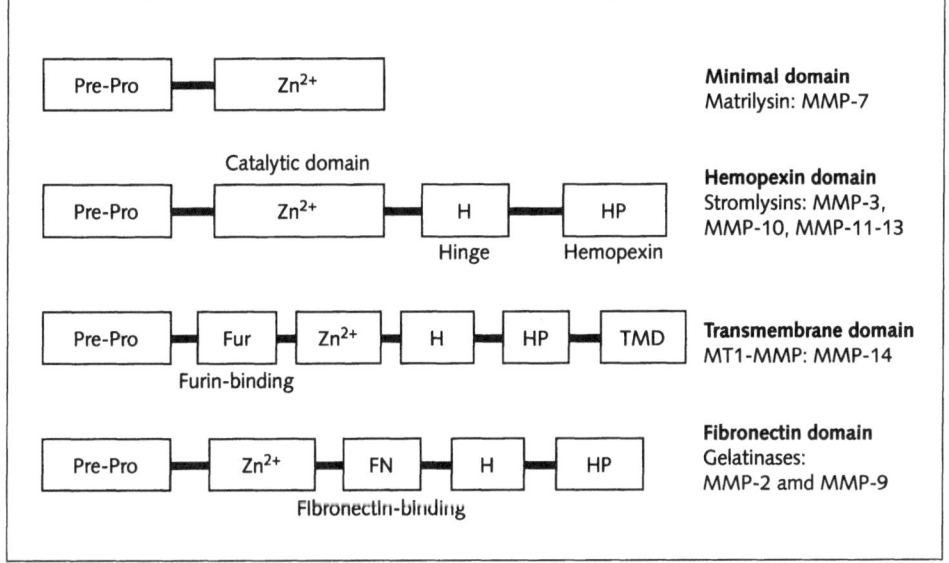

Figure 1

Domain structure of the MMPs. All of the MMPs have a pre-propeptide (Pre-Pro) domain that maintains the latency. The hemopexin (HP) domain is present in the stromelysins and the membrane-bound MMPs. Furin-binding domain is found in the MT-MMPs, and fibronectin-binding domain in the gelatinases.

MMPs are tightly regulated at multiple sites to prevent unwanted proteolysis. Transcriptional control of the MMPs has been studied intensively in many tissues, but less is known about the factors controlling transcription of the MMPs in brain cells. Activator protein-1 (AP-1) binding sites are present in the promoter regions of the genes for MMP-1, MMP-3, and MMP-9, while a nuclear factor-κB (NF-κB) site is found in the MMP-9 gene (Tab. 2). MMP-2 is a constitutively expressed enzyme that is normally present in brain tissue and in the cerebrospinal fluid; the MMP-2 promoter region is poorly defined. The AP-1 site, which is referred to as the tumor promoter-responsive element (TRE), interacts with oncogenes, c-jun and c-fos [16]. Cytokines, growth factors, and other substrates induce the production of the proinflammatory MMPs. Of the proinflammatory MMPs much is known about the collagenases and the stromelysins. Many substances affect the transcription of these inflammatory MMPs. A partial list of the factors that stimulate or suppress the MMP-3 gene promoter region is given in Table 3 [17].

Plasminogen activators and MMPs act together to disrupt ECM in many normal and pathological processes (Fig. 2). They have been extensively studied in development, where PA is involved in the growth cones of neurons [18], and in the inva-

Table 2 - Major transcription factors located in the promoter region of several matrix metal-loproteinase genes present in the central nervous system.

	TATA[1]	Ets	TRE	TIE	AP-2	NF-κB
Collagenase-1 (MMP-1)	X	X	X (3)			
Stromelysin-1 (MMP-3)	X	X (2)	X	X		
Gelatinase B (MMP-9)	X	X	X		X (2)	X
Gelatinase A (MMP-2)	X					

[1]*See text for explanation of abbreviations.*

Table 3 - Factors that modulate synthesis of stromelysin-1

Stimulatory factors	Suppressive factors
Interleukin-1α, -1β, -6, -10	Retinoic acid
Tumor necrosis factor-α	Glucocorticoid
Epidermal growth factor	Transforming growth factor-β
Platelet-derived growth factor	Interleukin-4
Basic fibroblast growth factor	Tetracycline
Nerve growth factor	Progesterone
Transforming growth factor-α	Interferon-γ
Fibronectin fragments	High glucose
Phorbol esters	
Lipopolysaccharide	
Heat shock	
Viral transformation	
Cellular aging	
Mechanical injury	

siveness of cancer cells [19]. The serine protease, plasmin, is produced by PAs. Plasmin activates proMMP-3 and proMT-MMP [20]. Activated MT-MMP activates proMMP-2 [15]. Furin, which is a member of the convertase family, may also be involved in the activation of the proMT-MMP [21]. An important exception to the need to have an activator for the MMPs, is the release of an active form of MMP-9 by infiltrating neutrophils [22]. This is a source of MMPs in stroke [23]. Brain cells are another important source of MMPs. Astrocytes in culture normally form MMP-2, and under stressful situations, such as stimulation by lipopolysaccharide (LPS), they release MMP-9 in a latent form [24]. Microglia produce low levels of MMP-2

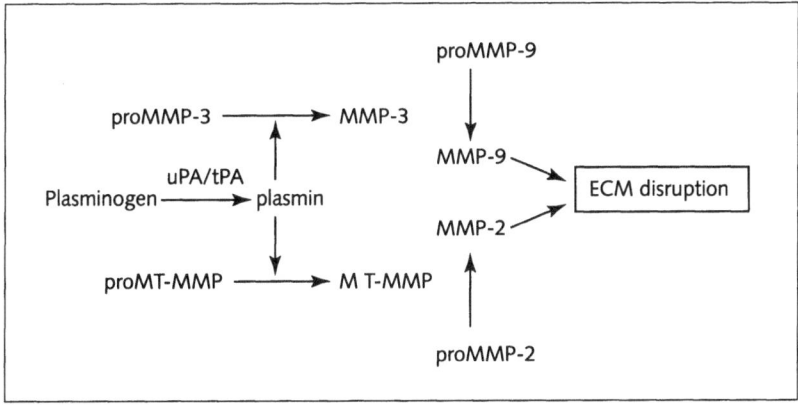

Figure 2
Plasmin is central to the activation of the activators of the gelatinases. Urokinase-type plas-
minogen activator (uPA), and tissue-type plasminogen activator (tPA) converts plasminogen
to plasmin. Plasmin acts on the proMMP-3 and proMT-MMP, and these convert the inactive
forms of the gelatinases to the active forms.

and are a major source of MMP-9 during LPS stimulation [25]. Endothelial cells produce MMP-9, which can be suppressed by dexamethasone [26, 27]. Steroids block the production of MMP-9 by interfering with the binding of the Fos/Jun dimer to the AP-1 site [28].

MMPs in cerebrovascular disease

Cytokines regulate the release of MMPs. Intracerebral injection of tumor necrosis factor-α (TNFα) leads to the delayed production of MMP-9 at 24 h. When the MMP-9 is elevated, the BBB is opened, and a synthetic inhibitor to the MMPs of the hydroxymate type reduced the damage to the BBB [29]. Similarly, LPS induces MMP-9 and opens the BBB, but the effect is seen earlier, and the BBB damage can be blocked with a MMP inhibitor [30].

Both permanent and temporary ischemia leads to MMP production, but the blood vessel undergoes a greater degree of damage during transient occlusion. Reperfusion causes a biphasic injury to the BBB, increasing the risk of brain edema and hemorrhage [31]. The MMPs, which are induced during reperfusion, participate in the BBB damage. Permanent occlusion of the middle cerebral artery in spontaneously hypertensive rats increased levels of MMP-9 within 24 h and MMP-2 at 5 days [4]. Confirmation of these observations have been made in mice and nonhuman primates [32–34]. Furthermore, autopsy studies of patients with cerebral infarction have shown increased levels of MMP-9 in regions of ischemia by immunohistochemistry and zymography [35, 36].

Increased levels of MMPs correspond to the BBB damage. Reperfusion injury results in a biphasic opening of the BBB [31, 37, 38]. We measured the levels of MMPs by zymography in normotensive rats subjected to a 2-h middle cerebral artery occlusion (MCAO) with reperfusion for 3 h to 21 days [39]. Measurement of BBB permeability with ^{14}C-sucrose 10 min prior to the end of the reperfusion time showed an initial injury after 3 h of reperfusion with the second opening at 48 h. The initial opening of the BBB correlated with an increase in MMP-2, while the delayed opening was associated with a rise in MMP-9. A second marked increase in MMP-2 occurred at 5 days and persisted for 3 weeks, which corresponded to the phase of wound healing and angiogenesis. MMP-2 has been shown to be associated with the early opening of the BBB in nonhuman primates, and MMP-9, which is increased at the time of the secondary opening at 48 h, is associated with hemorrhage [34].

Immunohistochemistry of MMPs in reperfusion injury

Immunohistochemistry with antibodies to MMP-9 showed localization to endothelial cells and infiltrating neutrophils in rats [23]. We studied the distribution of MMP-2, MMP-3, and MMP-9 by immunohistochemistry [42]. Rats had either a 90 or 120 MCAO by the suture method [40]. In sham-operated control rats, MMP-2 immunoreactivity was observed in astrocytic foot processes around cerebral blood vessels. The MMP-2+ cells were particularly prominent in the white matter, which has been seen in humans [41]. Reperfusion after 3 h increased immunostaining for MMP-2 in both astrocytic cell bodies as well as in astrocytic processes. The MMP-2 immunoreactivity was reduced at 24 h but reappeared in large, reactive astrocytes around the core of the infarction at 5 and 21 days.

MMP-9 is observed in endothelial cells and infiltrating neutrophils in the region of the infarct [23]. Immunohistochemistry was done for MMP-3 in ischemic tissues. We found MMP-3 immunostaining in reactive microglia, pericytes (perivascular microglia), and neurons in the ischemic zones at 16, 24, and 48 h. Cells containing MMP-3 were also positive for markers of apoptotic cell death, suggesting that MMP-3 participates in the cell death process [42]. Little is known about the role of MMP-3 in brain. We have used cell culture methods to explore this issue. Cultures of astrocytes and microglia were grown separately or in joint cultures. Enriched astrocyte cultures stimulated with LPS showed an activated form of MMP-2, but an inactive form of MMP-9. Enriched microglia cultures upon stimulation formed MMP-9 in both the latent and activated forms. Dual-labeling of enriched microglia cell cultures with markers for microglia and MMP-3 showed that microglia contained MMP-3, which was absent from astrocytes. This suggested that the MMP-3

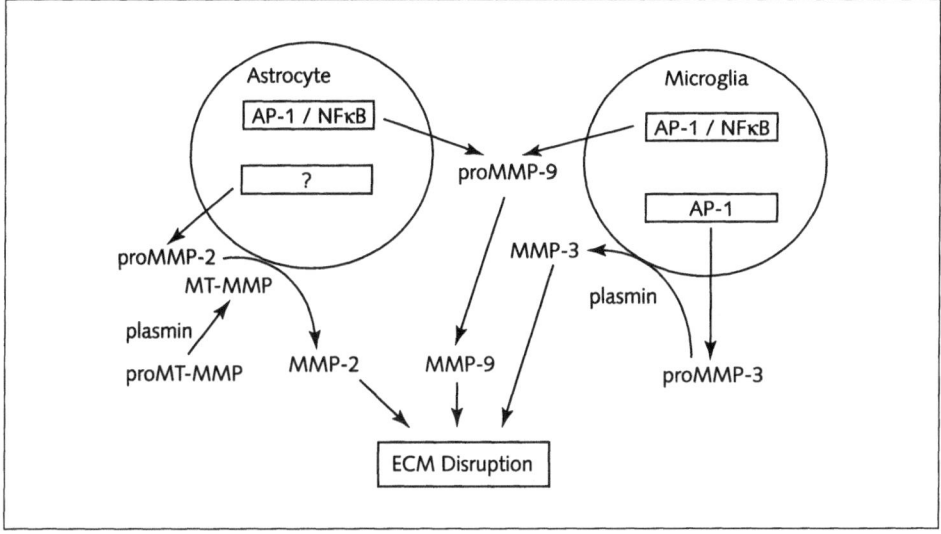

Figure 3
Schematic diagram of the interaction of the astrocytes and the microglia in the formation and activation of the gelatinases. Promoter regions of the MMP-9 gene contains both AP-1 and NF-κB sites, and the MMP-3 gene promoter region contains only the AP-1 site. Astrocytes are able to form and activate the MMP-2 during LPS stimulation, suggesting that they form both proMMP-2 and proMT-MMP. ProMMP-9 is formed by both astrocytes and microglia, but the activator, MMP-3, is derived from the microglia. The end result of the production and activation of the MMPs is the break down of the extracellular matrix (ECM).

derived from microglia was the factor involved in activation of MMP-9. Thus, each cell involved in forming the BBB has a separate MMP composition: endothelial cells form MMP-9, pericytes make both MMP-9 and MMP-3, and astrocytic foot processes contain the MMP-2. An interaction between the various cells in regard to the type of MMP released determines the permeability of the BBB. The interaction between the astrocytes and microglia in culture is shown schematically in Figure 3. Whether this is the manner in which these cells interact *in vivo* remains to be determined.

Proteolysis of the blood-brain barrier

Our biochemical and immunohistochemical observations suggest a possible mechanism to explain the biphasic opening of the BBB. The initial ischemic injury at 3 h was related to an increase in MMP-2, which could have been activated by MT-

MMP. The activator of the MT-MMP remains to be determined, but could have been either plasmin or furin. This could explain the increased propensity for hemorrhage that is seen during rtPA treatment of acute stroke. This initial opening, which sensitizes the brain for subsequent injury, is reversible. Because the released MMP-2 is constrained to the membrane by MT-MMP and TIMP-2, the damage is restricted to a focal region around the site of release. As the inflammatory response is amplified by the release of cytokines and the recruitment of neutrophils, a second opening occurs at 48 h. Other neuroinflammatory modulators act on the AP-1 and NF-κB sites in the promoter regions of the genes, leading to the induction and activation of MMP-3, probably by plasmin, and the activation of the MMP-9 by MMP-3. Since MMP-3 and MMP-9 are released and activated in the extracellular space, the damage caused would be more widespread, resulting in vasogenic edema with a heightened risk of hemorrhage.

These studies suggest possible therapeutic strategies for reduction of MMP-related disruption of the ECM. Previous studies have shown the efficacy in cerebrovascular diseases of agents that block MMPs; hydroxymate-type MMP inhibitors reduced the initial opening of the BBB during reperfusion and limited brain edema at 24 h [39]. An antibody to MMP-9 reduced the size of the infarct after a permanent middle cerebral artery occlusion [23]. Inhibitors of the hydroxymate type are nonspecific. Because they inhibit a wide range of MMPs, some of which are involved in normal processes, they may have unwanted side-effects. Since there is an interaction between the plasminogen/plasmin system and the MMPs, a potential strategy would be to reduce the activation of the plasminogen/plasmin system. Newer agents are under development that are more specific to the various MMPs [1]. Proper use of these agents, however, will require more information of the various roles for the MMPs in normal and pathological brain functions.

Acknowledgements
These studies were supported by a RO1 grant (NS-21169) from the National Institutes of Health. A number of people have contributed to these studies, including S. Alexander, L. Cunningham, J. Dencoff, E.Y. Estrada, M. Grossetete, D. Hofinger, M. Lukes, and J. Wallace.

Reference

1   Nelson AR, Fingleton B, Rothenberg ML, Matrisian LM (2000) Matrix metalloproteinases: biologic activity and clinical implications. *J Clin Oncol* 18: 1135–1149
2   Rosenberg GA, Kornfeld M, Estrada E, Kelley RO, Liotta LA, Stetler-Stevenson WG

(1992) TIMP-2 reduces proteolytic opening of blood-brain barrier by type IV collagenase. *Brain Res* 576: 203–207

3   Rosenberg GA, Dencoff JE, McGuire PG, Liotta LA, Stetler-Stevenson WG (1994) Injury-induced 92-kDa gelatinase and urokinase expression in rat brain. *Lab Invest* 71: 417–422

4   Rosenberg GA, Navratil M, Barone F, Feuerstein G (1996) Proteolytic cascade enzymes increase in focal cerebral ischemia in rat. *J Cereb Blood Flow Metabolism* 16: 360–366

5   Mignatti P, Rifkin DB (1996) Plasminogen activators and matrix metalloproteinases in angiogenesis. *Enzyme & Protein* 49: 117–137

6   Cuzner ML, Opdenakker G (1999) Plasminogen activators and matrix metalloproteases, mediators of extracellular proteolysis in inflammatory demyelination of the central nervous system, J. Neuroimmunol 94: 1–14

7   Anonymous. (1995) Tissue plasminogen activator for acute ischemic stroke. The National Institute of Neurological Disorders and Stroke rt-PA Stroke Study Group [see comments]. *N Engl J Med* 333: 1581–1587

8   Hornig CR, Dorndorf W, Agnoli AL. (1986) Hemorrhagic cerebral infarction – a prospective study. *Stroke* 17: 179–185

9   Hornig CR, Bauer T, Simon C, Trittmacher S, Dorndorf W (1993) Hemorrhagic transformation in cardioembolic cerebral infarction. *Stroke* 24: 465–468

10   Romanic AM, Madri JA (1994) Extracellular matrix-degrading proteinases in the nervous system. *Brain Pathol* 4: 145–156

11   Yong VW, Kerkoski CA, Forsyth PA, Bell R, Edwards DR (1998) Matrix metalloproteinases and diseases of the CNSs. *TINS* 21: 75–80

12   Mun-Bryce S, Rosenberg GA (1998) Matrix metalloproteinases in cerebrovascular disease. *J Cereb Blood Flow Metabolism* 18: 1163–1172

13   Lukes A, Mun-Bryce S, Lukes M, Rosenberg GA (1999) Extracellular matrix degradation by metalloproteinases and central nervous system diseases. *Mol Neurobiol* 19: 267–284

14   Nagase H (1995) Human stromelysins 1 and 2. *Meth Enzymol* 248: 449–470

15   Sato H, Takino T, Okada Y, Cao J, Shinagawa A, Yamamoto E, Seiki M (1994) A matrix metalloproteinase expressed on the surface of invasive tumour cells. *Nature* 370: 61–65

16   Fini ME, Cook JR, Mohan R, Brinckerhoff CE (1998) Regulation of matrix metalloproteinase gene expression. In: WC Parks, RP Mecham (eds.): *Matrix metalloproteinases*. Academic Press, San Diego, CA, 300–356

17   Nagase H, Woessner JF Jr (1999) Matrix metalloproteinases. *J Biol Chem* 274: 21491–21494

18   Krystosek A, Seeds NW (1981) Plasminogen activator release at the neuronal growth cone. *Science* 213: 1532–1534

19   Liotta LA, Goldfarb RH, Brundage R, Siegal GP, Terranova V, Garbisa S (1981) Effect of plasminogen activator (urokinase), plasmin, and thrombin on glycoprotein and collagenous components of basement membrane. *Cancer Res* 41: 4629–4636

20   Ramos-DeSimone N, Hahn-Dantona E, Sipley J, Nagase H, French DL, Quigley, JP

(1999) Activation of matrix metalloproteinase-9 (MMP-9) *via* a converging plasmin/stromelysin-1 cascade enhances tumor cell invasion. J Biol Chem 274: 13066–13076

21   Sato H, Kinoshita T, Takino T, Nakayama K, Seiki M (1996) Activation of a recombinant membrane type 1-matrix metalloproteinase (MT1-MMP) by furin and its interaction with tissue inhibitor of metalloproteinases (TIMP)-2. *FEBS Lett* 393: 101–104

22   Hibbs MS, Hasty KA, Seyer JM, Kang AH, Mainardi CL (1985) Biochemical and immunological characterization of the secreted forms of human neutrophil gelatinase. *J Biol Chem* 260: 2493–2500

23   Romanic AM, White RF, Arleth AJ, Ohlstein EH, Barone FC (1998) Matrix metalloproteinase expression increases after cerebral focal ischemia in rats: inhibition of matrix metalloproteinase-9 reduces infarct size. *Stroke* 29: 1020–1030

24   Deb S, Gottschall PE (1996) Increased production of matrix metalloproteinases in enriched astrocyte and mixed hippocampal cultures treated with beta- amyloid peptides. *J Neurochem* 66: 1641–1647

25   Colton CA, Keri JE, Chen WT, Monsky WL (1993) Protease production by cultured microglia: substrate gel analysis and immobilized matrix degradation. *J Neurosci Res* 35: 297–304

26   Herron GS, Werb Z, Dwyer K, Banda MJ (1986) Secretion of metalloproteinases by stimulated capillary endothelial cells. I. Production of procollagenase and pro-stromelysin exceeds expression of proteolytic activity. *J Biol Chem* 261: 2810–2813

27   Harkness KA, Adamson P, Sussman JD, Davies-Jones GA, Greenwood J, Woodroofe MN (2000) Dexamethasone regulation of matrix metalloproteinase expression in CNS vascular endothelium. *Brain* 123 (Pt 4): 698–709

28   Jonat C, Rahmsdorf HJ, Park KK, Cato AC, Gebel S, Ponta H, Herrlich P (1990) Antitumor promotion and antiinflammation: down-modulation of AP- 1 (Fos/Jun) activity by glucocorticoid hormone. *Cell* 62: 1189–1204

29   Rosenberg GA, Estrada EY, Dencoff JE, Stetler-Stevenson WG (1995) Tumor necrosis factor-alpha-induced gelatinase B causes delayed opening of the blood-brain barrier: an expanded therapeutic window. *Brain Res* 703: 151–155

30   Mun-Bryce S, Rosenberg GA (1998) Gelatinase B modulates selective opening of the blood-brain barrier during inflammation. *Am J Physiol* 274: R1203–R1211

31   Kuroiwa T, Ting P, Martinez H, Klatzo I (1985) The biphasic opening of the blood-brain barrier to proteins following temporary middle cerebral artery occlusion. *Acta Neuropathol* 68: 122–129

32   Gasche Y, Fujimura M, Morita-Fujimura Y, Copin JC, Kawase M, Massengale J, Chan PH (1999) Early appearance of activated matrix metalloproteinase-9 after focal cerebral ischemia in mice: a possible role in blood-brain barrier dysfunction. *J Cereb Blood Flow Metabol* 19: 1020–1028

33   Fujimura M, Gasche Y, Morita-Fujimura Y, Massengale J, Kawase M, Chan PH (1999) Early appearance of activated matrix metalloproteinase-9 and blood-brain barrier disruption in mice after focal cerebral ischemia and reperfusion. *Brain Res* 842: 92–100

34 Heo JH, Lucero J, Abumiya T, Koziol JA, Copeland BR, del Zoppo GJ (1999) Matrix metalloproteinases increase very early during experimental focal cerebral ischemia. *J Cereb Blood Flow Metabol* 19: 624–633

35 Clark AW, Krekoski CA, Bou S-S, Chapman KR, Edwards DR (1997) Increased gelatinase A (MMP-2) and gelatinase B (MMP-9) activities in human brain after focal ischemia. *Neurosci Lett* 238: 53–56

36 Anthony DC, Ferguson B, Matyzak MK, Miller KM, Esiri MM, Perry VH (1997) Differential matrix metalloproteinase expression in cases of multiple sclerosis and stroke. *Neuropathol Appl Neurobiol* 23: 406–415

37 Belayev L, Busto R, Zhao W, Ginsberg MD (1996) Quantitative evaluation of blood-brain barrier permeability following middle cerebral artery occlusion in rats. *Brain Res* 739: 88–96

38 Yang GY, Betz AL (1994) Reperfusion-induced injury to the blood-brain barrier after middle cerebral artery occlusion in rats. *Stroke* 25: 1658–64; discussion 1664–

39 Rosenberg GA, Estrada EY, Dencoff JE (1998) Matrix metalloproteinases and TIMPs are associated with blood-brain barrier opening after reperfusion in rat brain. *Stroke* 29: 2189–2195

40 Longa EZ, Weinstein PR, Carlson S, Cummins R (1989) Reversible middle cerebral artery occlusion without craniectomy in rats. *Stroke* 20: 84–91

41 Yamada T, Yoshiyama Y, Sato H, Seiki M, Shinagawa A, Takahashi M (1995) White matter microglia produce membrane-type matrix metalloprotease, an activator of gelatinase A, in human brain tissues. *Acta Neuropathol* 90: 421–424

42 Rosenberg GA, Cunningham LA, Wallace J, Alexander S, Estrada EY, Grossetete M, Razhagi A, Miller K, Gearing A (2001) Immunohistochemistry of matrix metalloproteinases in reperfusion injury to rat brain: activation of MMP-9 linked to stromelysin-1 and microglia in cell cultures. *Brain Res* 893: 104–112

Anti-oxidant strategies to treat stroke

Bernhard H.J. Juurlink

Department of Anatomy and Cell Biology, College of Medicine, University of Saskatchewan, 107 Wiggins Road, Saskatoon, SK, S7N 5E5, Canada

Introduction

There is an abundance of evidence that there is significant oxidative stress following stroke [1]. Human trials with therapies aimed at reducing oxidative stress have, however, been disappointing. The trials with the 21-aminosteroid tirilazad mesylate suggests that this anti-oxidant therapy does not result in better outcome following stroke [2] and may even result in worse outcome [3]. The reasons for these failures are understandable when pathways of oxidative stress are examined. A consideration of the consequences of oxidative stress at the cellular level and mechanisms used by the cell to minimize oxidative stress ought to provide the theoretical basis for rationally pursuing therapies directed towards minimizing oxidative stress.

Oxidative stress and cell dysfunction

Strong oxidants such as the hydroxyl radical [4] or peroxynitrous acid [5] can cause polyunsaturated fatty acid peroxidation that, in the presence of oxygen, initiates a self-perpetuating chain reaction of lipid peroxidation causing alterations in membrane fluidity [6], increased permeability of membranes [7] and decreased membrane ATPase activity [8]. This results in increased Na^+ and Ca^{2+} influx resulting in depletion of cellular ATP stores and all the problems associated with cellular Ca^{2+} overload [9, 10]. Lipid radicals and peroxides also break down (Fig. 1) forming pro-inflammatory isoprostanes [11] and isoleukotrienes [12] or strong oxidants including dicarbonyls such as malondialdehyde [13] and α,β-unsaturated aldehydes [14, 15]. The latter are strong oxidants that can interfere with critical cellular functions such as glutamate uptake [14, 16], alter membrane protein configuration [7], interfere with maintenance of ion homeostasis [17], as well as mitochondrial respiration [18]. In addition, other oxidants such as peroxynitrous acid inhibit the activity of the mitochondrial respiratory chain proteins [19].

Oxidative stress can promote activation of pro-inflammatory gene cascades activating nuclear factor κB (NF-κB), reviewed in [20]. NF-κB is a transcriptional

Inflammation and Stroke, edited by Giora Z. Feuerstein

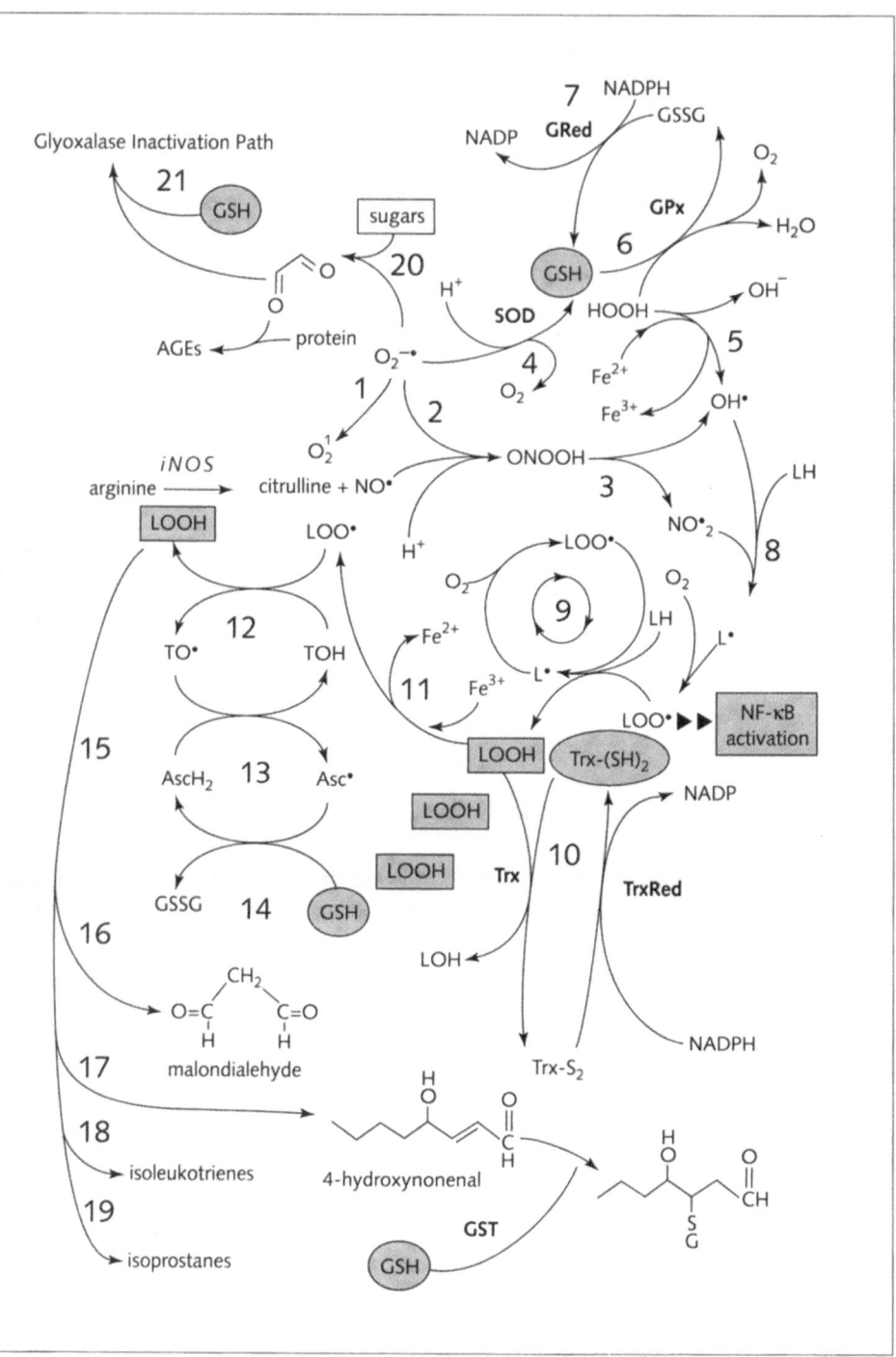

factor complex whose activation is required for maximal transcription of a wide array of pro-inflammatory proteins important in the generation of acute inflammation [21].

Mechanisms of strong oxidant production and scavenging

Glutathione (GSH)-dependent scavenging mechanisms

This is illustrated in Figure 1. References for these pathways can be found in [20, 22]. Note that GSH plays important roles in: (1) scavenging peroxides, both hydrogen peroxide and lipid peroxides, catalysed by the selenoproteins glutathione per-

---

Figure 1

Some pathways involved in generation and scavenging of strong oxidants. To reduce clutter, the reactions are not necessarily balanced and sometimes leave out intermediate steps. Superoxide can interact with another molecule of superoxide (#1) to form the strong oxidant, singlet oxygen. Superoxide can also interact with nitric oxide to give rise to peroxynitrous acid (#2) that in turn can give rise to strong oxidants such as the nitrogen dioxide and hydroxyl radicals (#3). Hence, superoxide is scavenged by superoxide dismutase (SOD) to form hydrogen peroxide and molecular oxygen (#4). In the presence of transition metal ions, hydrogen peroxide can give rise to the hydroxyl radical (#5). Hydrogen peroxide is scavenged by glutathione peroxidase (GPx) that requires GSH as the electron donor (#6). The oxidized-glutathione is reduced by glutathione reductase (GRed) that uses NADPH as the electron donor (#7). The hydroxyl radical can abstract an electron from a polyunsaturated fatty acid (LH) to form a carbon-centred lipid radical (#8). The lipid radical can interact with molecular oxygen to form a peroxyl radical that in turn can abstract an electron from a polyunsaturated fatty acid initiating a lipid peroxidation chain reaction (#9). The oxidative stress that ensues can activate NF-κB. The lipid peroxides that are formed are scavenged by either thioredoxin reductase using thioredoxin (Tr[SH]$_2$) as electron donor (#10) or glutathione peroxidase using GSH as the electron donor (not presented). It is necessary to scavenge the lipid peroxides since they can interact with transition metal ions to give rise to new lipid peroxyl radicals (#11) that can initiate new rounds of lipid peroxidation. Lipid peroxyl radicals are quenched by vitamin E (TOH) giving rise to an innocuous vitamin E radical (#12). The vitamin E radical is reduced by ascorbic acid (#13) and the oxidized ascorbate is reduced by GSH (#14). Lipid peroxides can also break down (#15) into: strong oxidants such as malondialdehyde (#16); 4-hydroxynonenal (#17) which is scavenged by glutathione S-transferase (GST) by formation of an adduct with GSH; isoleukotrienes (#18); and isoprostanes (#19). In the presence of transition metal ions, superoxide anion can also convert sugars to strong oxidants such as the dicarbonyl glyoxal (#20). Dicarbonyls are scavenged by the glyoxalase pathway that uses GSH as a cofactor (#21).

oxidases [23]; (2) the reduction of oxidized ascorbate [24], which is essential for the ultimate regeneration of vitamin E from the vitamin E radical; (3) in neutralizing strong oxidants including α,β-unsaturated aldehydes such as 4-hydroxynonenal by forming glutathione adducts catalyzed by various glutathione S-transferases (GSTs) [25]; (4) as an essential cofactor in the scavenging of α-oxo-aldehydes such as glyoxal and methylglyoxal [26]. Cellular levels of GSH typically vary from 2–10 mM [27].

Vitamin E, along with ascorbic acid, plays an important, albeit limited, role in peroxide scavenging by inactivating lipid peroxyl radicals, giving rise to innocuous vitamin E radicals plus lipid hydroperoxides. Inactivation of lipid peroxyl radicals does not eliminate the problems encountered with the lipid peroxidation cascade since lipid hydroperoxides can interact with transition metal ions giving rise to alkoxyl radicals, peroxyl radicals, α,β-unsaturated aldehydes or reactive aldehydes such as malondialdehyde and 4-hydroxyalkenals, as well as isoprostanes and isoleukotrienes: this is likely why anti-oxidant approaches such as administering tirilazad mesylate have not been proven to be efficacious treatments for oxidative stress.

Thioredoxin-dependent scavenging mechanisms

Thioredoxin(Trx)-dependent peroxidases (peroxiredoxins) [28] also scavenge peroxides; the significance of the peroxiredoxins in peroxide scavenging is still not clear. Oxidized-Trx is reduced by the selenoprotein Trx reductase (TrxRed). The typical concentration of Trx within cells is approximately 10 μM [29, 30]; hence, the efficiency by which Trx-dependent scavenging occurs is dependent upon the ability of the cell to reduce oxidized-Trx. TrxRed has been shown to have a number of other important anti-oxidant functions that include: (1) reduction of the ascorbyl radical [31] as well as oxidized-ascorbate [32] and lipoic acid [33]; and (2) with selenocyst(e)ine as a cofactor, TrxRed can also directly scavenge lipid peroxides [34] as well as peroxynitrite [35].

Central anti-oxidant players

GSH

During oxidative stress the ability to synthesize GSH is critical. Regulation of GSH synthesis is complex and involves the following two reactions [36]:

(1) l-glutamic acid + l-cysteine + ATP ↔ l-γ-glutamyl-l-cysteine + ADP + P_i
(2) l-γ-glutamyl-l-cysteine + ATP + glycine ↔ glutathione + ADP + P_i

The first reaction, catalyzed by 1-γ-glutamyl-1-cysteine synthase (GCS), is the rate-limiting reaction that is inhibited by GSH with the GSH-dependent inhibition alleviated by glutamate [37]. This first reaction is also rate-limiting in that cysteine is the rate-limiting amino acid. Cellular cysteine content is regulated principally by the uptake of cystine since cysteine is readily auto-oxidized. Cystine is taken up (or released) by the X^-_c antiporter in exchange for glutamate [38]; intracellularly, one molecule of cystine is reduced to two molecules of cysteine. The intracellular concentration of glutamate, thus, has a two-fold regulatory effect on intracellular GSH concentration: (1) alleviating the GSH inhibition of GCS, and (2) regulating uptake of cystine.

Phase 2 proteins

Another approach to increase intracellular GSH is to increase GCS activity. GCS is a heterodimeric enzyme whose 2 subunits are under the control of the anti-oxidant response element (ARE) [39]. The transcription of genes with an ARE in the promoter region can be induced by phase 2 protein inducers. There are a number of compounds (mainly Michael reaction acceptors, quinones and certain isothiocyanates) at low micromolar concentrations that selectively activate the anti-oxidant response; such phase 2 protein-inducing compounds can form components of our diet, see [22]. In addition to GCS, the following proteins belong to the phase 2 protein family: quinone reductase, GSTs, epoxide hydrolase, UDP-glucoronosyltransferase [40], TrxReds, both cytosolic and mitochondrial isoforms [41], inducible heme oxygenase, peroxiredoxin I, X^-c cystine/glutamate antiporter [42] and ferritin H [43].

There has been considerable study of phase 2 enzymes and their induction in the context of cancer prevention, e.g., [44, 45], but little attention has been paid in the context of other diseases. In principle, induction of phase 2 proteins ought to decrease oxidative stress.

Decreasing oxidative stress in the context of stroke

Stroke prevention

There is a link between diet and atherosclerosis, with diets high in fruits and vegetables being correlated with lower incidence of heart attacks and stroke [46, 47]. Factors that predispose one to atherogenesis all cause oxidative stress at the level of the endothelium, e.g., hypercholesterolemia, hypertension [48–50], homocysteine [51–55], hyperglycemia associated with diabetes increases the formation of advanced glycation endproducts [56, 57] which also causes increases in oxidative stress, while bacterial endotoxins activate pro-inflammatory gene expression in endothelial cells [58]. Therefore, decreasing oxidative stress ought to inhibit development of atherosclerosis. I have argued elsewhere [22] that a diet rich in phase 2 protein inducers will possibly inhibit atherogenesis; hence, I shall not dwell at length on this topic.

Decreasing oxidative stress once a stroke has occurred

One of the problems with nutritional studies in relationship to disease is that such studies tend to focus on one nutritional component without considering the interactions amongst nutritional components. For example, there are many studies on vitamin E which do not take into consideration the interaction between vitamin E radical and vitamin C, nor the importance of GSH and selenoproteins in the reduction of oxidized ascorbate and scavenging of the lipid hydroperoxides that are an endproduct of lipid peroxidation.

Nutritional intake of stroke patients is often suboptimal and malnutrition can occur secondary to stroke [59–61]. Following a stroke there is a rapid reduction of plasma anti-oxidants [62]. To date, nutritional support following trauma to the CNS been mainly targeted toward achieving caloric and nitrogen balance to prevent protein-energy malnutrition [63]. It is suggested that following a stroke there be aggressive nutritional intervention that not only targets caloric and nitrogen balance, but also promotes anti-oxidant activities of tissues.

Selenium and vitamins C and E
GPx's and TrxRed's are selenoproteins and the synthesis of these proteins is dependent upon the availability of selenium. Low serum selenium levels are associated with increased risk of stroke [64] and selenium supplementation has been shown to reduce the risk of stroke mortality in one trial [65]. The synthesis of selenoproteins is regulated by availability of dietary selenium [66]. Recommended daily allowance for selenium is 55 μg/day (National Academy of Sciences Institute of Medicine's Dietary Reference Intake value) with maximal safe intake being around 400 μg/day [67].

Vitamin E plays an important role in inactivating lipid peroxyl radicals while vitamin C plays an important role in reducing the vitamin E radical to vitamin E. The blood levels of these anti-oxidant vitamins decrease following a stroke [62]. The recommended daily allowance of vitamin is 15 mg/day of the RRR-α-tocopherol/day, while for vitamin C it is 75 and 100 mg/day for females and males respectively with an additional 35 mg/day for smokers.

It is recommended that stroke patients be administered selenium and vitamins C and E at a dose that is at least the daily recommended allowance.

GSH

Factors regulating GSH synthesis are (1) availability cysteine, (2) activity of GCS, and (3) cellular concentration of glutamate since glutamate can (a) promote cystine uptake and (b) alleviate the inhibition of GSH on GCS activity.

Cysteine delivery vehicles

Since cysteine auto-oxidizes and cystine has low solubility, an efficient way to increase intracellular cysteine is to administer cysteine-containing dipeptides that do not auto-oxidize readily. Thus, 1-γ-glutamyl-1-cysteine and especially 1-cysteinyl-glycine [68] have been shown to be efficient ways of increasing neuronal GSH by increasing intracellular cysteine. Dipeptides are increasingly used in clinical nutrition [69] and such dipeptides can be administered enterally or parenterally. A traditional nutritional approach might also be used. For example, an increase in GSH levels in tissues is seen following the consumption of whey [70–73]. The likely explanation for this is that bovine serum albumin has a high content of glutamyl cysteine residues that are released from the undenatured, but not denatured, protein as 1-γ-glutamyl-1-cysteine dipeptides in the gut. Pharmacological approaches might also be used by administering compounds that can be converted to cysteine intracellularly. Two such compounds are N-acetylcysteine (NAC) and 1-2-oxothiazolidine-4-carboxylate (OTC). We have shown that administration of OTC following spinal cord crush injury promotes GSH synthesis, decreases oxidative stress thereby minimizing tissue damage, enabling otherwise paraplegic rats to locomote [74]. OTC has been used in a number of small human clinical trials showing no untoward effects [75–78]. Although studies suggest that the procysteine compound NAC, unlike OTC [80], does not readily cross the blood-brain barrier [79], it has been shown to be neuroprotective following ischemia and reperfusion [81,82] in animal models. NAC is used clinically to treat acetaminophen-induced liver damage [83].

Increasing intracellular glutamate

Elevating intracellular glutamate promotes (1) cystine uptake and alleviates the glutamate-induced inhibition of GCS activity, and (2) ATP production since it protects against cataplerotic losses of Kreb cycle intermediates. An effective way to do this is to use glutamine as the delivery system since glutamine is readily taken up by cells and converted to glutamate by glutaminase. Since glutamine is somewhat unstable, it can be administered as the dipeptides 1-alanyl-1-glutamine or glycyl-1-glutamine [69]. Rats fed parenterally with glutamine or glutamine-containing dipeptides better maintained liver GSH than non-supplemented animals [84] and also had improved cardiac function following ischemia and reperfusion [85]. 1-Alanyl-1-glutamine supplementation parenterally has been demonstrated to be clinically safe and led to a better nitrogen balance in post-operative human patients with a significantly better clinical outcome in the supplemented patients as opposed to placebo controls [86]. Although increasing intracellular glutamate may be counter-intuitive, once a stroke has occurred it is not likely to exacerbate damage.

Induction of phase 2 protein

Increasing phase 2 enzyme proteins decreases oxidative stress *via* a large number of mechanisms. Inducers of phase 2 proteins are encountered in our diet and have been shown to increase phase 2 enzymes in rats, e.g., ellagic acid [87]; the isothiocyanate sulforaphane [88]; green tea polyphenolics [89]; soy meal [90], likely mediated by genistein [91]; certain polyphenolics in blueberries/cranberries [92]; the flavonol kaempferol [93]; curcumin, a component of turmeric [94]; and the lignan phytoestrogen enterolactone [91], the metabolite of the major flax seed lignan secoisolariciresinol diglucoside (SDG). Administration of dietary phase 2 protein inducers inhibits chemically-induced tumour formation (reviewed in [22]), suggesting that such dietary compounds might also decrease oxidative stress and accompanying inflammation.

Concluding remarks

There has been an enormous effort to develop drugs that block various glutamate receptors and calcium channels with little therapeutic effects seen in human clinical trials. There has been some effort directed toward minimizing oxidative stress following stroke and trauma; however, most of these efforts have been directed toward stopping the lipid peroxidation chain by scavenging lipid peroxyl radicals and, again, these approaches have not been promising. As can be seen from this review, scavenging lipid radicals does not eliminate the problems associated with lipid peroxides. Promoting scavenging of peroxides is an efficient way to decrease oxidative stress and this may be accomplished, in part, through a nutritional approach. It is suggested that there be an aggressive nutritional intervention following stroke to ensure that there is adequate intake of: (1) sulfur amino acids for glutathione synthesis, (2) vitamins E and C enabling efficient quenching of lipid peroxyl radicals, (3) selenium to ensure that there is optimal selenoproteins being synthesized, thus increasing peroxide scavenging efficiency.

It is also recommended that research be carried out on experimental animal models of stroke to determine whether administration of glutamine promotes glutathione synthesis and better maintains energy stores. It is also recommended that the therapeutic potential of phase 2 enzyme inducers be examined experimentally.

It seems most probable that a nutritional approach could be designed to better enable the vascular and the nervous tissues to cope with oxidative stress and decrease damage following a stroke.

Acknowledgements

I thank the Medical Research Council of Canada (now the CIHR), the Heart & Stroke Foundation of Saskatchewan, the Neurotrauma Initiative of Saskatchewan and the Saskatchewan Agriculture Development Fund for supporting my research.

References

1   Love S (1999) Oxidative stress in brain ischemia. *Brain Pathol* 9: 119–131
2   Scott P, Barsan W, Frederiksen S, Kronick S, Zink BJ, Domeier RM, Mitchiner JC, Judge FP, Levy RJ, Alexiou A et al (1996) A randomized trial of tirilazad mesylate in patients with acute stroke (RANTTAS). *Stroke* 27: 1453–1458
3   The Tirilazad Steering Committee (2000) Tirilazad mesylate in acute ischemic stroke: A systematic review. *Stroke* 31: 2257–2265
4   Braughler JM, Hall ED (1989) Central nervous system trauma and stroke. I. Biochemical considerations for oxygen radical formation and lipid peroxidation. *Free Rad Biol Med* 6: 289–301
5   Rubbo H, Radi R, Trujillo M, Telleri R, Kalyanaraman B, Barnes S, Kirk M, Freeman BA (1994) Nitric oxide regulation of superoxide and peroxynitrite-dependent lipid peroxidation. Formation of novel nitrogen-containing oxidized lipid derivatives. *J Biol Chem* 269: 26066–26075
6   McGrath LT, Douglas AF, McClean E, Brown JH, Doherty CC, Johnston GD, Archbold GP (1995) Oxidative stress and erythrocyte membrane fluidity in patients undergoing regular dialysis. *Clin Chim Acta* 235: 179–188
7   Subramaniam R, Roediger F, Jordan B, Mattson MP, Keller JN, Waeg G, Butterfield DA (1997) The lipid peroxidation product, 4-hydroxy-2-trans-nonenal, alters the conformation of cortical synaptosomal membrane proteins. *J Neurochem* 69: 1161–1169
8   Rauchova H, Ledvinkova J, Kalous M, Drahota Z (1995) The effect of lipid peroxidation on the activity of various membrane-bound ATPases in rat kidney. *Int J Biochem Cell Biol* 27: 251–255
9   Hossmann KA (1994) Glutamate-mediated injury in focal cerebral ischemia - the excitotoxin hypothesis revised. *Brain Pathol* 4: 23–36
10 Siesjö BK, Zhao Q, Pahlmark K, Siesjo P, Katsura K, Folbergrova J (1995) Glutamate, calcium, and free radicals as mediators of ischemic brain damage. *Ann Thorac Surg* 59: 1316–1320
11 Liu T-Z, Stern A, Morrow JD (1998) The isoprostanes: Unique bioactive products of lipid peroxidation. *J Biomed Sc* 5: 415–420
12 Harrison KA, Murphy RC (1995) Isoleukotrienes are biologically active free radical products of lipid peroxidation. *J Biol Chem* 270: 17273–17278
13 Esterbauer H, Zollner H, Schauer RJ (1990) Aldehydes formed by lipid peroxidation: mechanisms of formation, occurrence, and determination. In: C Vigo-Pelfrey (ed): *Membrane lipid peroxidation*. CRC Press, Boca Raton, FL, 239–268

14   Springer JE, Azbill RD, Mark RJ, Begley JG, Waeg G, Mattson MP (1997) 4-hydrox-ynonenal, a lipid peroxidation product, rapidly accumulates following traumatic spinal cord injury and inhibits glutamate uptake. *J Neurochem* 68: 2469–2476

15   Comporti M (1998) Lipid peroxidation and biogenic aldehydes: from the identification of 4- hydroxynonenal to further achievements in biopathology. *Free Radic Res* 28: 623–635

16   Blanc EM, Keller JN, Fernandez S, Mattson MP (1998) 4-hydroxynonenal, a lipid per-oxidation product, impairs glutamate transport in cortical astrocytes. *Glia* 22: 149–160

17   Mark RJ, Lovell MA, Markesbery WR, Uchida K, Mattson MP (1997) A role for 4-hydroxynonenal, an aldehydic product of lipid peroxidation, in disruption of ion home-ostasis and neuronal death induced by amyloid β-peptide. *J Neurochem* 68: 255–264

18   Picklo MJ, Amarnath V, McIntyre JO, Graham DG, Montine TJ (1999) 4-Hydroxy-2(E)-nonenal inhibits CNS mitochondrial respiration at multiple sites. *J Neurochem* 72: 1617–1624

19   Brown GC, Bolanos JP, Heales SJR, Clark JB (1995) Nitric oxide produced by activat-ed astrocytes rapidly and reversibly inhibits cellular respiration. *Neurosci Lett* 193: 201–204

20   Christman JW, Blackwell TS, Juurlink BHJ (2000) Redox regulation of nuclear factor kappa B: Therapeutic potential for attenuating inflammatory responses. *Brain Pathol* 10: 153–162

21   Blackwell TS, Christman JW (1997) The role of nuclear factor-kappa B in cytokine gene regulation. *Am J Respir Cell Mol Biol* 17: 3–9

22   Juurlink BHJ (2001) Therapeutic potential of dietary phase 2 enzyme inducers in ame-liorating diseases that have an underlying inflammatory component. *Can J Physiol Phar-macol* 79: 266–282

23   Flohé L (1989) The selenoprotein glutathione peroxidase. In: D Dolphin, O Avramović, R Poulson (eds): *Glutathione chemical, biochemical, and medical aspects. Part A.* Krieger Publishing, Malabar, FL, 643–731

24   Fornai F, Saviozzi M, Piaggi S, Gesi M, Corsini GU, Malvaldi G, Casini AF (1999) Localization of a glutathione-dependent dehydroascorbate reductase within the central nervous system of the rat. *Neuroscience* 94: 937–948

25   Goon D, Saxena M, Awasthi YC, Ross D (1993) Activity of mouse liver glutathione S-transferases toward trans,trans-muconaldehyde and trans-4-hydroxy-2-nonenal. *Toxi-col Appl Pharmacol* 119: 175–180

26   Thornalley PJ (1998) Glutathione-dependent detoxification of alpha-oxoaldehydes by the glyoxalase system: involvement in disease mechanisms and antiproliferative activity of glyoxalase I inhibitors. *Chem Biol Interact* 111–112: 137–151

27   Uhlig S, Wendel A (1992) The physiological consequences of glutathione variations. *Life Sci* 51: 1083–1094

28   Chae HZ, Kang SW, Rhee SG (1999) Isoforms of mammalian peroxiredoxin that reduce peroxides in presence of thioredoxin. *Methods Enzymol* 300: 219–226

29   Björnstedt M, Kumar S, Bjorkhem L, Spyrou G, Holmgren A (1997) Selenium and the thioredoxin and glutaredoxin systems. *Biomed Environ Sci* 10: 271–279

30   Das KC, White CW (1998) Detection of thioredoxin in human serum and biological samples using a sensitive sandwich ELISA with digoxigenin-labeled antibody. *J Immunol Methods* 211: 9–20

31   May JM, Cobb CE, Mendiratta S, Hill KE, Burk RF (1998) Reduction of the ascorbyl free radical to ascorbate by thioredoxin reductase. *J Biol Chem* 273: 23039–23045

32   May JM, Mendiratta S, Hill KE, Burk RF (1997) Reduction of dehydroascorbate to ascorbate by the selenoenzyme thioredoxin reductase. *J Biol Chem* 272: 22607–22610

33   Arner ES, Nordberg J, Holmgren A (1996) Efficient reduction of lipoamide and lipoic acid by mammalian thioredoxin reductase. *Biochem Biophys Res Commun* 225: 268–274

34   Björnstedt M, Hamberg M, Kumar S, Xue J, Holmgren A (1995) Human thioredoxin reductase directly reduces lipid hydroperoxides by NADPH and selenocystine strongly stimulates the reaction via catalytically generated selenols. *J Biol Chem* 270: 11761–11764

35   Arteel GE, Briviba K, Sies H (1999) Function of thioredoxin reductase as a peroxynitrite reductase using selenocystine or ebselen. *Chem Res Toxicol* 12: 264–129

36   Meister A (1983) Glutathione. *Ann Rev Biochem* 79: 711–760

37   Deneke SM, Fanburg BL (1989) Regulation of cellular glutathione. *Am J Physiol* 257: L163–L173

38   Bannai S (1984) Transport of cystine and cysteine in mammalian cells. *Biochim Biophys Acta* 779: 289–306

39   Galloway DC, Blake DG, Shepherd AG, McLellan LI (1997) Regulation of human gamma-glutamylcysteine synthetase: co-ordinate induction of the catalytic and regulatory subunits in HepG2 cells. *Biochem J* 328: 99–104

40   Prestera T, Holtzclaw WD, Zhang Y, Talalay P (1993) Chemical and molecular regulation of enzymes that detoxify carcinogens. *Proc Natl Acad Sci USA* 90: 2965–2969

41   Eftekharpour E, Holmgren A, Juurlink BHJ (2000) Thioredoxin reductase and glutathione synthesis is upregulated by t-butylhydroquinone in cortical astrocytes but not in cortical neurons. *Glia* 31: 241–248

42   Ishii T, Itoh K, Sato H, Bannai S (1999) Oxidative stress-inducible proteins in macrophages. *Free Radic Res* 31: 351–355

43   Tsuji Y, Ayaki H, Whitman SP, Morrow CS, Torti SV, Torti FM (2000) Coordinate transcriptional and translational regulation of ferritin in response to oxidative stress. *Mol Cell Biol* 20: 5818–5827

44   Benson AM, Hunkeler MJ, Talalay P (1980) Increase of NAD(P):quinone reductase by dietary antioxidants: possible role in protection against carcinogenesis. *Proc Natl Acad Sci USA* 77: 5216–5220

45   Prestera T, Zhang Y, Spencer SR, Wilczak CA, Talalay P (1993) The electrophile counterattack response: protection against neoplasia and toxicity. *Advan Enzym Reg* 33: 281–296

46 Keli SO, Hertog MG, Feskens EJ, Kromhout D (1996) Dietary flavonoids, antioxidant vitamins, and incidence of stroke: the Zutphen study. *Arch Intern Med* 156: 637–642

47 Yochum L, Kushi LH, Meyer K, Folsom AR (1999) Dietary flavonoid intake and risk of cardiovascular disease in postmenopausal women. *Am J Epidemiol* 149: 943–949

48 Nakazono K, Watanabe N, Matsuno K, Sasaki J, Sato T, Inoue M (1991) Does superoxide underlie the pathogenesis of hypertension? *Proc Natl Acad Sci USA* 88: 10045–10048

49 Ohara Y, Peterson TE, Harrison DG (1993) Hypercholesterolemia increases endothelial superoxide anion production. *J Clin Invest* 91: 2546–2551

50 Quyyumi AA (1998) Endothelial function in health and disease: new insights into the genesis of cardiovascular disease. *Am J Med* 105: 32S–39S

51 Stamier JS, Osborne JA, Jaraki O, Rabbani LE, Mullins M, Singel D, Loscalzo LE (1993) Adverse vascular effects of homocysteine are modulated by endothelium-derived relaxing factor and related oxides of nitrogen. *J Clin Invest* 91: 308–318

52 Loscalzo J (1996) The oxidant stress of hyperhomocyst(e)inemia. *J Clin Invest* 98: 5–7

53 Welch GN, Upchurch GR, Jr., Loscalzo J (1997) Homocysteine, oxidative stress, and vascular disease. *Hosp Pract (Off Ed)* 32: 81–82, 85, 88–92

54 de Jong SC, van den Berg M, Rauwerda JA, Stehouwer CD (1998) Hyperhomocysteinemia and atherothrombotic disease. *Semin Thromb Hemost* 24: 381–385

55 Hempel SL, Moses BL, O'Malley YQ (1998) Mixed disulfides of homocysteine and cysteine inhibit cystine uptake, decreasing intracellular glutathione. *Free Rad Biol Med* 25: S33

56 Brownlee M (1995) Advanced protein glycosylation in diabetes and aging. *Ann Rev Med* 46: 223–234

57 Cooper ME, Gilbert RE, Jerums G (1997) Diabetic vascular complications. *Clin Exp Pharmacol Physiol* 24: 770–775

58 Seitz CS, Kleindienst R, Xu QB, Wick G (1996) Coexpression of heat-shock protein 60 and intercellular-adhesion molecule-1 is related to increased adhesion of monocytes and T cells to aortic endothelium of rats in response to endotoxin. *Lab Invest* 74: 241–252

59 Paterson PG, Juurlink BHJ (1999) Nutritional regulation of glutathione in stroke. *Neurotoxicity Res* 1: 99–112

60 Gariballa SE (2000) Nutritional factors in stroke. *Br J Nutr* 84: 5–17

61 Finestone HM (2000) Safe feeding methods in stroke patients. *Lancet* 355: 1662–3

62 Cherubini A, Polidori MC, Bregnocchi M, Pezzuto S, Cecchetti R, Ingegni T, di Iorio A, Senin U, Mecocci P (2000) Antioxidant profile and early outcome in stroke patients. *Stroke* 31: 2295–2300

63 Roberts PM (1995) Nutrition in the head-injured patient. *New Horiz* 3: 506–517

64 Virtamo J, Valkeila E, Alfthan G, Punsar S, Huttunen JK, Karvonen MJ (1985) Serum selenium and the risk of coronary heart disease and stroke. *Am J Epidemiol* 122: 276–282

65 Mark SD, Wang W, Fraumeni JF, Jr., Li JY, Taylor PR, Wang GQ, Dawsey SM, Li B, Blot

WJ (1998) Do nutritional supplements lower the risk of stroke or hypertension? *Epidemiology* 9: 9–15

66   Burk RF, Hill KE (1993) Regulation of selenoproteins. *Ann Rev Nutr* 13: 65–81

67   Yang GQ, Xia YM (1995) Studies on human dietary requirements and safe range of dietary intakes of selenium in China and their application in the prevention of related endemic diseases. *Biomed Environ Sci* 8: 187–201

68   Dringen R, Pfeiffer B, Hamprecht B (1999) Synthesis of the antioxidant glutathione in neurons: supply by astrocytes of CysGly as precursor for neuronal glutathione. *J Neurosci* 19: 562–569

69   Fürst P, Kuhn KS (2000) Amino-acid substrates in new bottles: implications for clinical nutrition in the 21st century. *Nutrition* 16: 603–606

70   Bounous G, Gervais F, Amer V, Batist G, Gold P (1989) The influence of dietary whey protein on tissue glutathione and the diseases of aging. *Clin Invest Med* 12: 343–349

71   Zommara M, Toubo H, Sakono M, Imaizumi K (1998) Prevention of peroxidative stress in rats fed on a low vitamin E-containing diet by supplementing with a fermented bovine milk whey preparation: effect of lactic acid and beta lactoglobulin on the antiperoxidative action. *Biosci Biotechnol Biochem* 62: 710–717

72   Lands LC, Grey VL, Smountas AA (1999) Effect of supplementation with a cysteine donor on muscular performance [published erratum appears in *J Appl Physiol* 2000 Jan; 88 (1): following table of contents]. *J Appl Physiol* 87: 1381–1385

73   Lothian B, Grey V, Kimoff RJ, Lands LC (2000) Treatment of obstructive airway disease with a cysteine donor protein supplement: a case report. *Chest* 117: 914–916

74   Kamencic H, Griebel RW, Lyon A, Paterson PG, Juurlink. BHJ (2001) Promoting glutathione synthesis following spinal cord trauma decreases secondary damage and promotes retention of function. *FASEB J* 15: 243–250

75   Kalayjian RC, Skowron G, Emgushov R-T, Chance M, Spell SA, Borum PR, Webb LS, Mayer KH, Jackson LB, Yen-Lieberman B et al (1994) A phase I/II trial of intravenous L-2-oxothiazolidine-4-carboxylic acid (Procysteine) in asymptomatic HIV-infected subjects. *J Acquir Immune Defic Syndr* 7: 369–374

76   Barditch-Crovo P, Noe D, Skowron G, Lederman M, Kalayjian RC, Borum P, Buier R, Rowe WB, Goldberg D, Lietman P (1998) A phase I/II evaluation of oral L-2-oxothiazolidine-4-carboxylic acid in asymptomatic patients infected with human immunodeficiency virus. *J Clin Pharmacol* 38: 357–363

77   Bernard GR, Wheeler AP, Arons MM, Morris PE, Paz HL, Russell JA, Wright PE (1997) A trial of antioxidants N-acetylcysteine and procysteine in ARDS. The Antioxidant in ARDS Study Group. *Chest* 112: 164–172

78   Vita JA, Frei B, Holbrook M, Gokce N, Leaf C, Keaney JF (1998) L-2-oxothiazolidine-4-carboxylic acid reverses endothelial dysfunction in patients with coronary artery disease. *J Clin Invest* 101: 1408–1414

79   McLellan LI, Lewis AD, Hall DJ, Ansell JD, Wolf CR (1995) Uptake and distribution of N-acetylcysteine in mice: tissue-specific effects on glutathione concentrations. *Carcinogenesis* 16: 2099–2106

80 Anderson ME, Meister A (1989) Marked increase of cysteine levels in many regions of the brain after administration of 2-oxothiazolidine-4-carboxylate. *FASEB J* 3: 1632–1636

81 Carroll JE, Howard EF, Hess DC, Wakade CG, Chen Q, Cheng C (1998) Nuclear factor-kappa B activation during cerebral reperfusion: effect of attenuation with N-acetylcysteine treatment. *Brain Res Mol Brain Res* 56: 186–191

82 Cuzzocrea S, Mazzon E, Costantino G, Serraino I, Dugo L, Calabro G, Cucinotta G, De Sarro A, Caputi AP (2000) Beneficial effects of N-acetylcysteine on ischaemic brain injury. *Br J Pharmacol* 130: 1219–1226

83 Speeg KV, Bay MK (1995) Prevention and treatment of drug-induced liver disease. *Gastroenterol Clin North Am* 24: 1047–1064

84 Matilla B, Ortiz J, Gonzalez P, Garcia-Diez F, Jorquera F, Culebras JM, Gonzalez-Gallego J, Tunon MJ (2000) Effects of parenteral nutrition supplemented with glutamine or glutamine dipeptides on liver antioxidant and detoxication systems in rats. *Nutrition* 16: 125–128

85 Khogali SE, Harper AA, Lyall JA, Rennie MJ (1998) Effects of L-glutamine on postischaemic cardiac function: protection and rescue. *J Mol Cell Cardiol* 30: 819–827

86 Jian ZM, Cao JD, Zhu XG, Zhao WX, Yu JC, Ma EL, Wang XR, Zhu MW, Shu H, Liu YW (1999) The impact of alanyl-glutamine on clinical safety, nitrogen balance, intestinal permeability, and clinical outcome in postoperative patients: a randomized, double-blind, controlled study of 120 patients. *JPEN J Parenter Enteral Nutr* 23: S62–S66

87 Barch DH, Rundhaugen LM, Pillay NS (1995) Ellagic acid induces transcription of the rat glutathione S-transferase-Ya gene. *Carcinogenesis* 16: 665–668

88 Fahey JW, Zhang Y, Talalay P (1997) Broccoli sprouts: an exceptionally rich source of inducers of enzymes that protect against chemical carcinogens. *Proc Natl Acad Sci USA* 94: 10367–10372

89 Khan SG, Katiyar SK, Agarwal R, Mukhtar H (1992) Enhancement of antioxidant and phase II enzymes by oral feeding of green tea polyphenols in drinking water to SKH-1 hairless mice: possible role in cancer chemoprevention. *Cancer Res* 52: 4050–4052

90 Appelt LC, Reicks MM (1997) Soy feeding induces phase II enzymes in rat tissues. *Nutr Cancer* 28: 270–275

91 Wang W, Liu LQ, Higuchi CM, Chen H (1998) Induction of NADPH:quinone reductase by dietary phytoestrogens in colonic Colo205 cells. *Biochem Pharmacol* 56: 189–195

92 Bomser J, Madhavi DL, Singletary K, Smith MA (1996) *In vitro* anticancer activity of fruit extracts from *Vaccinium* species. *Planta Med* 62: 212–216

93 Uda Y, Price KR, Williamson G, Rhodes MJ (1997) Induction of the anticarcinogenic marker enzyme, quinone reductase, in murine hepatoma cells *in vitro* by flavonoids. *Cancer Lett* 120: 213–216

94 Dinkova-Kostova AT, Talalay P (1999) Relation of structure of curcumin analogs to their potencies as inducers of Phase 2 detoxification enzymes. *Carcinogenesis* 20: 911–914

Inflammatory adhesion molecules, kinins, nitric oxide complement factors and lipid mediators in stroke

Selectin- and complement-mediated mechanisms of tissue injury in stroke

David J. Pinsky and E. Sander Connolly Jr.

Columbia University College of Physicians and Surgeons, 630 W. 168th St., New York, NY 10032, USA

Overview of inflammatory mechanisms in stroke

When blood flow is interrupted to regions of the brain, even for very limited periods of time, a number of pathological mechanisms are set in motion which elicit adverse sequelae. Neurons are among the cells most vulnerable to relatively brief periods of ischemia, due to their exquisite and constant need for oxygen and glucose. The causes of neuronal death are multiple, but regardless of cause, once a neuron dies, it is irrevocably lost from the substance of the brain. The focus of this chapter is on inflammatory reactions triggered in neurons or adjacent vascular cells, which contribute to the neuronal demise and tissue injury in stroke.

Blood vessels in an organism respond to periods of interrupted blood flow with a limited number of paradigms. One of the strongest environmental influences which modulates the vascular response to periods of interrupted blood flow is that elicited by low oxygen tension in the blood [1]. Low levels of oxygen induce glucose transporter upregulation in endothelial cells, as well as increased levels of expression of glycoprotein adhesion receptors such as ICAM-1, P-selectin, and E-selectin [2, 3]. During the reperfusion period, there is also an important loss in endothelium-derived relaxation factor (nitric oxide [4, 5]), which also participates in the inflammatory upregulation of the ischemic cerebrovascular milieu. P-selectin, which is stored within the membranes of intracellular organelles called Weibel-Palade bodies, can be rapidly translocated to the endothelial surface following an abrupt reduction in oxygen tension [3, 6]. Of particular importance in this regard is the rise in intracellular calcium which comes about due to reduced levels of available oxygen, and which is further exacerbated by a decline in available nitric oxide.

P-selectin, an integral membrane adhesion receptor glycoprotein expressed on platelets and endothelial cells, is one of the earliest molecules which serves to capture leukocytes during their rapid transit in the circulation [7]. Neutrophils in particular, and monocytes as well, are captured in a series of rapidly forming and breaking calcium-dependent bonds, which cause the leukocyte to come to a rolling stop along the endothelial surface. This places the leukocyte in the proper steric rela-tionship so as to be firmly engaged by ICAM-1/β_2 integrin interactions [8]. At later times during the postischemic phase, increased expression of other adhesion recep-tors, such as E-selectin, which is not expressed constitutively on the endothelial cell, also contributes to leukocyte recruitment and tissue injury. Recruited leukocytes exacerbate cerebral injury by several mechanisms, which may include release of hydrolytic enzymes, reactive oxygen species, acids, and other injurious substances, as well as by physically obstructing the lumina of microvessels. Activated neu-trophils become stiff, thus further exacerbating their propensity to cause microvas-cular occlusion.

An additional important and deleterious effect is a mechanism which is activat-ed by ischemia, the complement cascade [9, 10]. Complement, a multi-protein cas-cade which is a quite primitive defense mechanism in terms of evolutionary time, is activated by fragments of dying cells as well as by specific receptor components, especially when immunoglobulins participate in inflammatory processes [11]. Complement activation can be deleterious for a variety of reasons. Most widely recognized is the fact that the terminal components of the complement cascade deposit on cell membranes near their site of activation, effectively punching deep holes in the membrane, causing the cell to become functionally eviscerated in terms of intracellular ionic gradients and intracellular organelles [12]. Another means by which complement can kill cells is by triggering receptor-mediated phagocytosis by adjacent cells. In the case of the brain, microglia are the predominant phagocytic scavenger cell types responsible for complement-mediated cell death [13]. Indirect-ly, the production of biologically active fragments of complement components termed anaphylotoxins, C3a and C5a in particular, may be responsible for ampli-fying leukocyte recruitment and eliciting deleterious leukocyte effector mechanisms in stroke.

There are a number of important reasons to investigate and understand deleteri-ous inflammatory effector mechanisms in stroke. Although thrombolytic therapy with rtPA is effective in certain cases of nonhemorrhagic stroke, especially when treatment begins within a narrow 3-h window, this therapy has only been adminis-tered to a small number of patients. In a community hospital setting, less than 1% of all patients presenting with acute stroke received this therapy [14]. ICAM-1, which presents a logical target for stroke therapy based on efficacy studies in rodents, has been a disappointing initial target based on preliminary results of an as yet unpublished clinical trial which was terminated several years ago. It is also like-ly that these disappointing results were not due to an inappropriate choice of target molecule for inhibition, but rather due to the type of therapy which was chosen. The anti-ICAM-1 antibody which was used [15] very likely activated complement in humans, and as complement was subsequently shown to be a deleterious effector mechanism in stroke [16], this could potentially explain the negative outcomes observed.

Evidence for a role of neutrophils and glycoprotein adhesion receptors in the pathogenesis of evolving stroke

Human epidemiologic studies indicate that neutrophils injure brain tissue and exacerbate clinical outcome following stroke [17]. In humans, neutrophils accumulate in areas of low cerebral blood flow, especially early during the post-ischemic period [18–21]. This may explain their potential role in postischemic hypoperfusion, neuronal dysfunction, and scar formation [22–25]. There is considerable experimental evidence suggesting that neutrophils exacerbate tissue damage following stroke [21, 26–30], although there is some discordant data on the subject. For instance, antibody-mediated depletion of neutrophils prior to stroke in dogs [31] or cyclophosphamide-induced leukocytopenia [32] in gerbils resulted in no beneficial effects following cerebral ischemia. On the other hand, in mice, immunodepletion of neutrophils prior to cerebral ischemia results in marked functional improvements, corresponding to reduction in infarct volumes, improved cerebral blood flow, and reduced mortality early after stroke [30]. Experimental therapy targeted at interfering with neutrophil-endothelial interactions has also produced dichotomous results. In a feline model of reperfused stroke, treatment with an antibody to CD18, the common subunit of heterodimeric β_2 integrins, did not alter recovery of cerebral blood flow, return of evoked potentials, or infarct volume [33]. Other experiments in primates, however, have found that microvascular patency following transient focal ischemia is improved by antibodies to CD18 [34]. In a rat model of stroke, anti-CD11b/CD18 antibody has also been shown to reduce both neutrophil accumulation and ischemia-related neuronal damage [35]. Some of this discordant data can be explained by the recent observation that CD18-mediated leukocyte recruitment participates in cerebral tissue injury only in the setting of reperfused, but not nonreperfused stroke [36]. Although data are too limited to comment on this with any degree of certainty, it is logical that therapies directed against neutrophil-mediated inflammatory mechanisms will be most likely to positively impact on outcome if they are administered in settings in which neutrophils typically have access to the injured region of the brain. Ultimate therapies may actually combine anti-inflammatory approaches with those which reestablish vascular patency.

P-selectin and stroke

Initial studies in a primate model of stroke demonstrated early upregulation of P-selectin expression in the ipsilateral ischemic hemisphere, particularly in ischemic cerebral microvessels. More recently, a mouse model of stroke was used to elucidate the role of the P-selectin gene [37]. Mice were subjected to reperfused stroke by threading a small intraluminal suture up the internal carotid artery, to occlude the origin of the middle cerebral artery [38]. This suture was left in place for 45 min, during which time near complete cessation of blood flow was documented using a laser Doppler flow probe placed over the ischemic zone. After this 45-min ischemic period, the suture was withdrawn, and reperfusion allowed to proceed. At 24 h, neurological examination was performed in order to determine functional deficits. After this, mice were sacrificed and the brains harvested for infarct volume or immunohistochemical analysis. Initial immunohistochemical examination at 24 h revealed a strong increase in expression of P-selectin in microvessels restricted to the ipsilateral, i.e. ischemic, cerebral cortex. Using another technique in which radiolabeled control anti-P-selectin antibodies were administered, the ischemic upregulation of P-selectin was confirmed at an even earlier observation point. By 30 min of reperfusion, there was a significant increase in the accumulation of radiolabeled anti-P-selectin IgG detected in the ischemic cortex [37]. The functional significance of the observed increase in ipsilateral microvascular P-selectin expression was examined using radiolabeled leukocytes. Leukocytes, specifically neutrophils, accumulated within minutes after reperfusion had commenced and continued throughout the 24-h observation period (Fig. 1).

Accumulation of leukocytes at sites of vascular injury can not only wreak havoc by products generated during release of reactive chemical species and by their respiratory burst and release of their lysosomal complement of lytic enzymes, but they stiffen as they become activated and obstruct microvascular flow. To evaluate the role of P-selectin expression on ischemia-driven changes in cerebral blood flow, experiments were performed in which blood flow was measured using a laser Doppler or flow probe, with serial measurements obtained at the same neuroanatomic region of the brain. Following removal of the occluding suture in wild type mice which express the P-selectin gene, blood flow increased to 50 to 60% of initial baseline value, but declined thereafter, a phenomenon known as postischemic no-reflow (this is both thrombosis- and leukocyte-dependent, and probably entails an element of local vasospasm as well) (Fig. 2). Although absence of the P-selectin gene did not completely abrogate postischemic no-reflow, it was markedly attenuated. These studies show that P-selectin-mediated neutrophil recruitment to ischemic foci participates in a major way in postischemic cerebral hypoperfusion.

Expression of P-selectin is also an important participant in adverse sequelae following stroke, at least in experimental animals. Infarct size following stroke in P-selectin null mice, quantified by serial staining of triphenyltetrazolium chloride-stained serial cerebral sections, was significantly smaller than infarct size in wild-type control mice which possessed the P-selectin gene [37] (Fig. 3). Additional studies were performed to prove that a pharmacological strategy could also be used to block deleterious P-selectin-mediated effector mechanisms. Use of a functionally blocking anti-P-selectin antibody caused a marked improvement in stroke outcome in mice. This was true even if the antibody was given after the ischemic period, at the onset of reperfusion. This is especially important in that clinical stroke therapy is generally only possible if it is effective after stroke onset.

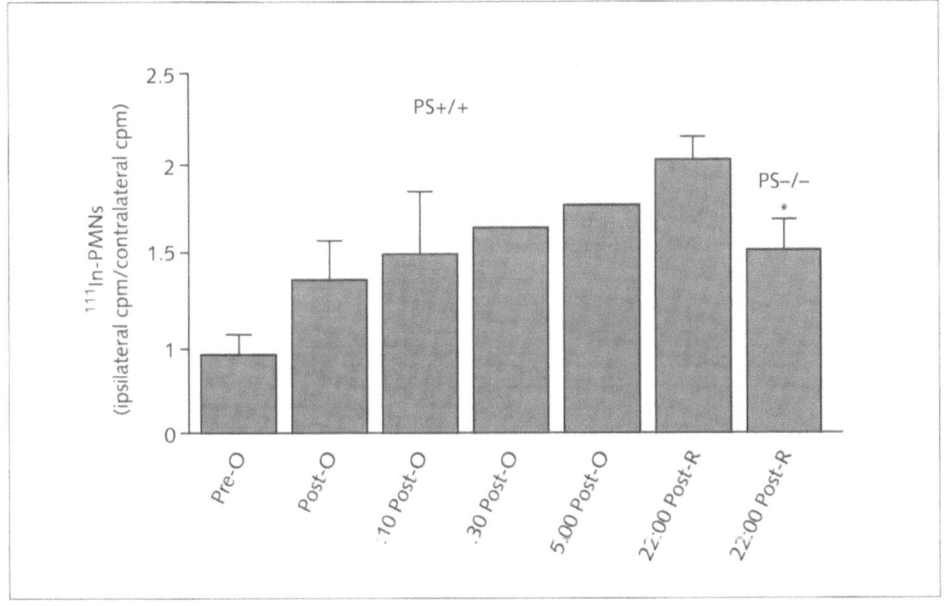

Figure 1
Accumulation of radiolabeled leukocytes, administered immediately prior to middle cerebral artery occlusion in mice. PS=P-selectin; genotype is indicated. Adapted from [47].

E-selectin and stroke

Compared with P-selectin, which may be rapidly expressed on hypoxic endothelial cells secondary to translocation from the Weibel-Palade body membrane to the cell surface [3], E-selectin is expressed at somewhat later time points during stroke, presumably due to the requirement for *de novo* synthesis of E-selectin mRNA. One of the earliest studies to identify the role of increased E-selectin expression in the ischemic brain showed that in rats, permanent occlusion of the middle cerebral artery resulted in a marked increase in E-selectin mRNA levels in the ischemic cortex, with very low contralateral expression, peaking at 12 h, but remaining elevated for up to 2 days [39]. In a murine model of stroke, E-selectin expression was noted to be upregulated by 4 h with continued increase in expression over the ensuing 20-h period [40]. This increase in E-selectin expression was associated with an increase in cerebral tissue leukocyte recruitment, quantified by measuring myeloperoxidase activity in the ischemic cortex. A functionally blocking anti-E-selectin antibody is, as for P-selectin, associated with an improved post ischemic period of blood flow and reduced cerebral infarct volume, compared with administration of a non-immune control antibody [40]. Neurological deficit following stroke was consider-

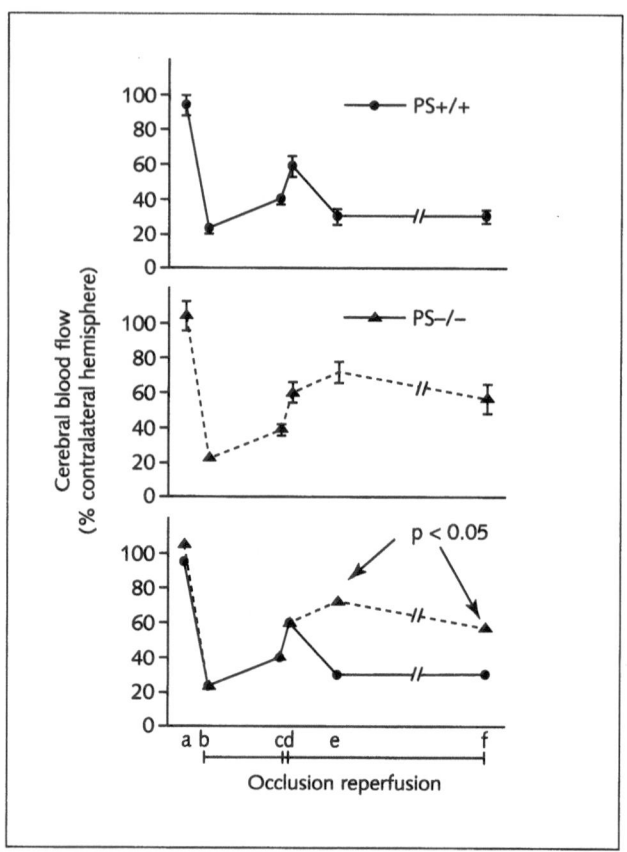

Figure 2
Role of P-selectin in cerebrovascular no-reflow. Cerebral blood flow was measured in PS+/+ (top panel) and PS–/– (middle panel) mice using a laser Doppler flow probe, and expressed as the percentage of contralateral (nonischemic) hemispheric blood flow (± SEM). Blood flow was measured at the following time points: (a) prior to middle cerebral artery occlusion; (b) immediately following middle cerebral artery occlusion; (c) 10 min following middle cerebral artery occlusion but still prior to reperfusion; (d) immediately following reperfusion; (e) 30 min following reperfusion; and (f) 22 h following reperfusion. The bottom panel represents an overlay of the top two panels (error bars omitted for clarity). Adapted from [47].

ably reduced following administration of the anti-E-selectin antibody. Again, as for the anti-P-selectin approach, blocking E-selectin at later time points following reperfusion also proved to be effective for reducing cerebral infarct volume and adverse sequelae, albeit less so than pre-ischemic administration. In a primate model of

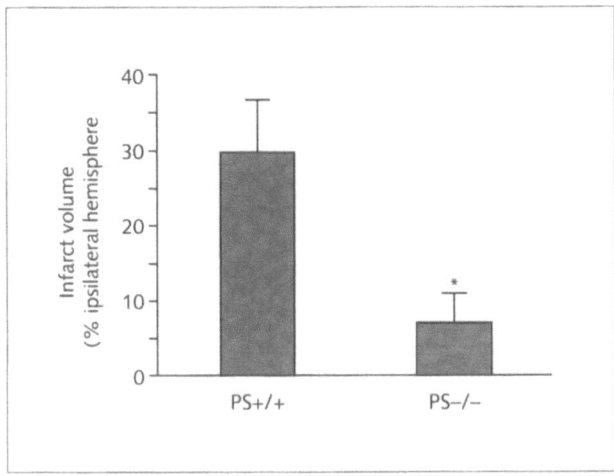

Figure 3
Effect of the P-selectin gene on cerebral infarct volume following transient middle cerebral artery occlusion in mice. PS, P-selectin; genotype is indicated. Adapted from [47].

reperfused stroke [41], E-selectin expression is also increased [42]. Preliminary data in non-human primates show that a humanized antibody which blocks both P-selectin and E-selectin may be especially useful in stroke [42].

Combination anti-selectin therapy in stroke

As both P- and E-selectin expression have been shown to contribute to deleterious outcomes in stroke, there has been some interest in the development of compounds which can simultaneously inhibit leukocyte-endothelial interactions mediated by both selectins. One such approach, which has held out modest experimental promise, is in the use of oligosaccharide or oligopeptide agents which compete with the sialyl-Lewis x (sialyl Le^x) carbohydrate epitope which covalently decorates specific glycoprotein ligands integral to the leukocyte membrane. These carbohydrate epitopes, particularly the sialyl Le^x oligosaccharide motif, given therapeutically as sugars, have been shown to mitigate ischemia-reperfusion injury in other model systems, as well as to reduce inflammation [43]. In stroke, there is the possibility that such approaches may also provide success, although significantly more work remains to be performed in this area. In a rodent model of focal cerebral ischemia, treatment with a synthetic oligopeptide corresponding to the lectin domain of selectins appeared to be efficacious [44]. An alternative approach, using a human-

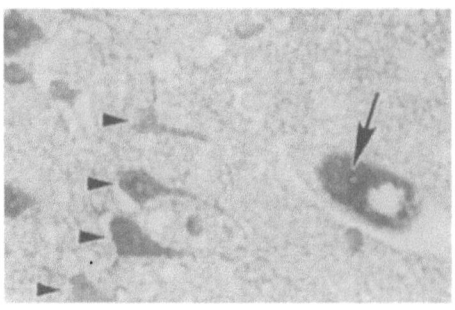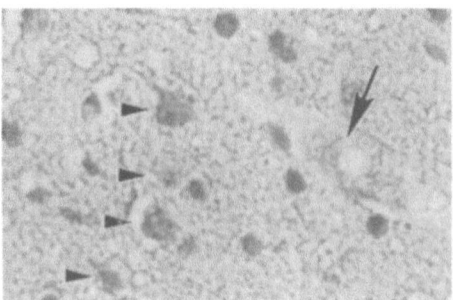

Figure 4
Neuronal expression of C1q in stroke, and complement activation in the microvasculature.
Mice were given sCR1 prior to stroke, and then adjacent ipsilateral (ischemic) brain sections
were immunostained with an anti-sCR1 (left panel) or an anti-C1q (right panel) primary
antibody. sCR1 binds to C1q expressed on neurons (arrowheads) as well as in microvessels
(arrows). Colocalization of staining (arrowheads), is shown. Adapted from [45].

ized antibody which blocks both P- and E-selectin mediated inflammatory events, has shown promise in a pilot study in a baboon model of stroke [42]. As discussed below, a selectin-blocking covalent carbohydrate modification of an inflammatory protein also appears to increase the parent compounds' efficacy in the setting of reperfused stroke [45].

Role of the complement system in stroke

Until recently, there was little indication that the complement system was an important pathological mediator in acute ischemic stroke. This was surprising given that complement had been identified as an important contributor toward other forms of ischemic injury in the heart, kidneys, lungs, and elsewhere. In a murine model of stroke, neurons were shown to express an early complement protein, C1q, along their entire membrane surface area, with neuronal cell bodies as well as axonal processes staining prominently for this protein after ischemia [45] (Fig. 4). The specificity of this staining was shown in histological sections, which used a purified C1q protein to block specific staining provided by the anti-C1q antibody. When this blocking procedure was used, it completely abrogated C1q immunoreactivity in neurons in the ipsilateral ischemic cerebral cortex. Additional confirmation of the ischemia-driven neuronal C1q expression was shown using Western blot analysis; these experiments demonstrated a prominent band of immunoreactivity in the C1q positive control lane as well as in lanes loaded with tissue extracts taken from the ischemic hemisphere of mice subjected to stroke (Fig.

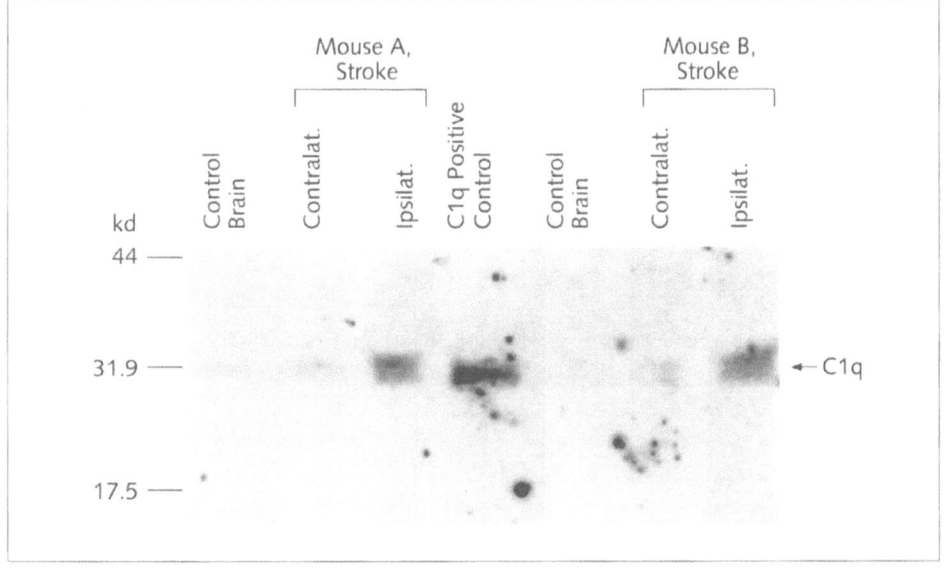

Figure 5
Ischemia drives cerebral expression of C1q. Immunoblot for C1q showing marked upregula-
tion of C1q protein in the ipsilateral (ischemic) cortex, with minimal expression seen in the
contralateral hemisphere. Control brain tissue was harvested from untreated and nonoper-
ated mice. The middle lane represents purified C1q protein, used as a positive control.
Adapted from [45].

5). However, immunoreactivity was virtually absent in the contralateral nonischemic cerebral cortex.

The next relevant question was what are the functional consequences of
ischemia-driven C1q expression? This was answered in experiments in which the
complement cascade was blocked using a protein called sCR1, which is the extracellular domain of soluble complement receptor-1. Modest cerebroprotection was
conferred using this potent complement inhibitory protein [45]. However, knowing
that complement mediated events are also pathophysiologically relevant in the setting of stroke, this sCR1 parent molecule was covalently modified to confer bifunc-
tionality [46]. SCR1 was expressed in the CHO-LEC 11 cells, which incorporate the
sLe^x tetrasaccharide as a post-translational modification, the glycoprotein product
of which (sCR1sLe^x) was purified for use in these experiments. SCR1sLe^x includes
between 10–15 sLe^x moieties per sCR1 molecule. *In vitro* experiments showed that
this hybrid molecule was capable of binding to both E- and P-selectins. When
sCR1sLe^x was given to mice prior to stroke, subsequent immunostaining at 24 h

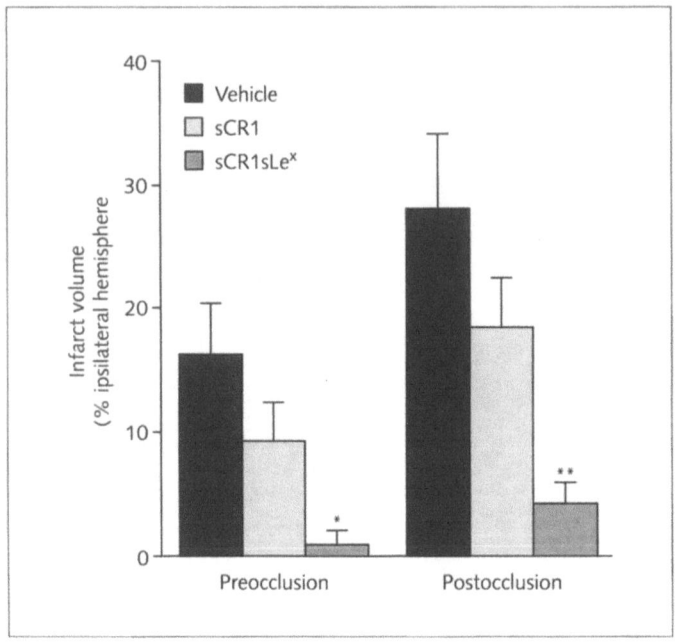

Figure 6
Effect of timing of complement blockade or simultaneous complement/selectin blockade on cerebral infarct volume. sCR1 or sCR1sLe^x were given immediately preoperatively, or following reperfusion, to mice subjected to intraluminal middle cerebral artery occlusion. Infarct volumes were calculated at 24 h from planimetered serial cerebral sections, stained with triphenyltetrazolium chloride. Adapted from [45].

revealed that this molecule colocalized both to ischemic neurons, as well as the microvessels in the ischemic zone (Fig. 4). These are the expected sites of colocalization, as these are the sites of C1q expression and complement activation.

The functional properties of sCR1sLe^x in terms of cerebroprotection were quite striking. Infarct volumes were reduced by sCR1sLe^x in a dose-dependent fashion [45] (Fig. 6). At the highest dose tested there was an 11-fold reduction in cerebral infarct volume. Neurological function was also significantly improved after sCR1sLe^x administration (Fig. 7). The level of protection conferred by the non-sLe^x-glycosylated sCR1 was intermediate, in that it was modestly effective compared to vehicle, but sLe^x-glycosylation conferred a more potent advantage. In determining the mechanisms by which sCR1sLe^x confer cerebroprotection, the accumulation of radiolabeled leukocytes and radiolabeled platelets was examined. sCR1sLe^x potently suppressed the accumulation of both of these hematological cells in the infarcted tissue (Figs. 8 and 9). The degree of suppression for both was more striking than that

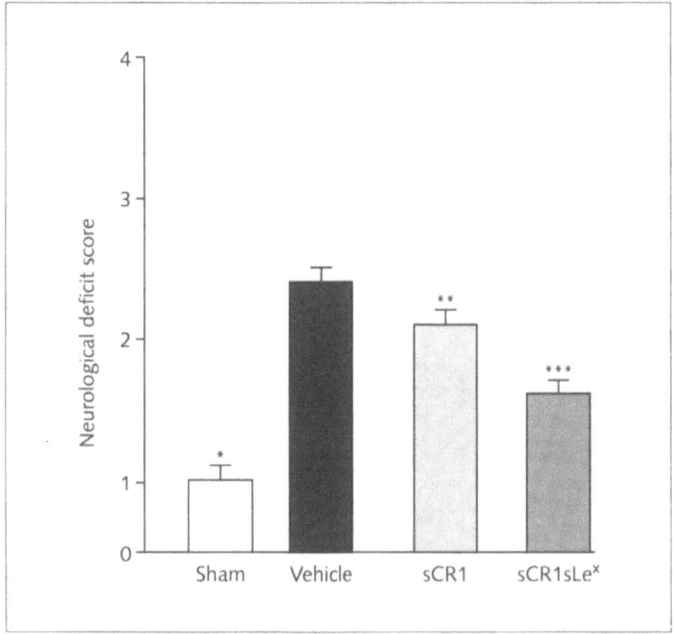

Figure 7
Effect of sCR1 or sCR1sLe^x on neurological deficit in mice after intraluminal middle cerebral artery occlusion (45 min) followed by reperfusion (23 h). Larger numbers indicate poorer neurological function. Adapted from [45].

observed with the non-sLe^x-glycosylated version of sCR1. Blood flow to the ischemic zone was also improved significantly by sCR1sLe^x. It is important to note that intracerebral hemorrhage, a feared consequence of stroke, was not increased by treatment with this selectin-inhibiting form of sCR1. Another important point of note is that the beneficial effects of this combined anti-complement and anti-selectin therapy were not only observed when inhibition occurred prior to stroke onset, but also when therapy was delayed for 45 min after the occlusive event (Fig. 6). The beneficial effects were sustained for up to 72 h of observation, and presumably beyond, although 72 h was the latest time point examined in these experiments.

Conclusions

These data show that activation of inflammatory mechanisms following ischemic stroke can have grave consequences. Inhibition of any single inflammatory mechanism appears to confer benefit in terms of improving neurological function and

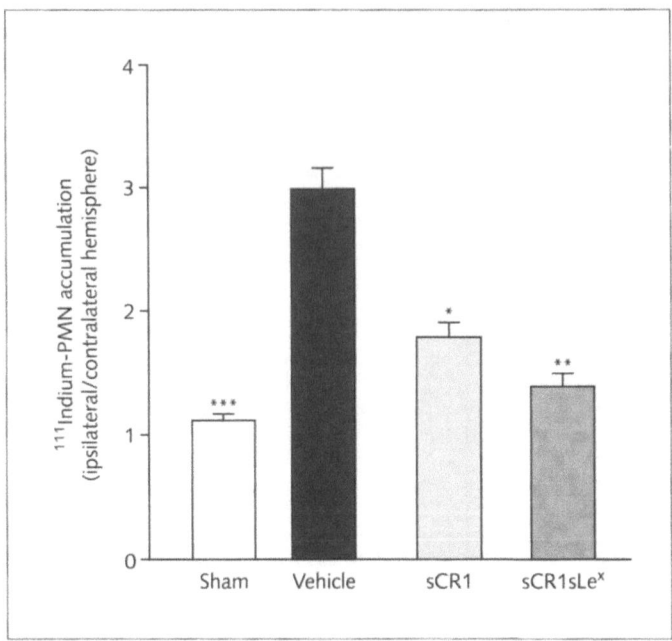

Figure 8
Effect of sCR1 or sCR1sLe^x on radiolabelled leukocyte accumulation in mice after intralumi-
nal middle cerebral artery occlusion (45 min) followed by reperfusion (23 h). Adapted from
[45].

reduced tissue injury, although strategies which seek to inhibit multiple effector mechanisms may be superior. This is not entirely unexpected, as there is considerable redundancy between adhesion receptor and other inflammatory mechanisms. Although this chapter did not cover the large body of experimental data demonstrating that coagulation reactions also play a critical role in stroke, *in vivo*, it is often hard to separate inflammatory from coagulant reactions, because of the considerable intersection between these axes. It is interesting to note that the most potent therapeutic agent described in this chapter, sCR1sLe^x, inhibits both complement- and selectin-mediated events, and it is known that selectins also participate in coagulation reactions, because P-selectin is rapidly translocated to the platelet cell surface during activation. Therefore, this single therapy actually acts as a triple therapy, inhibiting complement activation, leukocyte adhesion, and platelet accumulation.

Admittedly, there have been some disappointing results in terms of the use of certain anti-inflammatory agents to treat human stroke. However knowledge of the

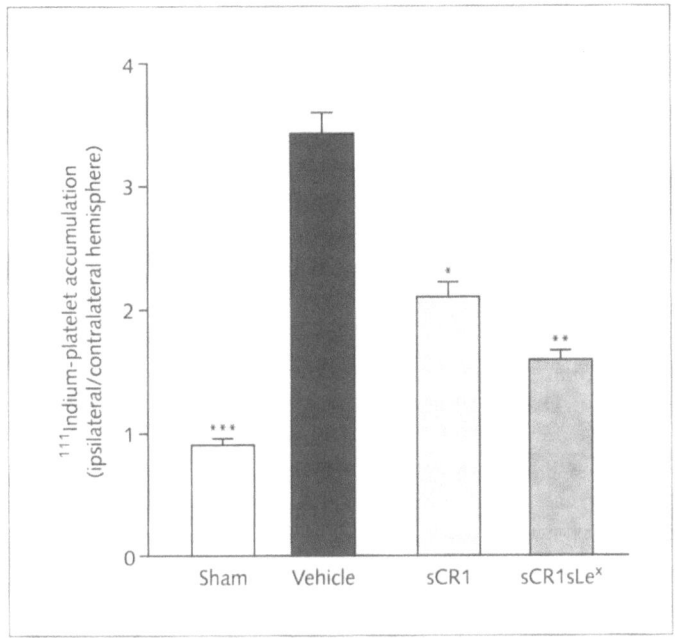

Figure 9
Effect of sCR1 or sCR1sLe^x on radiolabelled platelet accumulation in mice after intraluminal middle cerebral artery occlusion (45 min) followed by reperfusion (23 h). Adapted from [45].

underlying mechanisms provides a basis for moving forward to translate preclinical knowledge into effective clinical treatments. Because of differences in collateral blood supply to the brain in rodents and primates, and perhaps more subtle differences between prevailing pathways of inflammatory activation, it may become necessary to test therapies which have been proven effective in rodents and in primates before their application to human beings. Future studies will hopefully define the precise mechanisms that are operative in human stroke, so that new opportunities emerge for therapeutic intervention. The time is ripe and the need is great for new and effective treatments for acute ischemic stroke to emerge from the scientific caldron.

Acknowledgements

This work was supported in part by the National Institutes of Health grants NS 02038 (to ESC) and NS41460, HL-59488, and HL-55397 (to DJP).

References

1   Pinsky DJ, Yan S-F, Lawson C, Naka Y, Chen J-X, Connolly ESJ, M Stern D (1995) Hypoxia and modification of the endothelium: implications for regulation of vascular homeostatic properties. *Semin Cell Biol* 6: 283–294

2   Shreeniwas R, Koga S, Karakurum M, Pinsky DJ, Kaiser E, Brett J, Wolitzky BA, Norton C, Plocinski J, Benjamin W et al (1992) Hypoxia-mediated induction of endothelial cell interleukin 1-alpha: an autocrine mechanism promoting expression of leukocyte adhesion molecules on the vessel surface. *J Clin Invest* 90: 2333–2339

3   Pinsky DJ, Naka Y, Liao H, Oz MC, Wagner DD, Mayadas TN, Johnson RC, Hynes RO, Heath M, Lawson CA, Stern DM (1996) Hypoxia-induced exocytosis of endothelial cell Weibel-Palade bodies A mechanism for rapid neutrophil recruitment after cardiac preservation. *J Clin Invest* 97: 493–500

4   Pinsky DJ, Oz MC, Koga S, Taha Z, Broekman MJ, Marcus AJ, Liao H, Naka Y, Brett J, Cannon PJ et al (1994) Cardiac preservation is enhanced in a heterotopic rat transplant model by supplementing the nitric oxide pathway. *J Clin Invest* 93: 2291–2297

5   Pinsky DJ, Naka Y, Chowdhury NC, Liao H, Oz MC, Michler RE, Kubaszewski E, Malinski T, Stern DM (1994) The nitric oxide/cyclic GMP pathway in organ transplantation: Cricital role in successful lung preservation. *Proc Natl Acad Sci USA* 91: 12086–12090

6   Patel KD, Zimmerman GA, Prescott SM, McEver RP, McIntyre TM (1991) Oxygen radicals induce human endothelial cells to express GMP-140 and bind neutrophils. *J Cell Biol* 112: 749–759

7   Larsen E, Celi A, Gilbert G, Furie BC, Erban J, Bonfanti R, Wagner DD, Furie B (1989) PADGEM protein: a receptor that mediates the interaction of activated platelets with neutrophils and monocytes. *Cell* 59: 305–312

8   Springer, T A 1990 Adhesion receptors of the immune system Nature 346: 425–434

9   Rossen RD, Michael LH, Kagiyama A, Savage HE, Hanson G, Reisberg MA, Moake JN, Kim SH, Self D, Weakley S (1988) Mechanism of complement activation after coronary artery occlusion: evidence that myocardial ischemia in dogs causes release of constituents of myocardial subcellular origin that complex with human C1q *in vivo*. *Circ Res* 62: 572–584

10 Crawford MH, Grover FL, Kolb WP, McMahan CA, O'Rourke RA, McManus LM, Pinckard RN (1988) Complement and neutrophil activation in the pathogenesis of ischemic myocardial injury. *Circulation* 78: 1449–1458

11 Kagiyama A, Savage HE, Michael LH, Hanson G, Entman ML, Rossen RD (1989) Molecular basis of complement activation in ischemic myocardium: indentification of specific molecules of mitochondrial origin that bind human C1q and fix complement. *Circ Res* 64: 607–615

12 Ohanian SH, Schlager SI (1981) Humoral immune killing of nucleated cells: mechanisms of complement-mediated attack and target cell defense. *Crit Rev Immunol* 1: 165–209

13 Korotzer AR, Watt J, Cribbs D, Tenner AJ, Burdick D, Glabe C, CotmanCW (1995) Cultured rat microglia express C1q and receptor for C1q: implications for amyloid effects on microglia. *Exp Neurol* 134: 214–221

14 Chiu D, Krieger D, Villar Cordova C, Kasner SE, Morgenstern LB, Bratina PL, Yatsu FM, Grotta JC (1998) Intravenous tissue plasminogen activator for acute ischemic stroke: feasibility, safety, and efficacy in the first year of clinical practice. *Stroke* 29: 18–22

15 Vuorte J, Lindsberg PJ, Kaste M, Meri S, Jansson SE, Rothlein R, Repo H (1999) Anti-ICAM-1 monoclonal antibody R65 (Enlimomab) promotes activation of neutrophils in whole blood. *J Immunol* 162: 2353–2357

16 Vannucci SJ, Seaman LB, Vannucci RC (1996) Effects of hypoxia-ischemia on GLUT1 and GLUT3 glucose transporters in immature rat brain. *J Cereb Blood Flow Metabolism* 16: 77–81

17 Pozzilli C, Lenzi GL, Argentino C, Bozzao L, Rasura M, Giuabilei F, Fieschi C (1985) Peripheral white blood cell count in cerebral ischemic infarction. *Acta Neurol Scand* 71: 396–400

18 Obrenovitch TP, Kumaroo KK, Hallenbeck JM (1984) Autoradiographical detection of indium-111-labelled platelets in brain tissue section. *Stroke* 15: 1049–1056

19 Hallenbeck JM, Dutka AJ, Tanishima T, Kochanek PM, Kumaroo KK, Thompson CB, Obrenovitch TP, Contreras TJ (1986) Polymorphonuclear leukocyte accumulation in brain regions with low blood flow during the early postischemic period. *Stroke* 17: 246–253

20 Pozzilli C, Lenzi GL, Argentino C, Caroli A, Rasura M, Signore A, Bozzao L, Pozzilli P (1985) Imaging of leukocytic infiltration in human cerebral infarcts. *Stroke* 16: 251–255

21 Clark RK, Lee EV, White RF, Jonak ZL, Feuerstein GZ, Barone FC (1994) Reperfusion following focal stroke hastens inflammation and resolution of ischemic injured tissue. *Brain Res Bulletin* 35: 387–392

22 Ernst E, Matrai A, Paulsen F (1987) Leukocyte rheology in recent stroke. *Stroke* 18: 59–62

23 Grogaard B, Schurer L, Gerdin B, Arfors KE (1989) Delayed hypoperfusion after incomplete forebrain ischemia in the rat: the role of polymorphonuclear leukocytes. *J Cereb Blood Flow Metab* 9: 500–505

24 Kintner DB, Kranner PW, Gilboe DD (1986) Cerebral vascular resistance following platelet and leukocyte removal from perfusate. *J Cereb Blood Flow Metab* 6: 52–58

25 Mercuri M, Ciuffetti G, Robinson M, Toole J (1989) Blood cell rheology in acute cerebral infarction. *Stroke* 20: 959–962

26 Matsuo Y, Onodera H, Shiga Y, Nakamura M, Ninomiya M, Kihora T, Kogure K (1994) Correlation between myeloperoxidase-quantified neutrophil accumulation and ischemic brain injury in the rat: effects of neutrophil depletion. *Stroke* 25: 1469–1475

27 Dutka AJ, Kochanek PM, Hallenbeck JM (1989) Influence of granulocytopenia on canine cerebral ischemia induced by air embolism. *Stroke* 20: 390–395

28 Clark RK, Lee EV, Fish CJ, White RF, Price WJ, Jonak ZL, Feuerstein GZ, Barone FC

(1993) Development of tissue damage, inflammation and resolution following stroke: an immunohistochemical and quantitative planimetric study. *Brain Res Bulletin* 31: 565–572

29 Lindsberg PJ, Sirén AL, Feuerstein GZ, Hallenbeck JM (1995) Antagonism of neutrophil adherence in the deteriorating stroke model in rabbits. *J Neurosurg* 82: 269–277

30 Connolly ES Jr, Winfree CJ, Springer TA, Naka Y, Liao H, Yan SD, Stern DM, Solomon RA, Gutierrez-Ramos J-C, Pinsky DJ (1996) Cerebral protection in homozygous null ICAM-1 mice after middle cerebral artery occlusion Role of neutrophil adhesion in the pathogenesis of stroke. *J Clin Invest* 97: 209–216

31 Schott RJ, Natale JE, Ressler SW, Burney RE, Alecy LG (1989) Neutrophil depletion fails to improve outcome after cardiac arrest in dogs. *Ann Emerg Med* 18: 517–522

32 Aspey BS, Jessimer C, Pereira S, Harrison MJG (1989) Do leukocytes have a role in the cerebrovascular no-reflow phenomenon? *J Neurol Neurosurg Psychiatry* 52: 526–528

33 Takeshima R, Kirsch JR, Koehler RC, Gomoll AW, Traystman RJ (1992) Monoclonal leukocyte antibody does not decrease the injury of transient focal cerebral ischemia in cats. *Stroke* 23: 247–252

34 Mori E, del Zoppo GJ, Chambers JD, Copeland BR, Arfors KE (1992) Inhibition of polymorphonuclear leukocyte adherence suppresses no-reflow after focal cerebral ischemia in baboons. *Stroke* 23: 712–718

35 Chopp M, Zhang RL, Chen H, Li Y, Jiang N, Rusche JR (1994) Postischemic administration of an anti-Mac-1 antibody reduces ischemic cell damage after transient middle cerebral artery occlusion in rats. *Stroke* 25: 869–876

36 Prestigiacomo CJ, Kim SC, ConnollyES Jr, Pinsky DJ (1999) CD18-mediated neutrophil recruitment contributes to the pathogenesis of reperfused but not nonreperfused stroke. *Stroke* 30: 1110–1117

37 Connolly ES Jr, Winfree CJ, Prestigiacomo CJ, Kim SC, Choudhri TF, Hoh BL, Naka Y, Solomon RA, Pinsky DJ (1997) Exacerbation of cerebral injury in mice that express the P-selectin gene: identification of P-selectin blockade as a new target for the treatment of stroke *Circ Res* 81: 304–310

38 Connolly ES Jr, Winfree CJ, Stern DM, Solomon RA, Pinsky DJ (1996) Procedural and strain-related variables significantly affect outcome in a murine model of focal cerebral ischemia. *Neurosurgery* 38 (3): 523–532

39 Wang X, Yue TL, Barone FC, Feuerstein GZ (1995) Demonstration of increased endothelial-leukocyte adhesion molecule-1 mRNA expression in rat ischemic cortex. *Stroke* 26: 1668–1669

40 Huang J, Choudhri TF, Winfree CJ, McTaggert RA, Mocco J, Kim LJ, Protopsaltis TS, Zhang Y, Pinsky DJ, Connolly ES Jr (2000) Postischemic cerebrovascular E-selectin expression mediates tissue injury in murine stroke. *Stroke* 31: 3047–3053

41 Huang J, Mocco J, Choudhri TF, Poisik A, Popilskis SJ, Emerson R, Delapaz R, Khandji AG, Pinsky DJ, Connolly ES Jr (2000) A modified transorbital baboon model of reperfused stroke. *Stroke* 31: 3054–3063

42 Choudhri TF, Huang J, Mocco J, Harfeldt E, Efros L, Klingbeil C, Vexler V, Zhang Z,

Khandji A, Delapaz R et al (2000) Simultaneous E- and P-selectin blockade improves outcomes in a double-blinded, placebo-controlled study of primate stroke. *Stroke* 31: 341–(Abstr)

43 Mulligan MS, Paulson JC, de Frees S, Zheng Z-L, Lowe JB, Ward PA (1993) Protective effects of oligosaccharides in P-selectin-dependent lung injury. *Nature* 364: 149–151

44 Morikawa E, Zhang S-M, Seko Y, Toyoda T, Kirino T (1996) Treatment of focal cerebral ischemia with synthetic oligopeptide corresponding to lectin domain of selectin. *Stroke* 27: 951–956

45 Huang J, Kim LJ, Mealey R, Marsh HCJ, Zhang Y, Tenner AJ, Connolly ES Jr, Pinsky DJ (1999) Neuronal protection in stroke by an sLe^x-glycosylated complement inhibitory protein. *Science* 285: 595–599

46 Rittershaus CW, Thomas LJ, Miller DP, Picard MD, Geoghegan-Barek KM, Scesney SM, Henry LD, Sen AC, Bertino AM, Hannig G et al (1999) Recombinant glycoproteins which inhibit complement activation and also bind the selectin adhesion molecule. *J Biol Chem* 274: 11237

47 Connolly ES Jr, Winfree CJ, Prestiagiacomo C, Kim S, Naka Y, Solomon RA, Pinsky DJ (1997) Exacerbation of cerebral injury in mice which express the P-selectin gene: identification of P-selectin blockade as a new target for the treatment of stroke. *Circ Res* 81: 304–310

The kallikrein-kinin system in ischemic and traumatic brain injury

Nikolaus Plesnila[1] and Jane Relton[2]

[1]Massachusetts General Hospital, Harvard Medical School, Charlestown, MA 02129, USA and Institute for Surgical Research, Ludwig-Maximilians University, Marchioninistr. 15, 81366 München, Germany; [2]Biogen, Inc., 14 Cambridge Center, Cambridge, MA 02142, USA

Introduction

The surgeon Emil Karl Frey and the physiologist Heinrich Kraut, both working at the Ludwig-Maximilians University in Munich at that time, were first to describe the existence of the kallikrein-kinin system in 1928 [1]. The initial observation was that injection of urine into the circulation of anesthetized dogs had a marked hypotensive effect. The hypotension caused by peripheral vasodilation turned out to be induced by a family of proteins later named kinins [2]. Today we know that the most abundant kinins are the nonapeptide bradykinin (Arg^1-Pro^2-Pro^3-Gly^4-Phe^5-Ser^6-Pro^7-Phe^8-Arg^9), its degradation product des-Arg^9-bradykinin, and the dekapeptide kallidin (Lys^0-bradykinin) [3]. Bradykinin is mainly found in plasma where it is cleaved from its pre-cursor high molecular weight (HMW) kininogen (MW 120 kDa) by the plasma protease kallikrein (90 kDa) (Fig. 1). Kallidin is predominantly found in tissue and is cleaved from low molecular weight (LMW) kininogen (68 kDa) by a low molecular weight kallikrein (30 kDa) only found in tissue. Activation of the kallikrein-kinin system occurs by conversion of the inactive pre-kallikrein to active kallikrein by several proteins acting as kallikreinases, e.g., Hagman factor (blood clotting factor XII), trypsine, thrombin, plasmine, or C_1-esterase, which accumulate at the site of endothelial and tissue injury. Interestingly, kinin production can also occur independently of kallikrein activation by cellular proteases released from mast cells or granulocytes [4].

The main actions of kinins are mediated through two G-protein coupled receptors, named B_1 and B_2 (see below), and comprise all features of an acute inflammatory response, including pain, hyperemia and tissue swelling [5].

Most components of the kallikrein-kinin system are present in the brain [6, 7]. The 30 kDa low molecular weight, tissue-specific form of kallikrein was found

Inflammation and Stroke, edited by Giora Z. Feuerstein
© 2001 Birkhäuser Verlag Basel/Switzerland

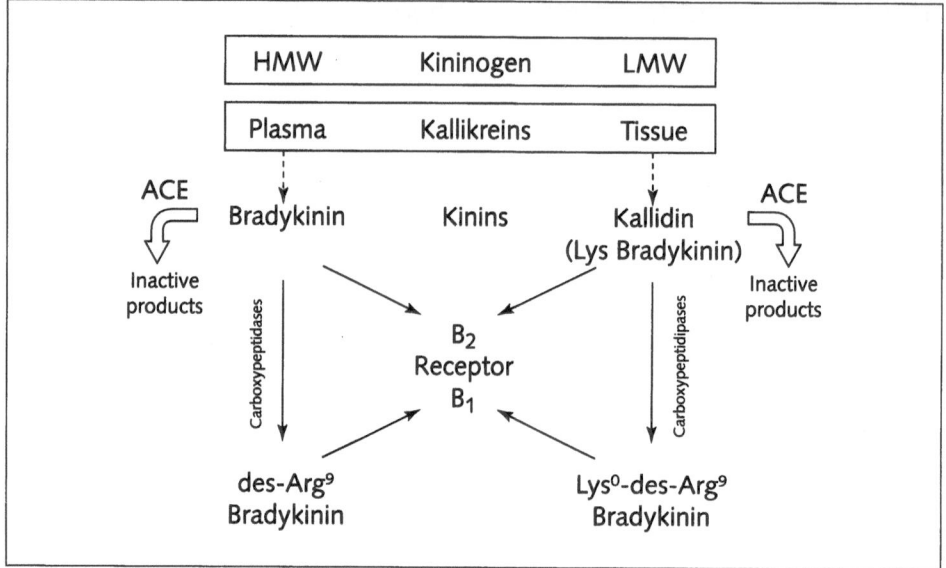

Figure 1
Schematic drawing of the organization of the kallikrein-kinin system

widespread and scattered in the brain and was preferentially located in neuronal cell bodies and their processes in both cerebral cortex and brainstem by immunohisto-chemistry [8].

Kininogen was found by the same method in neurons and axons of the brain stem, cerebellum (dentate nucleus), cerebral cortex (layers III and V), hippocampus (pyramidal cell layer), and corpus callosum. Glia and endothelial cells stained in all brain regions [9]. The levels of bradykinin in rat brain are reported to be about 0.6 pmol/g [10] and it shares a similar pattern of distribution to kininogen. Interestingly, the presence and location of kallidin in the brain has not been reported yet.

Kinin receptors

The actions of bradykinin and kallidin and their degradation products des-Arg^9-bradykinin and Lys^0-des-Arg^9-bradykinin are mediated *via* the receptors designated bradykinin B_2 and B_1 receptors, respectively [3, 11]. Human, mouse and rat receptors have been cloned and expressed [12–17]. Although B_2 and B_1 receptors only share 36% sequence homology [14], both are G protein coupled receptors and activate similar second messenger systems (outlined below) [11]. The B_2 receptor is expressed constitutively in many tissues whereas the B_1 receptor, with some exceptions, is not normally present but is rapidly and vigorously induced and upregulated in response to a wide variety of chemical, mechanical and inflammatory stimuli [11]. Inflammatory cytokines have been shown to be potent inducers of B_1 receptor expression [18] and ligand receptor binding at the B_1 receptor can result in homologous upregulation of the receptor [19]; the B_2, but not the B_1 receptor is rapidly desensitized, internalized and downregulated following activation [20].

The prevailing dogma is that the B_1 receptor is "pathological" and is induced by and exacerbates inflammatory responses, enhancing the effects of overactivation of the constitutive B_2 receptor in a disease setting. Both B_2 and B_1 receptor knockouts have been described and appear phenotypically normal but show attenuated disease pathology consistent with pharmacological inhibition of their respective receptors [11, 21].

B_2 receptors have been localized throughout the brain and spinal cord, in cortex, hippocampus, medulla and dorsal horn [22–24]. Initial studies suggested these binding sites were primarily located on cerebral blood vessels [22], but subsequent work has described B_2 receptor expression on neurons [25, 26], astrocytes [27], microglial cells and oligodendrocytes [28]. Autoradiographic and functional studies support their presence on the cerebrovasculature [22, 29, 30]. B_1 receptors are present on human neurons and astrocytes [31] and on neurons in rat spinal cord [32].

Function of the kinin system in the brain

Activation of B_1 or B_2 kinin receptors in the brain result in a wide variety of physiological and pathological responses [33]. Intraventricular or intraparenchymal injection of bradykinin induced a B_2 receptor dependent increase in blood pressure and heart rate [23]. This effect was considered to be mediated by a central action of bradykinin, because peripheral intravenous injection of bradykinin B_2 receptor antagonists in normotensive rats and disruption of the bradykinin B_2 receptor or kininogen gene did not have any influence on blood pressure or heart rate [34]. Intraparenchymal injection of bradykinin was also able to elevate nociceptive levels, most likely by releasing endogenous opioids [35].

However, the best studied effect of kinins in the brain is that on the cerebral vasculature [36]. Incubation with bradykinin *in vitro* relaxed ring segments of human cerebral arteries dose-dependently [37]. Perivascular microapplication of bradykinin dilated cat pial arterioles by 45% [38, 39]. A similar, but somewhat lower dilation was seen after superfusion of the brain with bradykinin [40]. Pial veins did not change their diameter after bradykinin superfusion [40]. Interestingly, intraarterial application of bradykinin did not have a vasomotor effect [40]. The bradykinin-induced vasodilation was not inhibitable by B_1 receptor antagonists [38], but could be reduced by B_2 receptor inhibition and was mediated by nitric oxide [41].

In addition to its vasodilatatory effect, bradykinin increases cerebrovascular permeability [36, 42, 43] and leads to formation of brain edema [44–46]. The opening of the blood brain barrier in cats occurred only to small molecular weight markers (Na-fluorescein) [44], while in mice the barrier opened also to bigger molecules (FITC-Dextran, 70 kDa). Opening of the BBB was observed after perivascular as well as after intracarotid application of bradykinin [44]. These effects were inhibited by B_2 receptors antagonists [43] and could be mimicked by application of B_2 receptor agonists [47]. Subsequent release of factors such as cytokines [48], eicosanoids [49], nitric oxide [29, 50] and free radicals [43] had been described as downstream mediators of B_2 receptor activation. Recent studies have demonstrated that also des-Arg^9-bradykinin, a B_1 receptor agonist, can result in an increase in cerebrovascular permeability, which is mediated by histamine [43].

Kinin receptors are also present on peripheral blood mononuclear cells [5] and the kinin system can be activated by granulocytes [4]. B_1 receptor blockade has been shown to attenuate IL-1β-induced leukocyte-endothelial cell interactions and leukocyte migration [18, 51, 52]. In B_1 knockout mice neutrophil infiltration into the pleural cavity is reduced in response to des-Arg^9-bradykinin or carageenan injection [21]. Similarly, B_2 receptor blockade inhibited neutrophil migratory activity in a model of peripheral inflammation [52].

Kinins in stroke

After experimental cerebral ischemia kinin and kininogen levels increase in the brain [53] and kininogen is consumed in the cerebral circulation in humans during brain ischemia and post-ischemic reperfusion [54]. Blockade of the kinin B_2 receptor has been shown to protect against ischemic brain injury after permanent or reversible middle cerebral artery occlusion in the rat [55, 56]. Paradoxically however, B_1 receptor blockade was not protective and was able to reverse the beneficial effect of B_2 receptor blockade [56]. These data may suggest opposing roles for B_1 and B_2 receptors after acute brain injury. The demonstration that blockade of the B_2 receptor inhibits ischemic brain injury supports the suggestion that B_2 antagonists may be of value in the treatment of stroke. However, our recent data suggests that the B_2 receptor is rapidly downregulated after ischemic injury in the rat [57] consistent with the predicted effect of over-activation of this G-protein coupled receptor. The value of B_2 antagonist therapy after brain ischemia therefore deserves further investigation.

Kinins in traumatic brain injury (TBI)

Early evidence for the involvement of the kallikrein-kinin system in the pathophysiology of brain injury was provided by the findings that significant amounts of plasma kininogen were found in the affected parenchyma after brain lesion [49, 58]. Seventy-five percent of kininogen found in the contused brain was subsequently converted to kinins [58]. Vascular reactivity to bradykinin was significantly reduced 24 and 48 h after a cortical lesion, indicating changes in vascular kinin receptor expression after brain injury [59]. In rabbits aprotinin, a kallikrein inhibitor, decreases posttraumatic brain swelling when given prior to or after the injury [60]. More recently, after the development of selective bradykinin receptor antagonists, a B_2 inhibitor (LF-16-0687) was found to reduce brain edema in a diffuse-closed and in an open-focal brain injury model in rats [61, 62, 62a]. In humans only one compound, CP-0127/deltibant/Bradycor™, has been evaluated so far after traumatic brain injury. After a preliminary study on 20 patients showed promising reductions in intracranial pressure (ICP), Glasgow Coma Score (GCS) and treatment intensity level (TIL) [63] a phase II prospective, randomized, double blind clinical trial was conducted at 31 centers within North America in 139 severely brain injured patients (GCS 3-8) [64]. The results published so far show consistent positive trends in ICP, TIL, neuropsychological tests, and, most importantly, 3- and 6-month outcome (neurological function and mortality). Although the results are not statistically significant yet, these data provide supportive evidence that a bradykinin antagonist may play a neuroprotective role in severe brain injury and further studies with this or similar compounds seem to be worthwhile. Particularly since all other clinical trials of therapeutics for traumatic brain injury to date have failed to demonstrate efficacy.

Taken together, the main effect of bradykinin studied so far in the pathophysiology of traumatic brain injury is that on brain edema. Specific inhibition of kinin B_2 receptors reduce brain edema after experimental and clinical brain trauma. However, these findings should not make us forget that knowledge about the pathophysiological role of kinins after trauma, e.g. receptor expression, is still very limited.

Conclusion

Outside the brain kinins are known to be among the first inflammatory mediators released after tissue injury and that they mediate vasodilation and tissue swelling. In the brain, where all components of the kallikrein-kinin system are present, kinins seem to have very similar effects. After cerebral ischemia and traumatic brain injury kinins mediate tissue injury and kinin B_2 receptor antagonists, have beneficial effects in experimental animals and, also in some patients. Although more detailed work needs to be done, especially on the physiological role of kinins in the brain, the kallikrein-kinin system is now an established component in the pathophysiology of brain injury.

References

1   Frey EK, Kraut H (1928) Ein neues Kreislaufhormon und seine Wirkung. *Arch Exp Pathol Pharmacol* 133: 1–56

2   Werle E, Berek K (1948) Zur Kenntnis des Kallikreins. *Angewandte Chemie* 60: 53–72

3   Regoli D, Barabe J (1980) Pharmacology of bradykinin and related kinins. *Pharmacol Rev* 32: 1–46

4   Proud D, MacGlashan DWJ, Newball HH, Schulman ES, Lichtenstein LM (1985) Immunoglobulin E-mediated release of a kininogenase from purified human lung mast cells. *Am Rev Respir Dis* 132: 405–408

5   Bhoola KD, Figueroa CD, Worthy K (1992) Bioregulation of kinins: kallikreins, kininogens, and kininases. *Pharmacol Rev* 44: 1–80

6   Scicli AG, Forbes G, Nolly H, Dujovny M, Carretero OA (1984) Kallikrein-kinins in the central nervous system. *Clin Exp Hypertens* [A] 6: 1731–1738

7   Walker K, Perkins M, Dray A (1995) Kinins and kinin receptors in the nervous system. *Neurochem Int* 26: 1–16

8   Kizuki K, Suzuki T, Kudo M, Noguchi T (1994) Immunohistochemical demonstration of tissue kallikrein in the neurons of rat brain. *Brain Res* 634: 305–309

9   Li Z, Tyor WR, Xu J, Chao J, Hogan EL (1999) Immunohistochemical localization of kininogen in rat spinal cord and brain. *Exp Neurol* 159: 528–537

10 Perry DC, Snyder SH (1984) Identification of bradykinin in mammalian brain. *J Neurochem* 43: 1072–1080

11 Marceau F, Hess JF, Bachvarov DR (1998) The B1 receptors for kinins. *Pharmacol Rev* 50: 357–386

12 McEachern AE, Shelton ER, Bhakta S, Obernolte R, Bach C, Zuppan P, Fujisaki J, Aldrich RW, Jarnagin K (1991) Expression cloning of a rat B2 bradykinin receptor. *Proc Natl Acad Sci USA* 88: 7724–7728

13 Hess JF, Borkowski JA, Young GS, Strader CD, Ransom RW (1992) Cloning and pharmacological characterization of a human bradykinin (BK-2) receptor. *Biochem Biophys Res Commun* 184: 260–268

14 Menke JG, Borkowski JA, Bierilo KK, MacNeil T, Derrick AW, Schneck KA, Ransom RW, Strader CD, Linemeyer DL, Hess JF (1994) Expression cloning of a human B1 bradykinin receptor. *J Biol Chem* 269: 21583–21586

15 Borkowski JA, Ransom RW, Seabrook GR, Trumbauer M, Chen H, Hill RG, Strader CD, Hess JF (1995) Targeted disruption of a B2 bradykinin receptor gene in mice eliminates bradykinin action in smooth muscle and neurons. *J Biol Chem* 270: 13706–13710

16 Pesquero JB, Pesquero JL, Oliveira SM, Roscher AA, Metzger R, Ganten D, Bader M (1996) Molecular cloning and functional characterization of a mouse bradykinin B1 receptor gene. *Biochem Biophys Res Commun* 224: 281

17 Ni A, Chai KX, Chao L, Chao J (1998) Molecular cloning and expression of rat bradykinin B1 receptor. *Biochim Biophys Acta* 1442: 177–185

18 McLean PG, Ahluwalia A, Perretti M (2000) Association between kinin B(1) receptor

expression and leukocyte trafficking across mouse mesenteric postcapillary venules. *J Exp Med* 192: 367–380

19   Schanstra JP, Bataille E, Marin CM, Barascud Y, Hirtz C, Pesquero JB, Pecher C, Gauthier F, Girolami JP, Bascands JL (1998) The B1-agonist [des-Arg10]-kallidin activates transcription factor NF-kappaB and induces homologous upregulation of the bradykinin B1-receptor in cultured human lung fibroblasts. *J Clin Invest* 101: 2080–2091

20   Faussner A, Proud D, Towns M, Bathon JM (1998) Influence of the cytosolic carboxyl termini of human B1 and B2 kinin receptors on receptor sequestration, ligand internalization, and signal transduction. *J Biol Chem* 273: 2617–2623

21   Pesquero JB, Araujo RC, Heppenstall PA, Stucky CL, Silva JAJ, Walther T, Oliveira SM, Pesquero JL, Paiva AC, Calixto JB et al (2000) Hypoalgesia and altered inflammatory responses in mice lacking kinin B1 receptors. *Proc Natl Acad Sci USA* 97: 8140–8145

22   Fujiwara Y, Mantione CR, Vavrek RJ, Stewart JM, Yamamura HI (1989) Characterization of [3H]bradykinin binding sites in guinea-pig central nervous system: possible existence of B2 subtypes. *Life Sci* 44: 1645–1653

23   Privitera PJ, Daum PR, Hill DR, Hiley CR (1992) Autoradiographic visualization and characteristics of [125I]bradykinin binding sites in guinea pig brain. *Brain Res* 577: 73–79

24   Murone C, Perich RB, Schlawe I, Chai SY, Casley D, MacGregor DP, Muller-Esterl W, Mendelsohn FA (1996) Characterization and localization of bradykinin B2 receptors in the guinea-pig using a radioiodinated HOE140 analogue. *Eur J Pharmacol* 306: 237–247

25   Raidoo DM, Ramchurren N, Naidoo Y, Naidoo S, Muller-Esterl W, Bhoola KD (1996) Visualisation of bradykinin B2 receptors on human brain neurons. *Immunopharmacology* 33: 104–107

26   Chen EY, Emerich DF, Bartus RT, Kordower JH (2000) B2 bradykinin receptor immunoreactivity in rat brain. *J Comp Neurol* 427: 1–18

27   Hösli L, Hösli E, Kaeser H, Lefkovits M (1992) Colocalization of receptors for vasoactive peptides on astrocytes of cultured rat spinal cord and brain stem: electrophysiological effects of atrial and brain natriuretic peptide, neuropeptide Y and bradykinin. *Neurosci Lett* 148: 114–116

28   Stephens GJ, Marriott DR, Djamgoz MB, Wilkin GP (1993) Electrophysiological and biochemical evidence for bradykinin receptors on cultured rat cortical oligodendrocytes. *Neurosci Lett* 153: 223–226

29   Onoue H, Kaito N, Tomii M, Tokudome S, Nakajima M, Abe T (1994) Human basilar and middle cerebral arteries exhibit endothelium-dependent responses to peptides. *Am J Physiol* 267: H880–H886

30   Xu J, Qu ZX, Moore SA, Hsu CY, Hogan EL (1992) Receptor-linked hydrolysis of phosphoinositides and production of prostacyclin in cerebral endothelial cells. *J Neurochem* 58: 1930–1935

31 Raidoo DM, Sawant S, Mahabeer R, Bhoola KD (1999) Kinin receptors are expressed in human astrocytic tumour cells. *Immunopharmacology* 43: 255–263

32 Wotherspoon G and Winter J (2000) Bradykinin B1 receptor is constitutively expressed in the rat sensory nervous system. *Neurosci Lett* 294: 175–178

33 Walker K, Perkins M, Dray A (1995) Kinins and kinin receptors in the nervous system. *Neurochem Int* 26: 1–16

34 Ellis EF, Heizer ML, Hambrecht GS, Holt SA, Stewart JM, Vavrek RJ (1987) Inhibition of bradykinin- and kallikrein-induced cerebral arteriolar dilation by a specific bradykinin antagonist. *Stroke* 18: 792–795

35 Raymond JJ, Robertson DM, Dinsdale HB (1986) Pharmacological modification of bradykinin induced breakdown of the blood-brain barrier. *Can J Neurol Sci* 13: 214–220

36 Wahl M, Whalley ET, Unterberg A, Schilling L, Parsons AA, Baethmann A, Young AR (1996) Vasomotor and permeability effects of bradykinin in the cerebral microcirculation. *Immunopharmacology* 33: 257–263

37 Toda N (1977) Actions of bradykinin on isolated cerebral and peripheral arteries. *Am J Physiol* 232: H267–H274

38 Whalley ET and Wahl M (1983) Analysis of bradykinin receptor mediating relaxation of cat cerebral arteries *in vivo* and *in vitro*. *Naunyn Schmiedebergs Arch Pharmacol* 323: 66–71

39 Wahl M, Young AR, Edvinsson L, Wagner F (1983) Effects of bradykinin on pial arteries and arterioles *in vitro* and *in situ*. *J Cereb Blood Flow Metab* 3: 231–237

40 Unterberg A, Wahl M, Baethmann A (1984) Effects of bradykinin on permeability and diameter of pial vessels *in vivo*. *J Cereb Blood Flow Metab* 4: 574–585

41 Görlach C, Wahl M (1996) Bradykinin dilates rat middle cerebral artery and its large branches *via* endothelial B2 receptors and release of nitric oxide. *Peptides* 17: 1373–1378

42 Wahl M, Unterberg A, Baethmann A, Schilling L (1988) Mediators of blood-brain barrier dysfunction and formation of vasogenic brain edema. *J Cereb Blood Flow Metab* 8: 621–634

43 Sarker MH, Hu D, Fraser PA (2000) Acute effects of bradykinin on cerebral microvascular permeability in the anaesthetized rat. *J Physiol* 528 Pt 1: 177–187

44 Unterberg A and Baethmann AJ (1984) The kallikrein-kinin system as mediator in vasogenic brain edema. Part 1: Cerebral exposure to bradykinin and plasma. *J Neurosurg* 61: 87–96

45 Unterberg A, Polk T, Ellis E, Marmarou A (1990) Enhancement of infusion-induced brain edema by mediator compounds. *Adv Neurol* 52: 355–358

46 Whittle IR, Piper IR, Miller JD (1992) The role of bradykinin in the etiology of vasogenic brain edema and perilesional brain dysfunction. *Acta Neurochir (Wien)* 115: 53–59

47 Bartus RT, Elliott P, Hayward N, Dean R, McEwen EL, Fisher SK (1996) Permeability

of the blood brain barrier by the bradykinin agonist, RMP-7: evidence for a sensitive, auto-regulated, receptor-mediated system. *Immunopharmacology* 33: 270–278

48 Ferreira SH, Lorenzetti BB, Poole S (1993) Bradykinin initiates cytokine-mediated inflammatory hyperalgesia. *Br J Pharmacol* 110: 1227–1231

49 Ellis EF, Chao J, Heizer ML (1989) Brain kininogen following experimental brain injury: evidence for a secondary event. *J Neurosurg* 71: 437–442

50 Tsutsui M, Onoue H, Iida Y, Smith L, O'Brien T, Katusic ZS (2000) Effects of recombinant eNOS gene expression on reactivity of small cerebral arteries. *Am J Physiol Heart Circ Physiol* 278: H420–H427

51 Ahluwalia A and Perretti M (1996) Involvement of bradykinin B1 receptors in the polymorphonuclear leukocyte accumulation induced by IL-1 beta *in vivo* in the mouse. *J Immunol* 156: 269–274

52 Perron MS, Gobeil FJ, Pelletier S, Regoli D, Sirois P (1999) Involvement of bradykinin B1 and B2 receptors in pulmonary leukocyte accumulation induced by Sephadex beads in guinea pigs. *Eur J Pharmacol* 376: 83–89

53 Xu J, He YY, Chao J, Hsu CY (1990) Kinin and kininogen in the full reperfusion stroke model of brain. *FASEB J* 4: A998

54 Makevnina LG, Lomova IP, Zubkov Y, Semenyutin VB (1994) Kininogen consumption in cerebral circulation of humans during brain ischemia and postischemic reperfusion. *Braz J Med Biol Res* 27: 1955–1963

55 Relton JK, Beckey VE, Hanson WL, Whalley ET (1997) CP-0597, a selective bradykinin B2 receptor antagonist, inhibits brain injury in a rat model of reversible middle cerebral artery occlusion. *Stroke* 28: 1430–1436

56 Relton JK, Rothwell NJ, Whalley ET (1996) Blockade of the bradykinin B1 receptor reverses the neuroprotective effect of B2 receptor blockade after focal cerebral ischemia in the rat. *Br J Pharmacol* 120: C81

57 Sloan KE, Frew EM, Whalley ET, Relton JK (2000) Downregulation of the bradykinin B2 receptor after focal cerebral ischemia in the spontaneously hypertensive rat. *Soc Neurosci (Abstr)* 672.15

58 Maier-Hauff K, Baethmann AJ, Lange M, Schürer L, Unterberg A (1984) The kallikrein-kinin system as mediator in vasogenic brain edema. Part 2: Studies on kinin formation in focal and perifocal brain tissue. *J Neurosurg* 61: 97–106

59 Görlach C, Benyo Z, Wahl M (1998) Dilator effect of bradykinin and acetylcholine in cerebral vessels after brain lesion. *Kidney Int* (Suppl) 67: S226–S227

60 Unterberg A, Dautermann C, Baethmann A, Müller-Esterl W (1986) The kallikrein-kinin system as mediator in vasogenic brain edema. Part 3: Inhibition of the kallikrein-kinin system in traumatic brain swelling. *J Neurosurg* 64: 269–276

61 Pruneau D, Chorny I, Benkovitz V, Artru A, Roitblat L, Shapira Y (1999) Effect of LF 16-0687MS, a new nonpeptide bradykinin B2 receptor antagonist, in a rat model of closed head trauma. *J Neurotrauma* 16: 1057–1065

62 Stover JF, Dohse NK, Unterberg AW (2000) Significant reduction in brain swelling by

administration of nonpeptide kinin B2 receptor antagonist LF 16-0687Ms after controlled cortical impact injury in rats. *J Neurosurg* 92: 853–859

62a Plesnila N, Schulz J, Stoffel M, Eriskat J, Pruneau D, Baethmann A (2001) Effect of the non-peptide bradykinin B2-receptor antagonist LF 16-0687 on vasogenic brain edema in rats. *J Neurotrauma; in press*

63 Narotam PK, Rodell TC, Nadvi SS, Bhoola KD, Troha JM, Parbhoosingh R, van DJ (1998) Traumatic brain contusions: a clinical role for the kinin antagonist CP-0127. *Acta Neurochir (Wien)* 140: 793–802

64 Marmarou A, Nichols J, Burgess J, Newell D, Troha J, Burnham D, Pitts L (1999) Effects of the bradykinin antagonist Bradycor (deltibant, CP-1027) in severe traumatic brain injury: results of a multi-center, randomized, placebo-controlled trial. American Brain Injury Consortium Study Group. *J Neurotrauma* 16: 431–444

Nitric oxide, nitric oxide synthases and cyclooxygenase-2 in experimental focal stroke

Xinkang Wang[1], Costantino Iadecola[2] and Giora Z. Feuerstein[1]

[1]Department of Cardiovascular Sciences, DuPont Pharmaceuticals Company, Experimental Station E400/3420B, Wilmington, DE 19880-0400, USA; [2]Department of Neurology, University of Minnesota, Minneapolis, MN, USA

Nitric oxide and nitric oxide synthase

Nitric oxide (NO) is a unique messenger molecule involved in the regulation of diverse physiological processes including central and peripheral neurotransmission, smooth and cardiac muscle contractility, platelet aggregation, and immune cell functions. NO is crucial for many physiological functions; however, inappropriate release of this mediator is associated with a number of pathological conditions [1]. NO is synthesized from a guanidino group (by oxidation) of L-arginine by the enzyme NO synthase (NOS) in virtually all mammalian cells, including endothelial cells, neurons, glia, and cells of the immune system [2] (Fig. 1). Three isoforms of NOS have been characterized, including neuronal NOS (nNOS or type I), inducible or immunological NOS (iNOS or type II), and endothelial NOS (eNOS or type III). eNOS and nNOS are constitutively expressed. In contrast, iNOS is not normally expressed but its expression can be induced in many cell types by selected immunological stimuli [2]. The constitutive expression of eNOS and nNOS contributes to small but consistent amounts of NO production that are sufficient for signaling function. A massive induction of iNOS results in the production of large amounts of NO that may result in pathophysiological consequences [3].

Nitric oxide, nitric oxide synthase and cerebral ischemia injury

Cerebral ischemia is commonly the outcome of obstruction of blood flow in major cerebral vessels, which, if not resolved within a short period of time, will lead to a core of severely ischemic brain tissue that may not be salvageable. Ischemic stroke leads to depletion of energy (ATP, PCr) and hence to membrane voltage reduction leading to ionic fluxes across the cell membrane. The increase in extracellular potassium can reach levels sufficient to release neurotransmitters such as glutamate and aspartate and stimulate sodium/calcium channels coupled to glutamate receptors leading to cytotoxic edema. The calcium overload is believed to cause further mito-

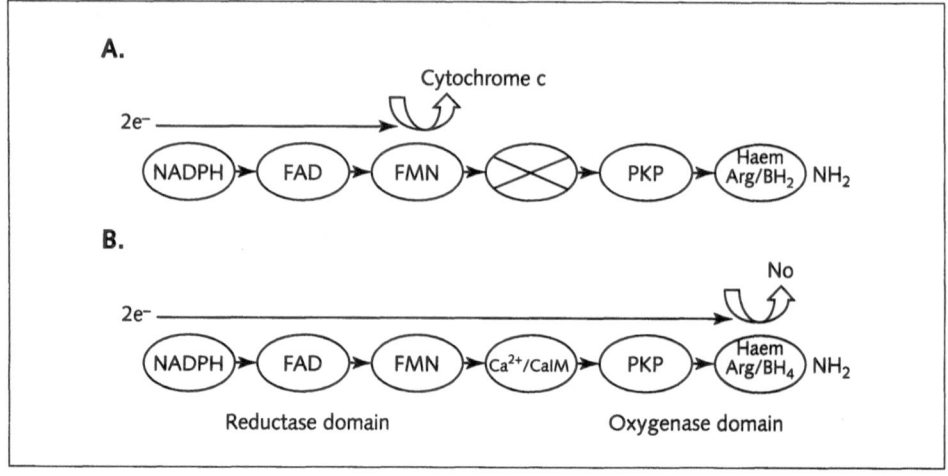

Figure 1

Schematic diagram of NO synthesis by NOS. Consensus sites for heam, L-arginine (Arg), tetrahydropterin (BH4), protein kinase phosphorylation (PKP), calcium/calmodulin (Ca^{2+}/CalM), flavin mononucleotide (FMN), flavin adenine dinucleotide (FAD) and nicotinamide adenine dinucleotide phosphate (NADPH) are indicated in order from the N-terminal to the c-terminal of the peptide. Electrons involved in NO production are donated by NADPH and transported through the reductase domain to the oxygenase domain. In the absence of Ca^{2+}/CalM, electrons do not flow to the oxygenase domain and are accepted by cytochrome c and other electron receptors (A). In the presence of Ca^{2+}/CalM, electrons will flow to the oxygenase domain and lead to the production of NO (B).

chondria damage and impairment in ATP production as well as extensive breakdown of cellular phopholipids, proteins and nucleic acids due to activation of phospholipases, proteases, and endonucleases. Free radicals are also produced during ischemia and contribute to membrane lipid peroxidation, protein and nuclear DNA toxic changes, and cellular injury (i.e., necrosis and apoptosis).

There is substantial evidence that NO is involved in ischemic brain injury (Fig. 2). The interaction of glutamate with its receptor can lead to NO formation [4]. This observation was supported by the blockade of NO surge by glutamate receptor antagonists, ketamine, dizocilpine maleate (MK801), or N(G)-nitro-L-arginine methyl ester (L-NAME) [5]. The levels of NO, and its stable metabolic breakdown products, nitrate and nitrite, are increased from < 10 nM (pre-ischemia) to approximately 2 μM within minutes of focal ischemia, after which NO concentration decreases slowly with a decay half-life of approximately 30 min [6]. The early production of NO is likely due to the upregulation of nNOS as well as eNOS by the ischemic event [6, 7]. These early events are followed by upregulation of iNOS

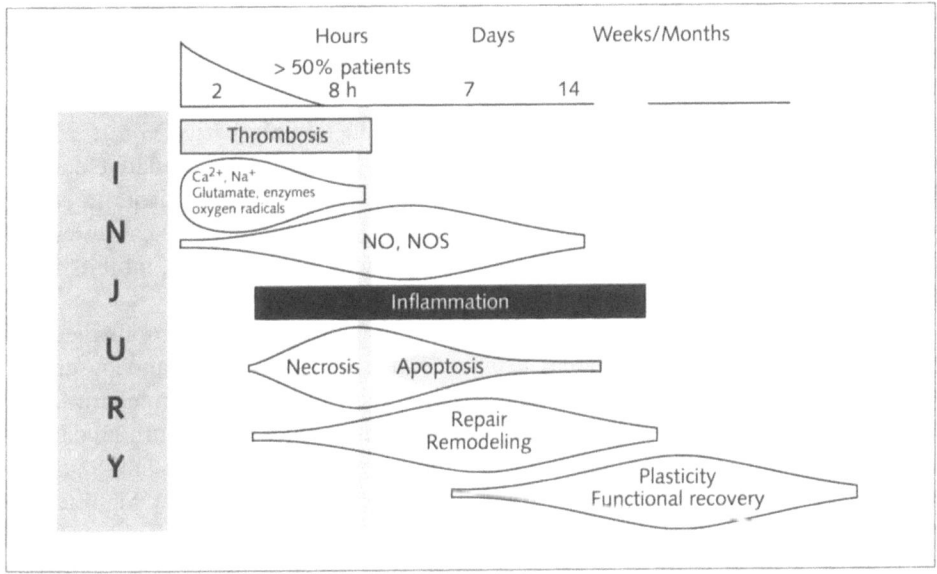

Figure 2
Schematic diagram depicts the dynamic changes following ischemic stroke.

which further contributes to the massive increases in NO production and results in progression of brain injury [7]. *De novo* expression of iNOS is part of an inflammatory reaction that evolves following brain ischemia. Following permanent or transient MCAO in rodents, iNOS mRNA, protein, and enzymatic activity are expressed in the ischemic brain tissue [7]. iNOS expression peaks 12–48 h after ischemia and occurs in inflammatory cells infiltrating the injured brain and in cerebral blood vessels. The expression of iNOS was also demonstrated in neutrophils and vascular cells in human brain after stroke [8]. Taken together, these studies suggest that early enhanced production of NO after cerebral ischemia is likely the product of nNOS and eNOS, while excessive production of NO at later stages is likely to be the result of iNOS induction.

The role of nitric oxide synthases in stroke

NO has beneficial as well as deleterious effects after brain ischemia, depending on its concentration, and its spatial and temporal distribution [6, 7]. NO produced at the low flow region by eNOS provides for vasodilation and therefore protects the brain by limiting the degree of flow reduction produced by the arterial occlusion [9]. At low levels NO might inhibit calcium influx through NMDA-receptor and therefore limit glutamate-mediated neurotoxicity in cerebral ischemia [7]. In addition, NO interacts and scavenges reactive oxygen species (O_2^-, superoxide) partially off-setting oxidative stress injury [10].

In general, however, excessive generation of NO (mainly by iNOS) after brain ischemia has been implicated in tissue damage [7]. NO promotes oxidative damage by avidly combining with superoxide anion (O_2^-) to form peroxynitrite (a strong oxidant) and by perturbing iron metabolism [3,11]. In addition, NO causes energy failure (inhibits cellular energy production), produces DNA damage, inhibits DNA synthesis, and triggers programmed cell death [6, 7].

Both protective and destructive roles of NO after brain ischemia are further supported by pharmacological studies using selective NOS inhibitors and by genetic approaches using knockout mice subjected to cerebral ischemia. Administration of selective inhibitors for nNOS or iNOS resulted in the reduction of neuronal damage and infarct volume [7, 12]. Similarly, disruption of either nNOS or iNOS gene in mice resulted in amelioration of brain damage after ischemia [13,14]. Significantly smaller infarct volume (38% reduction) was observed in mice deficient in nNOS than in the wild-type (Fig. 3) 24 h after MCAO [13]. In contrast, the significant reduction (24%) in the infarct was not observed in the iNOS deficient mice until 96 h after MCAO [14]. While there is no selective eNOS inhibitor available to date, mice with disrupted eNOS gene develop larger infarcts (28% increase) compared with their wild type counterparts after brain ischemia [15].

Cyclooxygenase gene expression and cerebral ischemia

Cyclooxygenases (COX) are rate-limiting enzymes in the synthesis of prostaglandins and thromboxanes. COX-2 expression is upregulated by a wide variety of stimuli, such as inflammatory mediators and mitogens [16]. Following cerebral ischemia, COX-2 mRNA and protein are upregulated, peaking 12–24 h after ischemia [17–20]. COX-2 is expressed in neurons and vascular cells located at the border of the ischemic territory [18, 19]. In neurons, COX-2 is expressed in cells that exhibit ischemic changes, as well as in neurons that appear structurally normal [19]. Recently, COX-2 was also found in the human brain after ischemic stroke [21]. Initial data suggest that the relatively selective COX-2 inhibitor NS-398 reduces infarct volume by 20–30% in a model of focal ischemia [19]. Furthermore, COX-2 inhibition also reduces neuronal damage in a model of global cerebral ischemia [22]. These observations raise the possibility that COX-2 reaction products contribute to cerebral ischemic injury.

iNOS and COX-2 are concomitantly expressed after stroke [19]. The spatial and temporal proximity of iNOS and COX-2 suggests that NO produced by iNOS could activate COX-2 and enhance the toxic output of the enzyme [23]. This possibility is supported by studies demonstrating that selective inhibition of iNOS reduces COX-

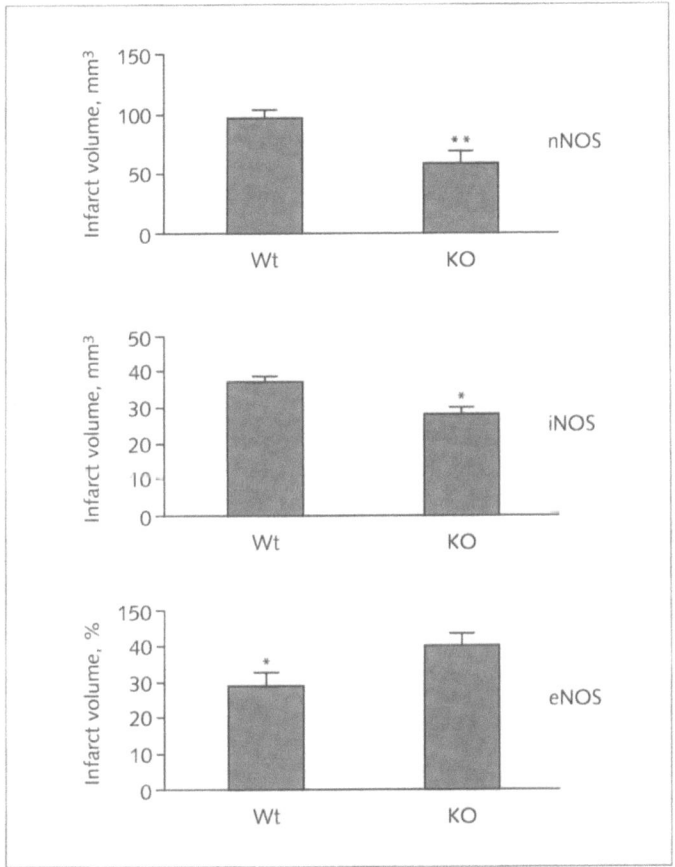

Figure 3
Infarct volume in wild-type and NOS deficient mice after occlusion of the middle cerebral artery. Mice deficient in nNOS and wild-type (SV-129) were subjected to permanent MCAO for 24 h [13]. The data for mice deficient in iNOS and wild-type (C57/B6) were obtained at 96 h after permanent MCAO [14], and deficient in eNOS and wild-type (SV-129) were obtained 24 h after MCAO [15].

2 reaction products in the post-ischemic brain [19]. Furthermore, COX-2 reaction products are reduced in iNOS null mice [19], which do not produce iNOS-derived NO after ischemia. These data, collectively, suggest that NO produced by iNOS may "drive" COX-2 activity in the post-ischemic brain and increase COX-2 reaction products.

Recent experiments have demonstrated that COX-2 null mice lack post-ischemic COX-2 expression and have reduced focal cerebral ischemic injury [24]. The protective effect of COX-2 deletion is likely to result from attenuation of post-ischemic inflammation and from reduced susceptibility to brain injury produced by activation of glutamate receptors, a process that contributes to the initiation of cerebral ischemic injury [24]. These data suggest that COX-2 may play a role both in the early and late stages of cerebral ischemia.

Conclusion

The evidence presented here indicates that NO plays a significant role in cerebral ischemia injury. Because both protective and destructive roles of NO have been characterized, the selective blockade of particular NOS activity in some spatial and temporal condition needs to be exercised to elucidate the best efficacy in the treatment of stroke and other CNS injury. A recent negative data [25] from clinical phase III trial for lubeluzole, an inhibitor for the glutamate-activated NOS pathway [26] that have been demonstrated for significant neuroprotection in animal models of stroke [27], in acute ischemic stroke treatment further revealed the complexity of NOS as therapeutic targets.

References

1   Hobbs AJ, Higgs A, Moncada S (1999) Inhibition of nitric oxide synthase as a potential therapeutic target. *Annu Rev Pharmacol Toxicol* 39: 191–220
2   Nathan C, Xie QW (1994) Nitric oxide synthases: roles, tolls, and controls. *Cell* 78: 915–918
3   Gross SS, Wolin MS (1995) Nitric oxide: pathophysiological mechanisms. *Annu Rev Physiol* 57: 737–769
4   Garthwaite J, Charles SL, Chess-Williams R (1988) Endothelium-derived relaxing factor release on activation of NMDA receptors suggests role as intercellular messenger in the brain. *Nature* 336: 385–388
5   Lin SZ, Chiou AL, Wang Y (1996) Ketamine antagonizes nitric oxide release from cerebral cortex after middle cerebral artery ligation in rats. *Stroke* 27: 747–752
6   Strijbos PJ (1998) Nitric oxide in cerebral ischemic neurodegeneration and excitotoxicity. *Crit Rev Neurobiol* 2: 223–243
7   Iadecola C (1997) Bright and dark sides of nitric oxide in ischemic brain damage. *Trends Neurosci* 20: 132–138
8   Forster C, Clark HB, Ross ME, Iadecola C (1999) Inducible nitric oxide synthase expression in human cerebral infarcts. *Acta Neuropathol* 97: 215–220
9   Huang Z, Huang PL, Ma J, Meng W, Ayata C, Fishman MC, Moskowitz MA (1996) Enlarged infarcts in endothelial nitric oxide synthase knockout mice are attenuated by nitro-L-arginine. *J Cereb Blood Flow Metab* 16: 981–987

10 Wink DA, Hanbauer I, Krishna MC, DeGraff W, Gamson J, Mitchell JB (1993) Nitric oxide protects against cellular damage and cytotoxicity from reactive oxygen species. *Proc Natl Acad Sci USA* 90: 9813–9817

11 Beckman JS, Beckman TW, Chen J, Marshall PA, Freeman BA (1990) Apparent hydroxyl radical production by peroxynitrite: implications for endothelial injury from nitric oxide and superoxide. *Proc Natl Acad Sci USA* 87: 1620–1624

12 Escott KJ, Beech JS, Haga KK, Williams SC, Meldrum BS, Bath PM (1998) Cerebroprotective effect of the nitric oxide synthase inhibitors, 1-(2-trifluoromethylphenyl) imidazole and 7-nitro indazole, after transient focal cerebral ischemia in the rat. *J Cereb Blood Flow Metab* 18: 281–287

13 Huang Z, Huang PL, Panahian N, Dalkara T, Fishman MC, Moskowitz MA (1994) Effects of cerebral ischemia in mice deficient in neuronal nitric oxide synthase. *Science* 265: 1883–1885

14 Iadecola C, Zhang F, Casey R, Nagayama M, Ross ME (1997) Delayed reduction of ischemic brain injury and neurological deficits in mice lacking the inducible nitric oxide synthase gene. *J Neurosci* 17: 9157–9164

15 Lo EH, Hara H, Rogowska J, Trocha M, Pierce AR, Huang PL, Fishman MC, Wolf GL, Moskowitz MA (1996) Temporal correlation mapping analysis of the hemodynamic penumbra in mutant mice deficient in endothelial nitric oxide synthase gene expression. *Stroke* 27: 1381–1385

16 Smith WL, Marnett LJ (1991) Prostaglandin endoperoxide synthase: structure and catalysis. *Biochim Biophys Acta* 1083: 1–17

17 Nogawa S, Zhang F, Ross ME, Iadecola C (1997) Cyclo-oxygenase-2 gene expression in neurons contributes to ischemic brain damage. *J Neurosci* 17: 2746–2755

18 Miettinen S, Fusco FR, Yrjanheikki J, Keinanen R, Hirvonen T, Roivainen R, Narhi M, Hokfelt T, Koistinaho J (1997) Spreading depression and focal brain ischemia induce cyclooxygenase-2 in cortical neurons through N-methyl-D-aspartic acid-receptors and phospholipase A2. *Proc Natl Acad Sci USA* 94: 6500–6505

19 Nogawa S, Forster C, Zhang F, Nagayama M, Ross ME, Iadecola C (1998) Interaction between inducible nitric oxide synthase and cyclooxygenase-2 after cerebral ischemia. *Proc Natl Acad Sci USA* 95: 10966–10971

20 Planas AM, Soriano MA, Rodriguez-Farre E, Ferrer I (1995) Induction of cyclooxygenase-2 mRNA and protein following transient focal ischemia in the rat brain. *Neurosci Lett* 200: 187–190

21 Iadecola C, Forster C, Nogawa S, Clark HB, Ross ME (1999) Cyclooxygenase immunoreactivity in the human brain following cerebral ischemia. *Acta Neuropathologica* 98: 9–14

22 Nakayama M, Uchimura K, Zhu RL, Nagayama T, Rose ME, Stetler RA, Isakson PC, Chen J, Graham SH (1998) Cyclooxygenase-2 inhibition prevents delayed death of CA1 hippocampal neurons following global ischemia. *Proc Natl Acad Sci USA* 95: 10954–10959

23 Salvemini D, Masferrer JL (1996) Interactions of nitric oxide with cyclooxygenase: *in vitro*, *ex vivo*, and *in vivo* studies. *Methods Enzymol* 269: 12–25

24 Iadecola C, Niwa K, Nogawa S, Zhao X, Nagayama M, Araki E, Morham S, Ross ME (2001) Reduced susceptibility to ischemic brain injury and NMDA-mediated neurotoxicity in cyclooxygenase-2 deficient mice. *Proc Natl Acad Sci USA* 98: 1294–1299

25 Diener HC, Cortens M, Ford G, Grotta J, Hacke W, Kaste M, Koudstaal PJ, Wessel T (2000) Lubeluzole in acute ischemic stroke treatment : A double-blind study with an 8-hour inclusion window comparing a 10-mg daily dose of lubeluzole with placebo. *Stroke* 31: 2543–2551

26 Lesage AS, Peeters L, Leysen JE (1996) Lubeluzole, a novel long-term neuroprotectant, inhibits the glutamate-activated nitric oxide synthase pathway. *J Pharmacol Exp Ther* 279: 759–766

27 De Ryck M, Keersmaekers R, Duytschaever H, Claes C, Clincke G, Janssen M, Van Reet G (1996) Lubeluzole protects sensorimotor function and reduces infarct size in a photochemical stroke model in rats. *J Pharmacol Exp Ther* 279: 748–758

The PIR-Series
Progress in Inflammation Research

Homepage: http://www.birkhauser.ch

Up-to-date information on the latest developments in the pathology, mechanisms and therapy of inflammatory disease are provided in this monograph series. Areas covered include vascular responses, skin inflammation, pain, neuroinflammation, arthritis cartilage and bone, airways inflammation and asthma, allergy, cytokines and inflammatory mediators, cell signalling, and recent advances in drug therapy. Each volume is edited by acknowledged experts providing succinct overviews on specific topics intended to inform and explain. The series is of interest to academic and industrial biomedical researchers, drug development personnel and rheumatologists, allergists, pathologists, dermatologists and other clinicians requiring regular scientific updates.

Available volumes:
T Cells in Arthritis, P. Miossec, W. van den Berg, G. Firestein (Editors), 1998
Chemokines and Skin, E. Kownatzki, J. Norgauer (Editors), 1998
Medicinal Fatty Acids, J. Kremer (Editor), 1998
Inducible Enzymes in the Inflammatory Response, D.A. Willoughby, A. Tomlinson (Editors), 1999
Cytokines in Severe Sepsis and Septic Shock, H. Redl, G. Schlag (Editors), 1999
Fatty Acids and Inflammatory Skin Diseases, J.-M. Schröder (Editor), 1999
Immunomodulatory Agents from Plants, H. Wagner (Editor), 1999
Cytokines and Pain, L. Watkins, S. Maier (Editors), 1999
In Vivo *Models of Inflammation*, D. Morgan, L. Marshall (Editors), 1999
Pain and Neurogenic Inflammation, S.D. Brain, P. Moore (Editors), 1999
Anti-Inflammatory Drugs in Asthma, A.P. Sampson, M.K. Church (Editors), 1999
Novel Inhibitors of Leukotrienes, G. Folco, B. Samuelsson, R.C. Murphy (Editors), 1999
Vascular Adhesion Molecules and Inflammation, J.D. Pearson (Editor), 1999
Metalloproteinases as Targets for Anti-Inflammatory Drugs, K.M.K. Bottomley, D. Bradshaw, J.S. Nixon (Editors), 1999
Free Radicals and Inflammation, P.G. Winyard, D.R. Blake, C.H. Evans (Editors), 1999
Gene Therapy in Inflammatory Diseases, C.H. Evans, P. Robbins (Editors), 2000
New Cytokines as Potential Drugs, S. K. Narula, R. Coffmann (Editors), 2000
High Throughput Screening for Novel Anti-inflammatories, M. Kahn (Editor), 2000
Immunology and Drug Therapy of Atopic Skin Diseases, C.A.F. Bruijnzeel-Komen, E.F. Knol (Editors), 2000
Novel Cytokine Inhibitors, G.A. Higgs, B. Henderson (Editors), 2000
Inflammatory Processes. Molecular Mechanisms and Therapeutic Opportunities, L.G. Letts, D.W. Morgan (Editors), 2000

Cellular Mechanisms in Airways Inflammation, C. Page, K. Banner, D. Spina (Editors), 2000
Inflammatory and Infectious Basis of Atherosclerosis, J.L. Mehta (Editor), 2001
Muscarinic Receptors in Airways Diseases, J. Zaagsma, H. Meurs, A.F. Roffel (Editors), 2001
TGF-β and Related Cytokines in Inflammation, S.N. Breit, S. Wahl (Editors), 2001
Nitric Oxide and Inflammation, D. Salvemini, T.R. Billiar, Y. Vodovotz (Editors), 2001
Neuroinflammatory Mechanisms in Alzheimer's Disease. Basic and Clinical Research, J. Rogers (Editor), 2001
Disease-modifying therapy in vasculitides, C.G.M. Kallenberg, J.W. Cohen Tervaert (Editors), 2001

Index